STUDIES IN IMPERIALISM

general editor John M. MacKenzie

Established in the belief that imperialism as a cultural phenomenon had as significant an effect on the dominant as on the subordinate societies, Studies in Imperialism seeks to develop the new socio-cultural approach which has emerged through cross-disciplinary work on popular culture, media studies, art history, the study of education and religion, sports history and children's literature. The cultural emphasis embraces studies of migration and race, while the older political, and constitutional, economic and military concerns will never be far away. It incorporates comparative work on European and American empire-building, with the chronological focus primarily, though not exclusively, on the nineteenth and twentieth centuries, when these cultural exchanges were most powerfully at work.

AVAILABLE IN THE SERIES

Propaganda and empire
The manipulation of British public opinion, 1880–1960 John M. MacKenzie

Imperialism and popular culture
ed John M. MacKenzie

'At duty's call'
A study in obsolete patriotism W. J. Reader

Images of the army
The military in British art, 1815–1914 J. W. M. Hichberger

The empire of nature
Hunting, conservation and British imperialism John M. MacKenzie

Imperial medicine and indigenous societies
ed. David Arnold

Imperialism and juvenile literature
ed. Jeffrey Richards

Asia in Western fiction
ed. Robin W. Winks, James R. Rush

Empire and sexuality
The British experience Ronald Hyam

Imperialism and the natural world
ed. John M. MacKenzie

Emigrants and empire
British settlement in the dominions between the wars ed. Stephen Constantine

Revolution and empire
English politics and the American colonies in the seventeenth century Robert M. Bliss

Air power and colonial control
The Royal Air Force, 1919–39 David E. Omissi

Acts of supremacy
The British Empire and the stage, 1790–1930 J. S. Bratton *et al.*

Policing the Empire
Government, authority and control, 1830–1940 ed. David Anderson, David Killingray

Policing and decolonisation
Nationalism, politics and the police, 1917–65 ed. David Anderson, David Killingray

Popular imperialism and the military, 1850–1950
ed. John M. MacKenzie

The language of empire
Myths and metaphors of popular imperialism, 1880–1918 Robert H. MacDonald

Travellers in Africa
British travelogues, 1850–1900 Tim Youngs

Unfit for heroes
Reconstruction and soldier settlement in the empire between the wars Kent Fedorowich

Colonial masculinity
The 'manly Englishman' and the 'effeminate Bengali' Mrinalini Sinha

Geography and imperialism, 1820–1940
ed. Morag Bell, Robin Butlin, Michael Heffernan

'An Irish Empire?'
Reading colonialism through children's books and magazines Keith Jeffery

Britannia's children
Aspects of Ireland and the British Empire Kathryn Castle

Western medicine as contested knowledge

edited by Andrew Cunningham
and Bridie Andrews

MANCHESTER UNIVERSITY PRESS
Manchester and New York

Distributed exclusively in the USA by
ST. MARTIN'S PRESS

Published by **MANCHESTER UNIVERSITY PRESS**
OXFORD ROAD, MANCHESTER M13 9NR
and ROOM 400, 175 FIFTH AVENUE, NEW YORK, NY 10010, USA

Distributed exclusively in the USA
by **ST. MARTIN'S PRESS, INC.**
175 FIFTH AVENUE, NEW YORK, NY 10010, USA

British Library Cataloguing-in-Publication data

A catalogue record for this book is available from the British Library

Library of Congress Cataloguing-in-Publication Data
Western medicine as contested knowledge / edited by Andrew Cunningham and Bridie Andrews
p. cm. — (Studies in Imperialism)
ISBN 0–7190–4673–4
1. Public health—Political aspects—Developing countries. 2. Imperialism. 3. Traditional medicine—Developing countries. 4. Social medicine—Developing countries. 5. Medicine—Political aspects—Developing countries. I. Cunningham. Andrew, Dr. II. Andrews, Bridie. III. Series: Studies in imperialism (Manchester, England)
RA441.5.W47 1997
306.4′61—dc20 96–34392
CIP

ISBN 0 7190 4673 4 *hardback*

Typeset in Trump Medieval
by Northern Phototypesetting Co Ltd, Bolton
Printed in Great Britain
by Bookcraft (Bath) Ltd

CONTENTS

GENERAL INTRODUCTION

The symbiotic relationship between imperialism and the development of Western intellectual disciplines and their practical application in the nineteenth and twentieth centuries has recently been subjected to increasing scrutiny. This has been particularly true of medical history, since Western medicine was both profoundly influenced by, and established hegemonic relationships through, encounters with the rest of the world during the imperial era. European medical practitioners, their methodologies still in the process of formulation, embarked upon their own patterns of social and scientific dominance. Through medicine and its related disciplines, the West assured itself that it was capable of diagnosing the bodily ills of the indigenous peoples of empire as part of its wider cultural, political and economic project.

Such a medical conquest far exceeded the formal boundaries of empire. Western doctors conceived a mission, scarcely less fervent than that of the Christian missionaries with whom they were often associated, to take their insights to the furthest corners of the world. Many missionaries – Livingstone was perhaps the most celebrated example – adopted medicine as a prime vehicle for imparting Christian values and ultimately beliefs. Within formal empire, medicine and its practitioners enjoyed high prestige, soon establishing powerful administrative networks and close connections with the armed forces, services associated with the environment, and educational institutions. It thus became both a significant cultural marker of imperial superiority and an acknowledged, if often exaggerated, facilitator of the white presence and dominance in the wider world.

It is, then, not surprising that its pervasive authority should have had little difficulty in surviving into the post-imperial age. Despite its comparatively limited focus in the understanding of health, illness, diagnosis and treatment, despite the modern fascination with alternative medical traditions, it is still invariably privileged as a superior 'scientific' system. This has had a profound influence on health-related international organisations and the social and cultural analysis of 'epidemics', of which AIDS is perhaps the best example.

This volume examines many of the issues associated with the relationship of medicine and power, together with the grappling of indigenous and Western medical systems. The studies that follow extend their concerns beyond the conventional boundaries of both empire and human medicine. They attempt some global comparative analysis. They embrace major Asian cultures where the contest between traditional methodologies and those of the West has been particularly acute. And they recognise that veterinary science, when applied to domestic stock, opens up fresh areas of conflict which can profoundly influence human health. Together they represent a significant stage in the recent highly rewarding research into the relationship between medicine and imperialism.

John M. MacKenzie

THE CONTRIBUTORS

BRIDIE ANDREWS, Department of History, School of Oriental and African Studies, University of London.

ANNE-EMANUELLE BIRN, Department of Health Policy and Historical Studies at the New School for Social Research in New York City.

ANDREW CUNNINGHAM, Wellcome Unit for History of Medicine, Department of History and Philosophy of Science, University of Cambridge.

ROSALIND J. HARRISON-CHIRIMUUTA, consultant ophthalmologist in south-east Staffordshire, co-author of *Aids, Africa and Racism* (1987).

KATHY HOMEWOOD, Department of Anthropology, University College, London.

DEEPAK KUMAR, National Institute of Science, Technology and Development Studies, New Delhi.

STEPHEN J. KUNITZ, Department of Community and Preventative Medicine, University of Rochester, New York.

HELEN LAMBERT, Department of Anthropology, London School of Hygiene and Tropical Medicine.

SUNG LEE, Stanford Medical School, Stanford, California.

JERROLD E. LEVY, Department of Anthropology, University of Arizona, Tucson.

ILANA LÖWY, INSERM, Unité 158, Hôpital des Infants Malades, Paris.

EMIKO OHNUKI-TIERNEY, Department of Anthropology, University of Wisconsin, Madison.

HELEN POWER, Department of Economic and Social History, University of Liverpool.

MARY PRESTON SUTPHEN, Department of the History of the Health Sciences, University of California, San Francisco.

ARMANDO SOLÓRZANO, Department of Family and Consumer Studies, and Ethnic Studies Program at the University of Utah, Salt Lake City.

RICHARD WALLER, Department of History, Bucknell University, Lewisburg, Pennsylvania.

ACKNOWLEDGEMENTS

For advice and assistance we are grateful to David Arnold, C. A. Bayly, Michael Bravo, Lionel Carter, Arne Hessenbruch, Tamara Hug, Christopher Pinney and Molly Sutphen. We are particularly grateful to the series editor, John MacKenzie, for his enthusiastic support of the project from the beginning.

INTRODUCTION

Western medicine as contested knowledge

Andrew Cunningham and Bridie Andrews

I

Investigating the relation of medicine and imperialism is a burgeoning area of academic research.[1] However, the present volume is the first to take quite such a wide perspective in examining the range and extent of non-Western responses to Western medicine across the whole spectrum of Western imperialist influence, from Japan in the east to the Navajo of the North American plains in the west, and is the first to put the issue of the contestation of knowledge at its centre. The volume treats imperialism as a distinct historical, political and cultural phenomenon; it similarly treats Western medicine as a distinct historical, political and cultural phenomenon. And it looks at the relations between the two, both as historical and as modern phenomena, finding that Western medicine, both metaphorically and literally, is imperialist as a form of knowledge and as a practice, and that this imperialist nature of Western medicine can be seen wherever it has been spread, both within and beyond the areas that were subject to political imperialism.

Medicine has always been a significant tool of empire.[2] In the nineteenth century Western missionaries were candid about the value of medicine for introducing the heathen first to Christianity and thence to trade with the West. Moreover, Western medicine, in the form of 'tropical medicine', was not only crucial to facilitating white settlement and colonisation of new territorial gains in the late nineteenth century, but was developed specifically with that aim in mind. The microbiology taught in the new Schools of Tropical Medicine of London and Liverpool, and in the Pasteur Institutes created throughout the French colonies, was built on the research conducted in these same institutions. As (Sir) Patrick Manson urged in 1897, the need to create institutions to teach and investigate malaria and other diseases was urgent:

> What, I would ask, does the student learn [in European medical schools] of practical value about beri-beri, a disease which, if he is to practise in the tropics, he is almost sure to encounter often enough, although he may not recognise it when he does come across it? Beri-beri is a very important malady. Occurring both endemically and epidemically, it annually kills its thousands and tens of thousands. It makes the settlement of many fertile lands almost impossible. It kills off the planter's coolies like flies and makes his plantations unprofitable. It fills the hospitals and is a downright scourge in some of the fairest lands of the earth.[3]

Amidst all the criticisms of colonisation and imperialism, Western observers have often assumed that the spread of Western medicine to the rest of the world was the one unambiguously beneficial effect of Western imperialist expansion over the last century and a half. This assumption is reinforced by the reduction, under the leadership of the World Health Organization, of the incidence of certain major infectious diseases which would have looked impossible only a century ago. Smallpox (at least at the time of writing) is a disease of the past, now eliminated in human populations; there is hope that polio and measles can be eliminated in the near future, and possibly also the cattle disease rinderpest. Moreover, the creation of public health programmes and of modern medical infrastructures in previously colonised countries seems to indicate that Western medicine has been adopted and continued on its merits, and those merits are very positive. And, even where there has been criticism of Western medicine, it has concentrated on the institutional arrangements (hospitals, expensive specialised training for doctors) and the difficulties of distributing care adequately, rather than on the nature of Western scientific medicine itself.

Recently historians have begun to challenge this view of the benefits of Western medicine to the previously colonised world. Their criticisms have been along two main lines. One is that Western colonialists and imperialist adventurers were primarily agents of disease rather than of health. They changed the disease ecology of the lands they laid claim to, by introducing diseases to which the native populations had no resistance, by spreading diseases across the world by their ships, or within colonies by their railways, canals and roads, and by altering the local habitat by introducing large-scale monoculture of crops or animals for the European market, and thus making conditions more favourable for the flourishing of microbial and insect agents of disease. The other main line of criticism is that Western medicine was imposed as an alien form of knowledge and an alien practice, and that it took no account of the cultures and medical systems already present. Not only was this an act of cultural condescension on a grand scale, but it meant that the settler communities and agents of imperialism wilfully dismissed even those aspects of local knowledge which might have assisted them in avoiding disease, or which could have helped them in coping with it.

We have a third kind of criticism to offer here, which involves the nature both of imperialism and of scientific medicine. We shall be arguing that an appreciation of the nature of imperialism, on the one hand, and of Western scientific medicine, on the other, will provide a general basis for understanding the origin of the contestation of Western medicine in the modern period in lands under imperialism, and will also throw light on the nature of the contested issues themselves.

In discussing the relationship of scientific medicine to imperialism we are dealing with two terms and concepts which are each of them very widely used, and equally difficult to define, since they are used with such a range of meanings. For our purposes here we shall take 'imperialism' in a relatively narrow sense, as referring to 'the use of the state power against foreign countries, for the purpose of winning economic advantage', by the use of 'overt or covert pressures by the agents of one state which infringe the independence of another', including the use of military force.[4] This is a working definition offered by Norman Etherington in his extensive discussion of theories of imperialism, and reflects historical usage of the term in the high period of European and American imperialism which occurred in the last decades of the nineteenth century and the first decades of the twentieth (approximately 1880 to 1930). Such a definition, of course, omits much of the colonial enterprise of European countries in earlier centuries which one might, on other occasions, want to refer to as imperialism. So it is an old term which was given new, relatively precise, meaning towards the end of the nineteenth century. The use of it in this sense here should help to concentrate attention on some of the special features of this imperialist episode.

One such feature of this form of imperialism was that it could be conducted without the formal take-over of other countries as colonies. Thus China in the late nineteenth century was subject to the imperialist attentions of the British, French, Germans, Japanese and Russians, all present in strength in the country and seeking economic advantage by their respective agents exerting covert and overt pressure which severely compromised the independence of the Chinese state. Yet China, though its autonomy was so tightly restricted by these other states, was never formally a colony of any of them. Similarly this use of the term allows us to speak of the behaviour of the Rockefeller

Foundation, a private health agency which sought to spread US scientific, cultural and economic values, especially in Latin America, as strictly imperialistic, even though it was never formally an agency of US colonialism. Another distinctive feature of such imperialism was that it was perceived, at the time, to be driven by the desire to develop markets for a capitalist system which was thought to be on the point of collapse owing to the 'congestion of capital' with nowhere to go.[5] Although the advent of this new version of imperialism had a significant effect on the old colonial powers, increasingly leading them to see their colonies primarily as economic resources to be exploited, it did not itself necessarily involve colonialism.[6] Imperialism was both an ideology and a practice, necessarily linked with Western capitalism, with the search for markets abroad and sources of raw materials, and concerned in practice as much with spreading the Western way of life and culture as with attaching the economies of other countries to the needs of the economies of the West.

For the terms 'science' and 'scientific medicine' we shall be taking the current position in history of science studies, according to which 'science', though an old term, was given precise new meanings in the course of the nineteenth century, and which (like imperialism) embraced both a new ideology and a new practice. This extended, of course, also to scientific medicine, which takes its definition from science.

It is striking to notice how the development of imperialism in the nineteenth century, from the 'scramble for Africa' of the 1870s to1890s, to the imperialist encroachments on countries such as China, Korea, Laos and Cambodia in the east, went hand in hand with the development of scientific medicine in Europe, particularly of laboratory medicine, with its unique focus on isolating, identifying and combating the pathogens of infectious disease. The two phenomena were products of the same political, industrial and social forces driving the expansion of the West and its economic and social development and reconstruction, and they had related characteristics. As Etherington has argued with respect to the term 'imperialism', the common element in its multifarous uses and applications over the last hundred years is always 'a reference to domination – domination of man over man, country over country, man over threatening circumstances. The subject then [of imperialism] is power …'.[7] It is similarly the case that the subject of Western scientific medicine is also power.

Historians of politics, imperialism and other subjects are usually deferential to science – and hence also to scientific medicine – in their history writing, and they tend to treat it at the evaluation of its own practitioners and advocates. Historians of politics and imperialism may be prepared to notice and comment on incidents where science or scientific medicine are evidently abused or misapplied or improperly withheld, and these they would regard as political events, but they rarely see science or scientific medicine themselves as political in their nature and structure, or as embodying and expressing an ideology. It may seem strange, therefore, for someone to claim that Western scientific medicine is a medicine of domination, given that it is based on 'value-free' science, and that it has achieved striking therapeutic successes. The view from today's disciplines of the history of science and the history of medicine, however, is different. For it is becoming increasingly clear that science and scientific medicine were new creations in the nineteenth century, and that they were the products of one particular society – western Europe and North America, especially France, the German states and Britain – at a particular time, and that they embody its values, both political and social. And while science and scientific medicine have been in a constant state of development since that period, they have both nevertheless continued to be centrally defined by the characteristics given them in the nineteenth century.[8]

Scientific medicine is based on two distinctive institutions: the hospital and the laboratory. The hospital is the centre of 'clinical' (bedside) medicine, where the correlation of symptoms and signs with internal changes is investigated, taught and practised. Empiricism and strict modes of reasoning are essential to the mental processes that make clinical medicine. The hospital is the centre of medical resources, and it is also where surgery and other high-technology interventions in the body take place. The laboratory has many roles in scientific medicine, but its original role is still the most important: as the place where the causes of diseases are tracked down, and where cures for them are sought or created, all by the deployment of scientific experiment. The correlation of cause with effect, especially of pathogen to disease in the case of infectious diseases, is the laboratory's primary *raison d'être*.

Taken together, the workers in the hospital and the laboratory isolate instances of disease, seek to understand their causes, and endeavour to supply cures for them, with the success of scientific medicine being assessed by its ability to deliver cure. This is the practice of scientific medicine. The process requires the 'objectification' of the patient, transforming the patient mentally from a whole suffering person into an integrated set of physiological processes, one or more of which is malfunctioning, which can be treated independently of the personality or the social position of the patient. In that sense scientific medicine treats the disease – more precisely, the cause of the disease – not the patient.

Above all, scientific medicine is premissed upon authority, the authority of qualified medical personnel over the patient, and indeed over the population at large. That authority, in turn, is itself premissed on the scientific basis of this medicine, on the rational, systematic, dispassionate, objective basis on which its knowledge has been built up and warranted true and effective. Thus the patient is not a participant in the diagnostic or curative processes, except in a trivial sense. The patient does not share the knowledge world of the doctor, for the patient has no scientific expertise. The patient has to take on the submissive 'patient's role' in order to receive treatment. There is no room for social negotiation of roles: doctor and patient do not come to a consensual conclusion about the nature of the illness or its treatment; the friends and relatives of the patient are not admitted as participants to discussion of the disease, its origin or its prognosis. Indeed, when talking about disease and cure, doctor and patient literally speak different languages. Scientific medicine is not open to alternative views, or to input from anyone not medically or scientifically qualified.

In scientific medicine, health is not just a matter of the care of individuals or small groups: health is a social matter, involving the whole community. Germ theory, the child of laboratory medicine, provides an understanding of disease causation which demands large-scale state involvement in medical care in times of epidemics, with military-style operations directed by doctors, in order to control the population and the spread of infection. It is again the scientific basis of the medicine which gives authority to such medical intervention on the large scale: public health and sanitary measures such as inoculation, health checks, sanitation, intrusive measures in epidemics, are all accepted without question in the modern Western state because they are premissed on the scientific viewpoint.

Its basis in the scientific approach also accounts for why scientific medicine is considered equally applicable to chronic conditions, even though it is relatively ineffective in this area by comparison with its successes in dealing with acute medical conditions. Based as it is on the true (that is, on the scientific) approach, scientific medicine is deemed applicable to all medical conditions, in all places, at all times, since scientific truth is one and indivisible and valid everywhere.

Finally, even when it comes to the provision of remedies for particular conditions, scientific medicine has a distinctive approach. For success in creating drugs in the laboratory – from Salvarsan (patented in 1909) to penicillin (discovered in 1928) to the drugs of today – has provided us with a view that, ideally, drugs are specific in their action: that one drug fights one condition. While the alleviation of symptoms is desirable as a palliative measure, drugs that effect cures are what are primarily sought in the modern pharmaceutical industry which supplies the practitioners of scientific medicine. The administration of drugs is not a hit-and-miss affair, with many possible ingredients being tried successively on a particular patient, nor are particular drugs seen as applicable in a wide range of conditions.

Scientific medicine, both as a concept and as a practice, has very positive connotations. Hence to call a medical system 'non-scientific' is virtually to damn it as arbitrary, irrational, unsystematic, misguided, ineffective and probably a danger to health. This indicates the ideological as well as the practical power that this particular medical system has acquired. Yet, looked at from a historical point of view, to describe a medical system as 'non-scientific' is not necessarily a condemnation, merely a description of it as not a product of this recent tradition in Western medicine. And this kind of Western medicine – its theory, practice, ideology, positive evaluation and all that goes with it – is very recent. We have had it for less than 200 years.

II

Scientific medicine, like science itself, is a defining characteristic of the modern world, and it is also a product of the modern world. Because we live in the modern world, and are brought up to take scientific values for granted, it is hard for us to see the goals and values of scientific medicine as having been *constructed*: curiously, we tend to look at them as timeless and even as 'natural', even if we are aware of how recently they were created.

Scientific medicine was begun in the French Revolution. First hospital (or clinical) medicine was created, in the great hospitals for the poor of Paris in the 1790s: systematic observation of the phenomena and course of diseases and their correlation with pathological findings from post-mortems allowed physicians to build up disease pictures while enabling them to visualise what pathological processes happening within the body were bringing about the visible phenomena. As an approach this 'hospital medicine' was built on Enlightenment theories of knowledge, especially the philosophy known as 'sensationalism'. This was the first kind of scientific medicine. From the 1860s there was welded to it, primarily in France, the German states and Britain, 'laboratory medicine': the techniques and practices of the laboratory dedicated to diagnosing disease and creating new modes of cure, and concerned in particular with pathogenic microbes. Laboratory medicine too was based on a distinctive theory of knowledge, especially with respect to the relation of cause and effect, depending, especially for its determinism, largely on the philosophy known as 'positivism', which flourished in mid-nineteenth-century Europe. Together these two elements gave us the scientific medicine which still prevails today, a medicine premissed on particular Western theories of knowledge, privileging systematic observation and experiment, aspiring to the models of physics and chemistry.

One can see the characteristics of this scientific medicine in the making, at the stage when they were still propagandist claims and not yet established facts, by looking at the promotional writings of the people trying to construct them. One very important such ideologist of scientific medicine was Claude Bernard, the French experimental physiologist (1813–78). Bernard lived at a time when the first element of scientific medicine – that is, clinical medicine – had been created, and he was one of the chiefs of those involved in adding the second, crowning element to this: laboratory medicine. Bernard famously wrote that:

> I consider hospitals only as the entrance to scientific medicine; they are the first field of observation which a physician enters; but the true sanctuary of medical science is a laboratory; only there can he seek explanations of life in the normal and pathological states by means of experimental analysis ... There, in a word, he will achieve true medical science.[9]

Bernard's celebrated book of 1865, *An Introduction to the Study of Experimental Medicine*, is a piece of propaganda, putting forward claims about what scientific medicine should be but was not yet. In this work Bernard not only argues that the hospital needs to be supplemented by the laboratory, he also argues for the experimental method to be seen as independent and impersonal, as above the limitations and fancies of the individual's mind, and hence as inherently authoritative – in short, as objective. He admits that the current state of affairs is evidence so far that 'the experimental method has by no means come into its own in medicine'.[10] The great advantage the experimental approach has over the merely empirical is that it reaches the *cause* of any disease, a cause which can either be removed or avoided. His example is the itch, caused by a mite not visible to the naked eye:

> Now that the cause of the itch is known and experimentally determined, it has all become scientific, and empiricism has disappeared ... We cure it *always*, without any exception, when we place ourselves in the known experimental conditions for reaching this goal.[11]

The claim that the laboratory was essential to medicine, and that only the combination of the hospital with the laboratory – of pathology with experiment – gave true medical knowledge, was made into fact over the next few decades through a series of profound conflicts, both between hospital clinicians and the men from the laboratory, and also between those advocating a joint experimental-and-clinical medicine and defenders of other approaches. Set-piece battles were contrived and won by doughty combatants such as Louis Pasteur and Robert Koch, the two greatest advocates of germ theory, in which they co-opted the forces of the state and the media to their side.

Modern sociology of knowledge is our key to understanding that truth – even scientific truth – is a product of fighting, or 'contestation'. We are beginning to appreciate that even 'objective' knowledge (so called) is itself something created out of struggle and contestation, at the personal, professional, class, national and disciplinary levels, and in that sense is itself contingent on rather than determined by nature. Truth is made, not found. And in the controversies which constitute this making, success goes to the strong, the persistent and the wily. Bruno Latour has demonstrated the Janus-facedness of scientific knowledge, how in process of the construction of facts about nature 'as long as controversies are rife, Nature is never used as the final arbiter since no one knows what she is and says. But *once the controversy is settled*, Nature is the ultimate referee.'[12] Equally, with respect to medicine, the question of which medical system is 'truer to nature' is settled by finding which medical system and its advocates have won the contest against other medical systems and their advocates. Within Western society the medical system that we call 'scientific medicine' won that contest in the nineteenth century and remains still the victor. Its status as victor is the reason why we regard it as truest to nature.

It may seem, however, that the curative success of scientific medicine indicates that, whether man-made or not, this kind of medicine has distinct claims to being in accord with nature, and hence true in an absolute sense. But we need to remember that one of the criteria established for this new kind of medicine by its creators was that its primary goal should be to regularly offer cure rather than amelioration, and that such cure should be statistically provable. That is, the cure of disease once contracted, and the systematic avoidance of the onset of disease, should be among the central criteria of the success of *any* medical system. If we treat scientific medicine as true to nature because it is usually successful in that way in cases of acute disease, we are simply judging it by the criteria it was created specifically to fulfil, rather than against any absolute criteria. After all, the relative incapacity of such medicine to cope with chronic illness is never held up as an indication of its *lack of* correspondence to nature!

The creators of the new medicine claimed for it (as we have already seen in the case of Claude Bernard) that it is – by its very nature – 'objective'. That is, that its doctrines and findings are free from human bias or interference, and that it is universally true: that its validity is not subject to local circumstances or to the individual proclivities of patient or practitioner but is the same wherever in the world it is practised. Scientific medicine came packaged complete with these values: they could not and cannot be detached from its practice, since they were the values it was constructed to embody and the goals it was constructed to fulfil. Hence the *values* of Western scientific medicine were exported to the rest of the world along with the theory, practice, institutions and social relations of that medicine.

We asserted earlier that scientific medicine is inherently imperialist by nature, and we went so far as to say that, like imperialism itself, its subject is power, that it is a medicine of domination, and that it expresses a political ideology in its very structure and nature. The claim is built on the use, origin and structure of scientific medicine.

First, with respect to its use, scientific medicine has been directly employed by imperialists to assist acts of imperialism and colonialism. Laboratory medicine in particular has been used to promote white settlement in areas hitherto shielded by 'tropical' diseases such as malaria, to protect colonial quarters from native diseases, to promote the efficiency of workers (against, for instance the 'germ of laziness' of hookworm disease) and the efficiency of animals and crops against insect-borne and microbial parasites.

In the second place, scientific medicine is historically the product of the imperialistic societies of nineteenth-century Europe and America, with all that goes with that in terms of industry, types of government, class interest. Karl Marx, though currently so unfashionable as a historical analyst, pointed out that the belief system or ideology of any society is that of its ruling elite, and that, when the ruling elite of a society changes, so does its ideology. As the industrial and intellectual middle class came to dominate nineteenth-century Europe and North America, so its values too came to dominate, and to be taken as natural. The middle-class ideology was based on liberal philosophical systems which idealised freedom of thought and individualism against despotism and the Church, which espoused free trade and the freedom of the market at the same time as they also promoted the monopolistic claims of expertise – that quintessentially middle-class attribute – and the cult of the expert in all domains, including that of medicine.

Simultaneously it was an ideology which promoted the development of the bureaucracies of centralising governments, where middle-class expertise, whether of civil servants or of sanitary police, was at a premium. These bureaucracies fostered the uniformity of institutions and values, and developed social and intellectual institutions to pursue the welfare of society as a whole, such as, in the case of medicine, hospitals and laboratories, and the superiority of reductionism in medical thinking over holism. This middle-class ideology promoted belief in progress as an unmitigated good, and in science as the embodiment of all good thinking and as the proper model for all other domains of human thought. Such belief extended to the dividing of human knowledge into science versus the rest (science versus art, science versus religion, science versus superstition, science versus opinion). Empiricism and experiment were made the watchwords of all sound reasoning, and the scientific method (although remaining impossible to define with precision) was presented as the arbiter of logical thinking.

And that leads on to the third dimension of scientific medicine which contributed and contributes to making it a medicine of domination: its very structure and nature, and the fact that modern Western society and its values are folded into it. Hence the authoritarian stance that the practitioners of Western medicine take as to its exclusive correctness: there is only one correct view, and it comes from the scientific basis of the medicine. This medicine is the domain of experts, whose writ runs everywhere. And, since the health of the people as a whole in any society is a society-wide issue, the concern of central governments, so health measures can and should be introduced forcibly if necessary. In such ways is scientific medicine a medicine of domination.

These characteristics of Western medicine have had very significant social and institutional ramifications wherever it has been spread. To operate properly, scientific medicine has to take with it, or replicate abroad, its instruments and its institutions, together with its inner social hierarchies of expertise. Scientific medicine can be practised only by true believers, since it is necessary to take its thought world with one. So where the medicine goes, so does Westernisation, and vice versa.

It should now be clear why the terms 'Western medicine' and 'scientific medicine' are interchangeable for the modern period; the more recently coined terms 'biomedicine' and 'allopathy' are also equivalent. They will be used interchangeably throughout this volume.

Thus Western medicine was being developed throughout the nineteenth century, that is, over the whole period of modern colonialism and imperialism. The hospital was central to it; the laboratory and its values came to dominate it, with their criteria of causation and cure; parasites, both visible insects and invisible germs, became an obsession of its practitioners; public health and sanitary safety, as defined by the laboratory men, demanded action on a militaristic model. And Louis Pasteur and Robert Koch, the two greatest innovators of laboratory medicine with respect to infectious diseases, were both strong supporters of empire and colonies, Koch in particular travelling out to them to deal with epidemics of human and animal disease which were inhibiting colonial and imperial expansion.

III

These and related criteria and values of scientific medicine are central to the issues dealt with in the present volume, for they have contributed to make scientific medicine different in kind from any other medical system. In particular, the general acceptance of these claims about the nature of scientific medicine has led to it being seen as the standard according to which all other medical systems should be judged. It is inevitable that, as a result, all other medical systems should have been found wanting, for the criteria of success in medicine are the criteria that scientific medicine (unlike any other medical system) was created to embody. From the point of view of its practitioners and supporters, scientific medicine is not one medical system among many: it is the standard to which all other medical systems should aspire (and which they inevitably must fail to meet). And the coincidence – taken literally – of the creation and practice of scientific medicine in the dominant European countries, simultaneously with the creation and practice of modern colonialism and imperialism by the same European states at the end of the nineteenth and the beginning of the twentieth centuries, means that the claims of this medicine to superiority were imposed on the populations subject to colonial and imperial influence.

From this perspective it can be seen that scientific medicine was a development in the native medicine of modern western Europe, which was then made universal by exportation – by the exporting of it to non-European countries as they became subject to imperialism and colonialism. As a contributor to this volume put it recently, 'science, a purely European enterprise, began to be exported to peripheral countries in the nineteenth century'.[13]

It is therefore not surprising that in lands subject to colonisation and imperialism in the nineteenth and twentieth centuries the local systems of medical understanding and treatment were judged inferior, stupid or merely superstitious in comparison with this scientific medicine. Similarly, the natives were in general regarded as dirty, lazy, and as reservoirs of disease, needing the imperialist to bring them health and civilisation. This view continues to be held. In such a climate it has been hard to broach the question whether medical systems other than the Western scientific one were based on criteria which were sensible and coherent in their own terms, since the only terms allowed for judgement were those of scientific medicine.

There was much resistance to the imposition of scientific medicine. For the most part such resistance has looked simply like that to Western eyes: resistance, based on nothing better than ignorance, cussedness, conservatism, wilful stubbornness. But looking from the point of view of those being colonised and imperialised, as our contributors do here, even 'passive resistance' (which Waller and Homewood discuss in Chapter Three below) can be a very positive act, sometimes the only avenue left to contest the claims of Western medicine and science in local contexts.

Episodes of 'resistance' to Western medicine can be used as means of listening to the 'native voice', as it is called, and hearing it say something sensible and reasonable, in its own terms. The need to listen to the voice of 'the other', if one is to give accounts which do not simply replicate the power relations of the observers to the observed, has come to be appreciated by anthropologists, and recently also by historians. It is a theme which runs through virtually every contribution in the present volume.

It requires a certain ingenuity for Western metropolitan intellectuals to hear such other voices. One way of doing so is to listen to disputes with a different ear – and hence with a different set of values – and that is what many of our contributors do. A valuable tool here is again the concept of 'contestation'. This concept has proved exceptionally useful in recent years, as one of the more accessible aspects of 'postmodernism' as applied to history, and it has been taken up in historical domains as varied as feminism, gay studies, ecology, new sociology, and even the functioning of the capitalist market; it has been of particular value in adding a new vigour to what used to be 'colonial' or 'imperial' history.[14] For the postmodern approach in general rejects the customary historical stories of victorious modernisation, such as the triumph of the West (however ambiguous or ironic a triumph it is taken to have been), or the advancement of science, or (in the present case) the diffusion of scientific medicine, all of which have a strong moral subtext about the inherent superiority of whatever Western, male, industrial, scientific or political thing it is that is taken to have triumphed. And, in saying farewell to the grand narratives, postmodernists replace them with histories which explore cultural difference, are alert to political, sexual and cognitive pluralism, and focus on locally situated disputes. Taking a postmodern stance is itself an act of contesting the values inherent in the traditional accounts of how we got where we are. And 'contestation' is proving to be a valuable tool to use when exploring the activities of people who were or are challenging or resisting existing cultural authorities and hegemony in general, without having to abandon attempts to reach larger historical pictures as some postmodernist historians do.

We have already seen something of the fruitfulness of the concept of contestation in allowing one to see how the values, ideology and practice of scientific medicine were themselves created. Now we turn it outward to the occasions and places where scientific medicine was spread by imperialism. The great advantage of the concept is that it allows us to look at both past and present disputes over attitudes, knowledge and cultural behaviour in a perfectly symmetrical way, without prejudging the issue in favour of one tradition of thinking or one set of cultural norms. It has allowed our contributors to look at disputes between Western and non-Western medical systems as potentially having equal rationality on each side, without leading them to place all the sense on the side of science and all the superstition on the side of other medical approaches, or setting up a dichotomy between 'tradition' and 'progress' in which 'tradition' is necessarily backward, and 'progress' necessarily enlightened. And, while the concept of contestation allows us to appreciate the rational grounds for protest against the imposition of Western medicine, it does not demand that this rationality should be Western-style scientific rationality. Moreover, the concept of contestation, especially as applied to everyday life, allows one to appreciate the social and political significance of attempts to challenge hegemony which stop short of open confrontation.[15]

As the studies in the following pages show, in fact just about every instance of the introduction of Western medicine into non-Western societies has been contested at some level. The contests have taken place over the presence, nature and causation of disease; over appropriate therapies; over the legitimacy of native, foreign and foreign-trained healers; over the imposition of police measures in the name of public health; over the need for the institutional infrastructure of Western medicine; over the intellectual presuppositions themselves of Western medicine.

The imperialist relationship with respect to medicine formally ceased to exist once individual colonies gained nominal independence during the central decades of the twentieth century, and the new post-colonial states have been able to modify the form and delivery of Western medicine to some extent in order to meet their own perceived needs. However, modern Western medicine's rapid rate of development presents the former colonies with the problems of staying abreast of new medical developments at the same time as having very little influence over their direction or appropriateness. Tensions have continued between traditional culture and modern medicine, and between states at the postcolonial periphery and those at the centre. Various solutions and compromises have been adopted, some of which are explored in the anthropological studies in the volume.

Historians writing today on reactions to medicine in colonised and imperialised countries are tending to lay great stress on how 'interactive' the relationship was, and how Western medicine (or at least its practice and its institutions) was not just unilaterally imposed but was actually modified as it confronted the many different cultures into which it was introduced. Such historians have argued that scientific medicine was not a monolithic entity but something open to negotiation or modification to meet the local circumstances in which it had to operate in colonised and imperialised lands.[16] They have introduced this view primarily in order to counter the older ('modernist') view that Western medicine spread by simple 'diffusion' or because of its inherent correctness or superiority. While this new approach certainly turns attention very constructively to the local circumstances of the contestation of Western medicine, it embodies a fond illusion. For, to someone coming from the discipline of the history of medicine – rather than being primarily a historian of one or other of the regions colonised or imperialised – it is evident that the intrinsic nature of the Western medicine that was being spread abroad, and being contested as it was spread, was not and is not amenable to being changed *in its nature* by contests outside its metropolitan circle of origin. Of course, the particular local conditions directly affected and continue to affect the forms and outcomes of local moments of contestation, and they affect also what kind of accommodation with Western medicine is reached in any particular place. But the fact that Western scientific medicine has been repeatedly contested is actually inherent in the very nature of that medicine, because it is itself hegemonic. And, whatever the consequences of any particular moment of contestation, the content and nature of scientific medicine were and are emphatically *not* changed as a result, though the extent to which scientific medicine is (or is not) adopted or assimilated or believed may well vary from case to case. As an analytical tool of history, the postmodern approach can deconstruct the making of scientific medicine and reveal the interests and values that went into its making, but it cannot remake it with different characteristics, values and properties from the ones it was actually historically given by those at the metropolitan and imperialist centre who constructed it.

IV

Such were among the considerations that led us to conceive the present volume and invite the contributions. In order to emphasise the historical continuities of the confrontation, we have in some cases been able to provide complementary anthropological and historical case studies, though reasons of space precluded extending this treatment to all regions. The contributors have been able to reconstruct several of the contests from a range of historical and anthrological perspectives. They have used local records as well as the records of international organisations and imperial administrators, newspaper reports, field studies and interviews, direct and indirect witness and even rumours.

In the early days of decolonisation in the twentieth century it was taken for granted that the aim of decolonised societies should be modernisation, that is, development on the Western model. Ideally, each new state would emerge from its former dependent status with respect to the economies of the West, and be autonomous in developing its own agriculture and industry and its own medical system, as well as its own political institutions. In Chapter One, Sung Lee shows that this first stage, with respect to medicine, consisted primarily of a 'donor–recipient' relationship being expected by the decolonised states, wanting Western medicine to be established with Western money. Although this was resisted by the WHO, whose leaders wanted to supply only technical assistance rather than medical equipment, the WHO nevertheless expected to guide such states in the full adoption and application of Western medical systems. Building hospitals and training medical personnel took priority, and this ideology was shared by all the Western member states of the WHO, from the United States to the Soviet Union. But, as Lee shows, this approach came to be seriously questioned in the 1970s, thirty years after the WHO was founded. Although the WHO had been founded on what seemed at the time to be the most liberal and anti-colonial of bases, its behaviour had in fact been neo-imperialistic. Lee shows that the new model of medical provision and ideological thinking came from the 'undeveloped' world itself – from China – but it was made into new Western ideology as a result of Cold War conflict between the Western powers. A lesson one might learn from this incident perhaps is that medicine on the world stage is political at all times, especially when it is apparently least political. In the course of these events a new concept – indeed, a new medical ideology – was created: 'primary health care'. This concept, basic to the 'barefoot doctors' scheme, that universal health care can be provided more efficiently and economically if health worker training and institutional provision are geared to successive levels of patient care, has had significant repercussions in Western health care delivery systems and around the world.

A similar contestation of accepted values and reversal of perspective is argued for by Rosalind Harrison-Chirimuuta in Chapter Two, where she claims that current discussion of the origin of the most prominent of modern diseases, AIDS, is itself a piece of neo-imperialistic racism. AIDS has been given an origin in Africa by Western medical scientists. Harrison-Chirimuuta shows that the evidence on which the claim is based is tenuous in the extreme. However, it would seem that no kind of evidence or argument will remove this view from Western minds, since the contesting of the assertion by argument by Africans is simply dismissed and ignored by Western doctors. The attribution of an African origin to AIDS – of all modern diseases – is not arbitrary, Harrison-Chirimuuta argues, but related to how Western scientists view the disease as epidemic and sexually threatening, and how they have unthinkingly absorbed a historical racist image of 'darkest Africa'. Racism, she claims, at least as applied to Africans, is an historical product of the exploitative economic relation of Western colonialists towards Africans, which was necessary as an underpinning of the slave trade, and which was subsequently given pseudo-scientific justification. The same justifications are still at work in AIDS science today. At the heart of modern scientific medicine a contestation thus exists in which the contestants' voices are unequally audible, owing to the experience of the colonial and imperialist past.

The voices of the African pastoralists, the Maasai, whose attitudes to disease control in their cattle are discussed by Richard Waller and Kathy Homewood, were equally inaudible to the colonialists and continue to be so today. The health and management of cattle have long been a nodal point of conflict in some colonised territories, since the requirements placed on them by colonisers and natives have been at such variance. Waller and Homewood show that in the case of the Maasai traditional lands, pastoral herd management was the enemy of land enclosure and efficient land use in the eyes of the colonisers, militating not only against effective disease control and herd improvement but also against colonial authority. They portray a classic area of contestation between two forms of knowledge, 'equally but differently expert', one from a culture superior in power, whose knowledge therefore ought to prevail, the other superior in time and resistance. They show that to the Maasai elders disease is something natural and managed; to Western veterinary experts it is something to be excluded, kept at bay – leading to the imposition of controlled zones, quarantine and other impediments to the Maasai way of effectively managing cattle diseases. These areas of contestation over cattle disease management persist, since meat supply has become part of the way in which the Maasai lands have become incorporated into postcolonial international capitalism. Scientific veterinary medicine, Waller and Homewood imply, simply will not, cannot, listen to other world views, even if they function adequately, because the 'perfectly well' of the elders (keeping cattle alive, large herds) is not the 'perfectly well' of the vets (cash crops, small herds but better animals).

Similar difficulties over hearing native voices were experienced in the attempt to bring the remnants of the original native population of the United States under the administration of Western medicine on the reservations. It was a curious situation: a swamped original population was provided with its own modern health care system, initially intended to help assimilate them, and expected to wither away from its own success. Changes in state attitudes to the Indian Medical Service in successive administrations led to its continued existence but with changing aims. The Indians were only ever marginal participants in the delivery or shaping of this health care. As Stephen Kunitz and Jerrold Levy show in Chapter Four, throughout all the years the image of the ignorant native persisted, deriving from 'the perception of things Indian as being somehow less than things White'. On the other side, the Navajo passively resisted Western medicine by never giving up their own religion-medicine. Only through persistent attempts to provide good translation and training in cultural differences did the rationale behind Navajo acceptance or rejection of Western medicine in particular circumstances come to be understood by the administrators.

Although Brazil was an independent state, the campaigns to eradicate yellow fever there in the early twentieth century were certainly imperialist in mode and tone, especially with the involvement of the Rockefeller Foundation. The changing focus and procedures of the sanitary campaigns that Ilana Löwy describes in Chapter Five themselves reflected contests within scientific medicine as to what was the most significant reservoir of the disease. In turn, these changing views seemed to demand progressively tighter disciplining both of the natives (alive and dead) and of the sanitary service personnel themselves. The sanitary campaigns were repeatedly experienced as 'violence mediated through sanitary measures', as a Rio de Janiero newspaper claimed in 1903, and as the 'tyranny of new doctrines', as a local physician complained in the same year. The direct involvement of the Rockefeller Foundation led to the campaign being portrayed explicitly as a struggle between superstition and civilisation. Local populations were seen in racist terms as backward and ignorant, and their reasonable objections to particularly offensive and insensitive policing procedures had to be ignored in the name of medical progress.

The activities of the Rockefeller Foundation, that great charitable arm of the spread of Western medical knowledge and the American way of life, is the theme also of the chapter by Anne-Emanuelle Birn and Armando Solórzano – but this time in Mexico. They describe the imperialistic way in which the Rockefeller Foundation's International Health Board got itself invited in by the government of Mexico to eradicate hookworm, a chronic human intestinal condition caused by a parasite. They detail also how (as in Brazil) the Rockefeller Foundation retained all the authority, while the host country was placed in the junior position of the relationship, and met the costs of the campaign. The hookworm campaign was a 'hook' – Birn and Solórzano also describe it as an 'entering wedge' or 'lever' – by which the foundation intended to introduce public health on the Western model to Mexico. Hookworm was deliberately chosen as an easy target, not even being experienced as a disease as such by the natives. When natives died of poisoning under the treatment the problems were 'systematically blamed on the habits of Mexican peasants rather than on the campaign's adminstration'.

It must be stressed that what is being said in these chapters about the imperialistic behaviour of those introducing Western medicine is not that it was simply cynical. For, while it is relatively easy to find instances where the health of the Westerners or of the Westerners' animals was the prime goal, the health and well-being of the native populations were also often an aim. The activities and actions of the Rockefeller Foundation show the ambiguities in the situation most starkly. While the Foundation's tactics often appear cynical and authoritarian when re-examined today, its motivations (particularly those of its local administrators) were often clearly philanthropic and honourable. The points at issue here, however, are that, whatever its motives (and, indeed, whatever its successes), the activities of the Rockefeller Foundation were imperialist by their very nature, and that the scientific medicine it was seeking to introduce was equally imperialist in its nature. Inspection of moments of contestation of Rockefeller Foundation activities therefore allows us to see the political nature of the encounter, rather than rehearse the interpretations of the imperialists and see it as an encounter between knowledge and superstition, sense and nonsense, progress and conservative resistance.

India, long a colony of the British, exemplifies the difference between the impact of pre-imperial and imperial medicine. Deepak Kumar shows in Chapter Seven how until the 1860s Western physicians and Indian practitioners of both indigenous and pre-scientific

Western medicine were open to syncretism in their medical practice, but the situation changed when the advocates of scientific medicine began to seek 'absolute supremacy'. The esteem in which indigenous medicine was held thereafter declined, even though it was the medicine of 90 per cent or more of the population. Only in the last decade of the century was there a significant response, provoked by the increasingly forceful way in which Western medicine was imposed in plague outbreaks and enforced vaccination. The revival of Ayurvedic medicine became inevitably bound up with issues of 'Indianisation' and nationalism.

After these decades of the contestation of Western medicine in one way or another, one might ask: how plural is medicine in India today? Helen Lambert raises this question with respect to the non-literate folk medicine of Rajasthan in north-west India. Here Western medicine is one of many kinds of medical system in simultaneous practice. The villagers themselves decide whether their illness is appropriate to treatment by Western medicine or whether it is a 'deity's illness'. The poorest will seek a deity's help first, because it is cheaper. Strikingly, as Lambert shows, adverse reaction to Western medicine is interpreted as meaning that the illness was caused by divine anger. Moreover, biomedicine can be used to correct conditions which have been diagnosed within the radically different thought worlds of indigenous medicine. For Western medicine is thought only to treat the symptoms, not the causes! Given how cause-based Western medicine actually is, this is a great irony: it shows how the Western concept of cause in medicine has not been accepted here. It is evident that, in rural India at least, Western medicine has not driven out indigenous forms of medicine. However, Lambert argues that the antiseptic surgery of Western medicine did replace a native tradition of surgery in the 1880s. Under the apparent co-option and accommodation of Western medicine into local medical systems, it seems, what has been contested in this instance in the world of everyday is precisely Western medicine's largest claim: its claim to 'inherent and general superiority'.

In Japan, according to Emiko Ohnuki-Tierney, what is contested is nothing less than the self. In Chapter Nine she points out that the use in high-technology medicine today of 'brain death' as the criterion of whether to allow the removal of organs from human bodies for transplantation threatens the sense of personhood experienced in many other cultures. The Japanese, even after more than a century of enthusiastic Westernisation, retain a folk religiosity which requires an 'intact body' at death. Consequently they have been remarkably resistant to the adoption of the transplant practices of modern scientific medicine, and indeed of surgery more generally. Moreover, the Japanese have continued to cultivate their traditional popular medicine, *kampō*, which fulfils a crucial role for them precisely at the point where scientific medicine denies or ignores unwell conditions experienced by the patient. Thus they effectively subvert the claim of scientific medicine to define disease states and their presence or absence. The social sensibilities of the Japanese lead them to contest scientific medicine in the subtlest of ways: by negotiating its appropriate realm of validity, and thereby refuting its claims to universality.

On the face of it, rumours are the least reliable form of evidence. In Chapter Ten, Mary Preston Sutphen argues that careful treatment of rumours can yield valuable insights into the nature of the relationship between colonisers and colonised. Her chapter is on the outbreak of plague in 1894 in Hong Kong and in Cape Town in 1901 as an index of reactions to Western medicine by the native population. Rumours have power, since they are impossible to refute, hence rumours of outrages in medical treatment can be a tool for contesting elite Western medical knowledge, and also for challenging the measures that practitioners of scientific medicine thought were required to combat plague. Sutphen shows that rumours about the way the British were dealing with plague were, quite rightly, taken to be threatening to the political hegemony of the British in Hong Kong. Similarly, in Cape Town a few years later, rumours about plague invoked discussion of the city's race and class hierarchies.

Finally we turn full circle to the WHO. Helen Power presents a case of contestation in medicine almost the reverse of those we have seen so far. Thailand had accepted Western medicine and had developed a teaching tradition, but had no tradition of research. It was also suffering the effects of severe drug resistance to the WHO treatment of choice in malaria: chloroquine. But a Thai researcher announcing this fact in 1962 was disbelieved and patronised: although she spoke the language of scientific medicine and had been trained in the West, she came from the wrong country to be taken seriously. The same condescension has been shown, Power claims, to the work of Chinese researchers who have recently produced the new anti-malarial drug qinghaosu. The West disdains it, but the Thais have had to take it up for practical reasons.

We hope that, by treating medicine as an emblem of the larger power relations involved, the studies of the contestation of Western medicine under imperialism presented here will make a contribution to the debate about the relationship between knowledge and political power, on a global scale.

Notes

1 Among the best recent work in English known to us and which is alert to the cultural and social issues, are David Arnold, ed., *Imperial Medicine and Indigenous Societies*, Manchester University Press, 1988; Roy MacLeod and Milton Lewis, eds, *Disease, Medicine and Empire: Perspectives on Western Medicine and the Experience of European Expansion*, London, Routledge, 1988; John Farley, *Bilharzia: a History of Imperial Tropical Medicine*, Cambridge University Press, 1991; David Arnold, *Colonizing the Body: State Medicine and Epidemic Disease in Nineteenth-Century India*, Berkeley, Cal., University of California Press, 1993; Mark Harrison, *Public Health in British India: Anglo-Indian Preventive Medicine, 1859–1914*, Cambridge University Press, 1994; Terence Ranger and Paul Slack, eds, *Epidemics and Ideas: Essays on the Historical Perception of Pestilence*, Cambridge University Press, 1992; David Arnold, 'Medicine and colonialism', in W. F. Bynum and Roy Porter, *Companion Encyclopedia of the History of Medicine*, London, Routledge, 1993, II, pp. 1393–416; Milton I. Roemer, 'Internationalism in medicine and public health', in Bynum and Porter, *Companion Encyclopedia* II, pp. 1417–35; Shirley Lindenbaum and Margaret Lock, eds, *Knowledge, Power and Practice: the Anthropology of Medicine and Everyday Life*, Berkeley, Cal., University of California Press, 1993; Michael Worboys, 'The emergence of tropical medicine: a study in the establishment of a scientific speciality', in Gerard Lemaine, Roy MacLeod, Michael Mulkay and Peter Weingart, eds, *Perspectives on the Emergence of Scientific Discipines*, The Hague, Mouton, 1976, pp. 75–98; E. E. Sabben-Clare, D. J. Bradley and K. Kirkwood, *Health in Tropical Africa during the Colonial Period*, Oxford, Clarendon Press, 1980; John Z. Bowers and Elizabeth F. Purcell, eds, *Medicine and Society in China*, New York, Josiah Macy Jr Foundation, 1974; N. G. Owen, ed., *Death and Disease in South East Asia: Explorations in Social, Medical and Demographic History*, Singapore, Oxford University Press, 1987; Maryinez Lyons, *The Colonial Disease: a Social History of Sleeping Sickness in Northern Zaire, 1900–40*, Cambridge University Press, 1992; D. Landy, ed., *Culture, Disease and Healing: Studies in Medical Anthropology*, New York, Macmillan, 1977; Paul Cranefield, *Science and Empire: East Coast Fever in Rhodesia and the Transvaal*, Cambridge University Press, 1991; and the public health essays in Dagmar Engels and Shula Marks, eds, *Contesting Colonial Hegemony: State and Society in Africa and India*, London, British Academic Press, 1994; Megan Vaughan, *Curing their Ills: Colonial Power and African Illness*, Cambridge, Polity Press, 1991. This listing is necessarily selective.

2 On this general theme see Daniel R. Headrick, *The Tools of Empire: Technology and European Imperialism in the Nineteenth Century*, London, Oxford University Press, 1981.

3 Patrick Manson, 'An introductory address on the necessity for special education in tropical medicine. Delivered at St George's Hospital [London] at the opening of the winter session, Oct. 1st., 1897', *Lancet*, 2 October 1897, pp. 842–5, at p. 843, col. 2.

4 Norman Etherington, *Theories of Imperialism: War, Conquest and Capital*, London, Croom Helm, 1984, p. 278. Our debt to this work will be evident.

5 Etherington, *Theories of Imperialism*, p. 15, citing *The Investor*, 1898.

6 Germany supposedly pioneered the 'new imperialism' as it affected colonies by establishing from the 1870s an empire of diverse but interlinked territories protected by tariff barriers and defended by military might. This was thought by some Britons to be a desirable model to copy. Etherington, *Theories of Imperialism*, p. 53.

7 Etherington, *Theories of Imperialism*, p. 5.

8 Although it is not usually formulated as directly as we have done here, this view underlies much modern work in the recent history of science and history of medicine. For further discussion with relation to the science underlying scientific medicine see Andrew Cunningham and Perry Williams, 'De-centring the 'big picture': *The Origins of Modern Science* and the modern origins of science', *British Journal for the History of Science* 26 (1993), pp. 407–32.

9 Claude Bernard, *An Introduction to the Study of Experimental Medicine*, first published in French in 1865, translated by Henry Copley Greene, New York, 1927, pp. 146–7.

10 Bernard, *Introduction*, pp. 28–32, chapter 2, part I: 'Experimental truths are objective or external'; quotation is from pp. 42–3.

11 Bernard, *Introduction*, p. 214.

12 Bruno Latour, *Science in Action: How to Follow Scientists and Engineers through Society*, Milton Keynes, Open University Press, 1987; the quotation is from p. 97, emphasis as in original.

13 Ilana Löwy, 'Yellow fever in Rio de Janeiro and the Pasteur Institute Mission (1901–1905): the transfer of science to the periphery', *Medical History* 34 (1990), 144–63, p. 144; for this view see also Andrew Cunningham and Perry Williams, eds, *The Laboratory Revolution in Medicine*, Cambridge University Press, 1992.

14 Academic works using the term in their title are appearing with great rapidity, for instance: Douglas Haynes and Gyan Prakash, eds, *Contesting Power: Resistance and Everyday Social Relations in South Asia*, Berkeley and Los Angeles, Cal., University of California Press, 1992; Roy Dilley, ed., *Contesting Markets: Analyses of Ideology, Discourse and Practice*, Edinburgh University Press, 1992; Frank M. Turner, *Contesting Cultural Authority: Essays in Victorian Intellectual Life*, Cambridge University Press, 1993; Steven Seidman, *Contested Knowledge: Social Theory in the Postmodern Era*, Oxford, Blackwell, 1994 (which appeared after the present volume was already in progress); Dagmar Engels and Shula Marks, *Contesting Colonial Hegemony: State and Society in Africa and India*, London, British Academic Press, 1994; Michael Zimmerman, *Contesting Earth's Future: Radical Ecology and Postmodernity*, Berkeley and Los Angeles, Cal., University of California Press, 1994. We have found the introductions by Haynes and Prakash, by Engels and Marks and by Zimmerman particularly helpful.

15 See Haynes and Prakash, *Contesting Power*, pp. 11–12.

16 David Arnold's recent book *Colonizing the Body* is a very good example of such writing.

CHAPTER ONE

WHO and the developing world: the contest for ideology

Sung Lee

I. WHO and uncontested Western medical paternalism

Today it seems obvious that the health of the people is subject to political and ideological contests. Yet, throughout the first thirty years of the World Health Organization, Western or Westernised medical doctors controlled its knowledge and practices, and the nature of 'world health' went uncontested. In 1948, during the first meeting of the World Health Organization's World Health Assembly, the delegate from India remarked that 'India has great hopes that the beneficent activities of this organization will spread throughout the countries of the world and especially to those unfortunate areas where the existing low standards of health are crying out for immediate assistance.'[1] That statement, loaded as it was with implicit acceptance of Western medicine's methods and standards of health care, was typical of the thinking of WHO delegates. No challenge to this ideology and WHO's corresponding practices arose until the 1970s, when WHO accepted the membership of China. The Chinese presented WHO with an astonishing example of successful, low-technology health care by 'barefoot doctors'. It was a programme born of China's socialist revolution. By 1978, as the Chinese challenge was absorbed, the Director General of WHO proclaimed, 'Gone are the days of donor–recipient relationships between WHO and its Member States; an era of real partnership has replaced them.'[2]

Throughout the first thirty years of its existence, the essence of WHO's programme had gone unquestioned. The conflicts were only over matters of degree and not substance, as WHO members haggled over how much aid must be delivered from the rich countries to the poor. The ideology of diffusion – of knowledge, practices, professional medicine generally – which lay at the heart of WHO's policies was a seeming boon for the developing world. It was China's entry into

WHO in 1973 that forced WHO to re-evaluate its aims. China contested the ideology of WHO's programmes, and helped steer it on to a course which would eventually include the promotion of 'traditional medical practices,' a de-emphasis on Western-style professional medicine, and attacks on corporate pharmaceutical interests.

The event which symbolised the eventual contest for the heart of WHO was the 1978 Declaration of Alma Ata, in which WHO affirmed that 'the existing gross inequality in the health status of the people, particularly between developed and developing countries as well as within countries, is politically, socially and economically unacceptable'. WHO declared that 'Governments have a responsibility for the health of their people.' And, as the overarching goal, Primary Health Care was to be the 'key to attaining [Health for All by the year 2000] as part of development in the spirit of social justice'.[3]

What was the route to WHO's new ideology? It was China that showed WHO a different model of health care, but it was the Soviets who spurred the contest that led WHO to Alma Ata. The purpose of this chapter is to trace the international political and professional agendas which have shaped WHO ideology regarding the developing world, from its foundation to the late 1970s.

Postcolonial paternalism and the origins of WHO

WHO was created in 1948 as an arm of the United Nations. The WHO constitution provided for the creation of three major organs: an Assembly of delegates from each member nation, the Executive Board, and the Secretariat, the latter under the head of a Secretary General. The Assembly acts as the supreme policy-making body; it sets policy, approves the budget, and instructs the Executive Board and the Director General. The Executive Board is charged with carrying out the decisions of the World Health Assembly; it also takes the initiative in proposing policies for approval by the Assembly, and in practice has considerable power. The Director General, nominated by the board and appointed by the Assembly, is the chief technical and administrative officer of WHO. He or she has numerous responsibilities and, although formally subject to the authority of the board, can exert considerable power in the selection of priorities and controversies.

WHO is an intergovernmental organisation with no supra-governmental authority. It cannot execute policies which override the will of its member governments. In that sense, all the historical, political and economic relationships among nations can play and have played themselves out in this arena. However – and this was true especially in the early years – WHO has been composed chiefly of medical professionals. As such they have tended to see problems and solutions in medical terms. WHO's pronouncements have thus had the weight, and indeed the baggage, of shared professional opinion. In general, then, the forces shaping WHO policy have tended to be of two kinds: the politics of nation states and the interests of professional medicine.

To understand the larger-scale political forces driving WHO's early policies, we must begin with decolonisation. It was in the shadow of retreating empires that WHO both identified its problems and offered its solutions. After World War Two the young leaders of the newly independent states found themselves with the enormous task of governance in the place of Europeans who had largely dictated their lives. Western techniques and ideologies – including those of medical science – had been adopted nearly wholesale in the colonies by their elites, and in large measure they assumed that their future path was to be one of development towards Western-style society. The indigenous way of life, having failed to withstand the overwhelming force of colonisation by Europe, was regarded as backward. There was no contest, no serious questioning of what the leaders of the former colonies wished to attain – wealth comparable to that of the developed world. Rather, disputes lay in questions of how, or from whom, that wealth was to be gotten.

The ideology and activities of WHO reflected the paternalistic assumptions of the days of empire, from its inception until the early 1970s. WHO saw itself alternately waging a war on disease and dispensing the know-how to lead the ex-colonial peoples on a road to Western-style society. The elites of the former colonies were fully reconciled to that mission. The modes of assistance were often hotly debated, but always within the paradigm of Western medicine. That is, the Western powers were adamant about restricting their aid to technical assistance; WHO should not become a supplier of medical equipment. From the former colonies, however, came a demand for as much assistance as possible – whether as supplies or funds. Thus, from the point of view of the ex-colonial people, WHO was an instrument through which they could exact aid from, and air grievances against, their former masters. Nursing a guilty conscience, the European powers tended to be in tacit agreement with that view. Thus there was an abiding tension within WHO between the rich and poor nations, and resentment of the former colonisers was obvious in the language of formerly colonial WHO delegates. The early leader of the former colonies, in WHO as in the world, was India. In the World Health Assembly the delegates from South Asia were keen to claim as much as possible from the Western-led organisation. The delegate from India pronounced in 1949 that 'there is only one royal road, and that is active field work ... the salvation of the backward countries lies in active work in their spheres'.[4] The delegate from Pakistan implored that 'special care should be bestowed on countries which lack the resources possessed by the more advanced and prosperous countries of Europe and America'.[5]

Aid must be unilateral and unconditional. The Indian delegate complained that 'I must confess that we are very disturbed about the proposal that medical supplies should be paid for by governments.'[6] The delegate from Ceylon: ' I stress it again ... We need medical supplies in all our countries, facilities for the obtaining of which we expect from an international organization like the WHO.'[7] The words of his successor two years later were even stronger:

> South East Asia is not receiving as much aid as it ought ... the European nations of the world owe to the South East Asian nations a duty that they shall undertake to raise the living conditions and the health conditions of the people [of] those areas, whom they have exploited for over 200 years.[8]

The new states of the Middle East followed suit. The Lebanese delegate argued that 'We need assistance on a larger scale ... Could we not suggest an international aid plan ...?'[9] Perhaps the bluntest demands of all came from the delegate representing Jordan:

> If the WHO adheres strictly to the approved principles governing the granting of its financial help to the backward and under-developed countries, it should immediately provide the necessary funds for starting work on these projects totally at its own expense. It may commence with one project at a time, and after its completion start with the next, and so on until the projects are completed to the entire satisfaction of my country and WHO.[10]

The delegate warned that his country would withdraw from WHO if the demand was not met, and the 'moral effect' of the withdrawal would be 'great'.

The demands of the ex-colonial lands were heard and were not denied. In his annual report for 1951 the Director General, Brock Chisholm wrote that the 'richly endowed' countries had a 'duty' to help the world's poor.[11] However, Western delegates were highly wary of massive material assistance, which the UK delegate likened to the dole, adding that 'some of us feel considerable anxiety as to whether we may not be casting our net too widely'.[12]

A paternalistic relationship was thus deeply embedded within the assumptions of WHO members, rich and poor alike. It was never questioned in those early years that WHO's assistance would be based on the superiority and universal applicability of Western medical science.

That outlook was perhaps as well stated in WHO's official history as anywhere:

> If new ideas or methods could be effectively introduced merely by training one or two receptive individuals in a country the problem would be relatively simple; but established tradition and inertia often bar the way of progress. It therefore becomes necessary to influence deep-rooted attitudes which is more difficult than imparting knowledge or skills.[13]

In its *First Report on the World Health Situation* WHO maintained that:

> The struggle against disease, ignorance and poverty has been retarded by the persistence of superstitious beliefs and practices ... the path from magic to medicine has often been slow and difficult ... Adjustment to the machine age is a long process of social education.[14]

To combat such superstition and remake the poor world in the image of the rich, WHO provided fellowships to natives of the ex-colonial and undeveloped lands. Fellows were to bring back European techniques and professional authority to their homelands. Formal medical training was the benchmark, though WHO noted that 'in some countries it has been customary, and ... probably necessary, to employ auxiliary personnel to do work which would ordinarily be entrusted only to professional health workers'. The WHO doctors soberly warned that auxiliary personnel 'should know their own limitations and be warned against taking on greater technical responsibilities than they are able to carry.'[15] Progress in health depended on bringing Western medicine to the world.

The war on disease

In terms of immediate action, WHO's earliest, highest priority was to engage in a war on disease.[16] The WHO sent its specialists around the world, bringing Western medical and public health techniques to bear wherever they went. In the first year of its existence WHO sent teams of medical officers, nurses, sanitary engineers, public health officers, bacteriologists and other personnel to China, Ethiopia, Haiti, India, Ceylon, North Korea, South Korea and the Philippines.[17] It set up 'health demonstration areas', model sites which were meant to be copied throughout the country.

The language of its members in the developed world was explicit in its military imagery. In his very first annual report Brock Chisholm declared that 'The World Health Organization, during the first few months of its existence, has prepared plans and begun operations for launching offensives against disease.'[18] Here was the legacy of the post-

World War Two origins of WHO. Squads of physicians, public health officers, sanitary engineers and other technicians were sent around the world to wage war against the agents of sickness. The WHO official history is steeped in activist military metaphors for WHO's campaign against malaria.

WHO's malaria campaign was its first project, and it was an immense failure.[19] Enormous sums were spent on the project. In 1960, when WHO's regular budget was US$16,330,900, the separately administrated malaria account was budgeted for US$18,197,726.[20] Brief successes were repeatedly followed by renewed outbreaks. By mid-decade the World Health Assembly had agreed to scale back its original goal of total victory over the disease. According to Harrison, 'WHO gave way ... But it was not easy either to abandon the old ways or to find new ones. Eradication had been a jealous idol.'[21]

The retreat marked the painful end of an era for the organisation and sowed misgivings which contributed to the upheavals in WHO's work during the 1970s. One former WHO official wrote in 1975 that:

> Unreality has been WHO's chief weakness, symbolized by the malaria eradication scheme upon which money, time and effort has [sic] been unstintingly spent in the belief, seemingly, that the basic laws of ecology and social-anthropology would be lifted to allow a magical disappearance of the disease.[22]

Yet confidence in Western methods and know-how had not disappeared; the problem was only that proper public health techniques had been supplanted by the 'emotionalism' of the mass campaign. And although there were charges that 'doctors trained in the traditional medical schools of the developed world were likely to be more of a hindrance than a help', that was only because they were 'ill-equipped to direct auxiliaries trained for house to house work'. In principle the necessity of medical leadership went unchallenged. *'Creating the infrastructure and training doctors and auxiliaries to work in it called urgently for attention, possibly before all else.'*[23] The model of health care still lay in *creating* a health care system, i.e. imitating a Western model of health care. By 1978 these assumptions had become untenable.

Decolonised Africa: looking back to Europe

The decade from the mid 1950s to the mid 1960s saw a great tide of new African nations created out of the dissolution of empire. Shades of decolonised Asia – poor and demanding – appeared quickly. The assumption of diffusion underlying WHO policy was to be reinforced by the pressures applied by the young African states. During the decade 1956–65 WHO's membership increased by about half.

The elder members of WHO treated the newcomers as so many new needy cases. WHO had co-ordinated the sending of medical teams as part of a UN relief effort during the crisis of total and immediate Belgian withdrawal from the Congo in 1960, and it seemed as though that event might be the exemplar of future WHO relations with Africa. In 1961, with WHO having admitted fifteen new African states in the preceding year alone, Upper Volta led the World Health Assembly to pass a resolution which noted 'with satisfaction the speedy assistance given by WHO to the Republic of Congo' and requested the Director General 'to continue to give such speedy assistance to all newly independent states which become members of WHO'.[24] The American delegate announced his 'strong support', and that sentiment was typical of the reaction from the Assembly at large.

During that same Assembly, the Soviet Union collaborated with Cuba, Ghana, Iraq, Mexico, New Zealand, Poland, South Africa and the United Arab Republic to submit what was to be WHO's first resolution detailing the nature of WHO's imminent assistance to the soon-to-be states of Africa. The assumption remained that health care was a function of medical personnel numbers. The Assembly resolved that:

> WHO has an important part to play in promoting the fundamental and inalienable right to freedom and independence ... and that one of WHO's urgent tasks is to help newly independent countries, and those preparing for independence, to overcome deficiencies in health programs and serious shortages in trained medical and health personnel.[25]

Thus WHO requested 'the Director-General to make all possible efforts to ... cooperate with [new members] in the training of local medical personnel technically qualified to undertake the responsibility of combating infectious and parasitic diseases and of improving national health services'.[26]

With WHO in consensus on the importance of aid, the Director General, Dr M. G. Candau, took the lead in presenting the Assembly with a vision of the form that aid should take. Candau presented the Assembly with a report in 1962 on 'Continued Assistance to Newly Independent States'. The report was yet another reflection of the paternalistic, universalistic medical assumptions embedded in WHO's activities; the agenda presented might have come die-cast from a mould for anywhere in the world. Candau wrote that 'the current WHO programme in newly independent states is, in many ways, like that which the organization is carrying out in other countries [i.e. Asia]'.[27] As he did in other reports, Candau outlined malaria eradication programmes, projects for the control of other communicable diseases, education, training, public health administration, environmental health. If there was a particular problem in Africa, it was the severe paucity of Western-style doctors: 'It has been estimated that the newly independent and emerging states in Africa alone will require something like 1100 physicians every year for twenty years.' As a major part of his report Candau had provided 'An Expanded and Accelerated Education and Training Program': a blueprint for the young nations to churn out as many physicians as possible. Like the resolution presented by Upper Volta the previous year, Candau's report was praised from all sides – Europe, America, the USSR, the developing nations of Asia and Africa alike.

Physicians, whether European or African, made the decisions at WHO, and the future of health care was considered in terms of the future of the medical profession. The delegate from Upper Volta, a physician, reported to the Assembly in 1967 that his country had only sixty-five physicians, forty-eight of whom were non-nationals on assignment, and thirty-six of whom were specialists in 'urban centres, with no benefit to the rural population', which represented over 95 per cent of the total population. The ratio of physician to patients, he deplored, was 1:73,000. And though he was 'grateful' for 'stopgap' technical assistance from France and other industrialised countries, he insisted that the 'real solution to the problem lies in training our own national staff'.[28] Upper Volta's long-term future health care lay in a kind of import substitution of professionals, replacing foreign physicians with native ones.

European policies, and perhaps more fundamentally European examples, had left the African leadership with scarcely even a conception of any future dissimilar from a European one.[29] In 1967 a bloc of twenty-six African countries pressed a resolution through WHO asking the Director General to report again on WHO's policy in the developing countries. In particular he was to study ways of increasing material assistance to the developing world (drugs, vaccines and serums), increasing the organisational resources available to member states (labs, electrotherapy, surgical sterilisation equipment, vehicles, refrigerators) and sharing in the operating expenses of programmes there (for staff). This resolution again reflected WHO's medical bias: the assumption that the organisation must transmit Western techniques worldwide.

When Europeans conquered Asia and Africa in the nineteenth century they imposed on Asians and Africans alien forms of economic organisation and governance. European statesmen carved out spheres of influence which in the age of decolonisation would become the *de facto* boundaries of new countries. European colonial administrators trained their subjects in European ways, and health was no exception.

The domination of WHO by medical professionals led to an understanding of health care whereby the physician lay at the centre. Through the late 1960s WHO members, African, Asian, American or European, saw the means of achieving a healthy world as the production of ever more physicians. This programme went uncontested.

II. 'Primary health care' as novel contest of ideology

As we have seen, the leaders of the developing countries had taken for granted the superiority of the Western mode of health care, and WHO was seen as the arena for them to exact aid from the West, to implement Western methods. The unquestioned status of that agenda was evident in the nature of the resolutions passed by the developing countries. At the same time there was growing frustration within WHO over the failure to bring greater health to the poor nations, expressed in the anguished remarks of the Director General and delegates at Assembly meetings, or more aseptically in technical reports: health manpower shortage, the 'inadequacy of the existing health infrastructure'. The world recession of the early 1970s heightened the sense of crisis.

In 1978, eleven years after the World Health Assembly had passed its major resolution on the need to seek new ways of increasing assistance to the developing countries, WHO issued its Declaration of Alma Ata, whose assumptions were far removed from notions of 'assistance'. WHO proclaimed at Alma Ata that 'the people have the right and duty to participate individually and collectively in the planning and implementation of their health care'.[30] The declaration proceeded to a lengthy description of primary health care, affirming first of all that it 'reflects and evolves from the economic conditions and socio-cultural and political characteristics of the country'.

What led WHO to Alma Ata? The declaration represented a radically new ideology, and to understand it we must understand the political changes on which it rested.[31] We must look to the politics and foreign policies of China, the USSR and the United States in the twentieth century. The investigation will be simultaneously an exploration of the underestimated importance of the Chinese revolution to the modern world and a portrayal of the ever-present, if sometimes concealed, reality of the Cold War in international activities, even those of a health organisation.

The arrival of the People's Republic of China in the World Health Organization in 1973 presented an implicit, profound challenge to WHO, at a time when the failure of malaria eradication had left it especially impressionable. Without any assistance from the agency, an 'undeveloped nation' comprising one-fifth of the world's population had created an outstanding system of basic health care for its massive peasantry. The manpower for that system had come not from professionals trained in Western medicine but from the very peasant populace it served.

China provided the example, but it was only the Soviet Union which spurred the Chinese success into a contest for WHO ideology. It was the Soviets that led WHO to create a new rhetoric at Alma Ata, which eschewed the former goal of diffusing Western techniques around the world in favour of a strident, politicised advocacy of primary health care.

The road to change: a failure in 'basic health services'

With expectations high, discontent ran deep over the failure of the newly independent nations to achieve Western standards of health care. Director General Candau had consistently championed what he perceived as the interests of the developing world, but as usual he was wary of doling out aid or materials, suspicious of WHO's 'becoming a supply organization instead of an organization providing technical assistance'.[32] In a report issued in 1968 he downplayed the importance of equipment and supplies in a list of newer forms of assistance. WHO's role remained that of benefactor, if an increasingly reluctant one.

In a complaint which was, again, to reflect the medical orientation of the WHO, Candau identified lack of medical manpower – the lack of interest among medical graduates in pursuing public health careers, in particular – as a serious problem. It was a sentiment reiterated by many member governments. In 1968 the delegate from Congo complained that 'everybody knows how difficult it is, in the developing countries, to get a young doctor fresh from a European medical faculty to accept the practice of preventive medicine'.[33]

It was this nagging discontent that led the Executive Board, in 1971, to recommend that the World Health Assembly should adopt 'Methods of promoting basic health services' as the topic of its next routine organisational study. The Assembly so voted. The study was to set in motion a series of resolutions which were to lead eventually to the ideology of Alma Ata. Yet that study might have died in committee like so many others. A desire for new approaches at WHO surely existed by the turn of the decade, but the catalyst of change at WHO was the entry of China.

China and the 'barefoot doctors'

From the founding of the UN and WHO, the delegate representing

China had hailed from the Republic of China, based on the island of Formosa. In 1972 the Sino-American *rapprochement* which had begun in the late 1960s culminated in the admission of the People's Republic to the UN and its agencies. The experiences of the most populous country on earth – the People's Republic of China – which had previously been practically invisible to WHO, were soon to arrive in full force on WHO's agenda.

Chinese society has undergone massive transformations in the twentieth century, and the Cultural Revolution of the 1960s and 1970s was to have important consequences for health care in the People's Republic. Anti-intellectualism was central to the Cultural Revolution, and Chairman Mao had harsh words for the medical profession. In 1965 Mao announced, in what was later to be memorialised as the '26 June Directive':

> Tell the Ministry of Public Health that it only works for fifteen per cent of the total population of the country and that this fifteen per cent is mainly composed of gentlemen, while the broad masses of the peasants do not get any medical treatment ... The Ministry of Public Health is not a Ministry of Public Health for the people, so why not change its name to the Ministry of Urban Health, the Ministry of Gentlemen's Health, or even the Ministry of Urban Gentlemen's health?[34]

The problem, Mao contended, lay in the vested interests of an urban medical profession. The solution was to train a new kind of doctor – the 'barefoot doctor'. Precedents for the barefoot doctors had existed as early as the 1920s, but they were not made the centrepiece of rural health care until the Cultural Revolution.[35] It has been estimated that by the late 1960s in China there were perhaps 150,000 doctors trained in Western medicine, 172,000 assistant doctors, 186,000 nurses, 42,000 midwives and 100,000 pharmacists. The training of barefoot doctors began in earnest in 1965, and within seven years there were probably over a million.[36]

Typically, barefoot doctors received three to six months of training, either in their commune or in a local hospital, in both traditional Chinese and Western therapeutic techniques.[37] They were also trained to take on responsibilities 'for environmental sanitation, for health education, for immunization, for first aid, and for aspects of personal primary medical care and post-illness follow-up.'[38] They were paid according to the 'work points' they accumulated, with their health work being remunerated at about the level of heavy labor.[39] The training was soon extended to include 'worker doctors' in the factories and 'Red Guard doctors' in urban neighbourhoods.

Crucially, barefoot doctors – and their counterparts in other settings

– continued to serve as labourers. They were peasants, factory workers or housewives who had an additional responsibility for the rudimentary preventive and curative health care of their fellow workers. They were generally selected by their peers. The barefoot doctor was not to be a medical professional.

The frank political rhetoric accompanying the barefoot doctor system was striking. Health care workers must serve the peasant masses. The Revolutionary Committee of the Shanghai First Medical College had declared in 1968 that doctors were 'bourgeois intellectual aristocrats who rode over the working people and thought of nothing else than personal fame, wealth and position. [Medical education] ignored the five hundred million peasants and served only the cities.'[40]

The instructions written on the wall of a health station in Peking outlined the working responsibilities of Red Guard doctors as follows:

> 1. Hold high the great banner of Mao Zedong's thought. Stand up for proletarian politics. Study Chairman Mao's philosophical works creatively. Change our world outlook. Practise and apply it in every day's work.
> 2. Strengthen revolutionary discipline. Do not be late to work, do not go home early, do not be 'thrice divorced': divorced from the mass movement, divorced from physical labor, or divorced from the masses.[41]

Other instructions stressed prevention, family planning and the 'three traditions: traditional doctors, traditional medicines, and traditional methods'. One Western visitor described Chinese policies as dedicated to 'deprofessionalization, demystification, decentralization, popular participation'.[42] The glorification of the barefoot doctor exemplified the aspirations of the Cultural Revolution: pragmatism, self-sacrifice, anti-intellectualism.

The Chinese challenge to WHO

With relations developing between the United States and China in the late 1960s, China gained membership of the United Nations in 1971, and to WHO in 1973. The communist Chinese were inexperienced in the ways of international organisations, but the sheer size of their nation and the indisputable success of their barefoot doctors were to initiate a revolution in WHO's basic understanding of health care and of the organisation's very mission. China's example led to a reorientation of the relationship between WHO and the developing countries. Some delegates from the developing world would take up China's rhetoric of the politics behind health; some were to assign new meanings to their traditional medicine. These were the changes which led to Alma Ata.

Chinese delegates spared no effort to impress upon their counterparts at WHO the success of the barefoot doctors, and they repeatedly stressed the political origins of their health care. In his country's first address to the World Health Assembly the communist Chinese delegate to WHO proclaimed:

> To develop national public health services and improve the people's health conditions is [sic] an important question bearing on the national prosperity and economic development of each country ... The most essential conditions for the realization of this desire are to shake off aggression and oppression by imperialism, colonialism, and neo-colonialism, combat big-power hegemonism and power politics, win and safeguard national independence and develop the national economy independently by relying on the broad masses of the people. To serve the worker-peasant masses – the majority of the people – is the fundamental orientation for public health in China ... A million 'barefoot doctors' are growing up sturdily in the vast rural areas in China. They form a new force in the medical contingent, who, while taking part in collective productive labor, prevent and treat diseases for the peasants.[43]

Like numerous delegates from the developing world before him, the Chinese delegate invoked the sins of great-power aggression, which China too had known since the nineteenth century. However, unlike them he declared that the solution lay not in redress but in self-reliance. Rather than invoke the time-worn politics of redistribution, he called for a revolutionary understanding of the people's health. It was this call to a new politicisation, based not on global transfers of wealth but on the reordering of domestic political priorities, that was to be such a profound lesson for WHO.[44]

The Chinese had given some aid to the new African states during the 1960s in an abortive attempt to create a non-aligned bloc of developing countries, and they surely induced some of those states to adopt China's line in WHO. During the 1973 Assembly the delegate from Dahomey announced that his government's 'new policy in the health field must basically be directed toward the masses ... to give preventive medicine priority over curative medicine, to associate modern and traditional medicine with one another'.[45] The Guinean delegate proclaimed that the 'health squads' of the 'local revolutionary authorities' were 'rooted in the people ... taking as their starting point the real needs of the people'.[46] In closing his speech he offered sincere thanks to the Chinese for the disinterested assistance rendered.

WHO reports began to acknowledge the Chinese challenge. According to a 1973 document:

> Change, it was thought, was much more likely to occur in the local set-

ting if it came from within the community itself ... the ability to utilize and build on local traditional methods of medicine that can be implemented at low cost and have their own degree of effectiveness is an example of good management.[47]

The Chinese example behind the report's high-flown universalistic language was unmistakable.

WHO's lean towards a new course was obvious by 1975, when it published a major study with the politely pluralistic title *Alternative Approaches to Meeting Basic Health Needs in Developing Countries*. The study opened with a claim that:

> [H]istory and experience show that conventional health services, organized along 'western' or other centralized lines, are unlikely to expand to meet the basic health needs of all people ... Some countries will need to make drastic or revolutionary changes in their approach to health services ... The remodeled approach must be linked to the prevailing human attitudes and values, which differ from community to community, and it will require a clear motivation and commitment on the part of the people who have the knowledge and political and economic power to make change.[48]

In spite of its many references to health systems and projects in a number of countries, the study was in essence, again, an acknowledgement of the success of the Chinese and a genuinely optimistic investigation of China's health care as a model for the developing countries.

The authors of the section on China had been deeply impressed. The Chinese example, they concluded, showed that:

> fundamental changes in health and health care may require fundamental changes in the social structure in which they are embedded ... But surely the greatest lesson China offers is that it can be done – that a nation can within one generation move from a starving, sickness-riddled, illiterate, elitist semi-feudal society to a vigorous, healthy, productive, highly literate, mass participation society. If China can accomplish it, other nations can too.[49]

The conclusion was firm:

> have the approaches described been really successful ...? In the cases of China and Cuba, a definite positive answer can be given ... What characterizes successful national programmes is a strong political will that has transformed a practicable methodology into a national endeavor.[50]

Changing meanings associated with the word 'traditional' illustrate the depth of the change wrought by the Chinese. In the late 1960s, in a short-lived period of nationalist pride, there had been calls from several developing countries for WHO to assist them in learning about the efficacy of their traditional medicines. In 1967 the delegates from Upper Volta and Nigeria requested WHO's Division of Pharmacology and Toxicology to analyse chemically plants which had been used 'traditionally for curative purposes'.[51]

Two years later the issue was raised again, this time in a joint resolution presented by the delegates of Congo (Brazzaville) and Guinea. By that time the national pride behind the 'tradition' had disappeared. On the one hand, the delegates emphasised not the benefits of traditional medicines but the 'hazards and economic wastage connected with such use'.[52] On the other hand, the delegates requested the Director General 'to assist governments in the study of the efficacy and safety of traditional medicines ... with a view to developing the production of drugs from naturally occurring raw materials'. The Ethiopian delegate complained of the 'burden' imposed by the practice of traditional medicine, while the Pakistani delegate bemoaned the 'problems' which traditional medicine posed in his country.

China definitively reoriented the question of traditional medicine back to one of national pride. The Chinese had no intention of demanding or even passively accepting Western medicine as the other developing nations had. They were instead emphatic about bringing their own health care practices into the world spotlight. Following the Chinese lead, during the World Health Assemblies of 1973 and 1974 delegations from Zaire, Dahomey, Congo, Guinea, the United Republic of Cameroon, Sri Lanka, India and Malawi, many of which had never before mentioned the topic, began speaking of their traditional medicine as a positive affirmation of their native cultures.

Traditional medicine and traditional health workers were to gain even more stock as the Assembly began to give shape to its Primary Health Care ideology. The delegate from Malawi asserted in 1975 that:

> in his country it was the traditional midwives and healers who offered primary health care to the great majority of the people. It would therefore be inappropriate for WHO to enhance such health care without taking the importance of traditional medicine into account.[53]

In the Director General's report for 1976–77 traditional medicine had become a category unto itself. In 1978 WHO arranged a study tour for members from twenty-nine countries to visit China; another was arranged the following year. That same year the delegations of Ghana, India, New Zealand, Rwanda, Sri Lanka and Thailand sponsored a major resolution on the 'Promotion and development of training and research in traditional medicine'. In sponsoring the resolution, the delegate from India stressed that 'in a number of countries, notably in

South East Asia and China, traditional systems of medicine had made spectacular contributions to the health of the people'.[54]

In 1978 WHO supported research into the efficacy of ayurvedic medicine in rheumatoid arthritis, and it sent a group of Africans to China to study acupuncture. Since 1979 it has opened numerous collaborating centres around the world for the study and practice of traditional medicine. The promotion of traditional medicines, healers and midwives has served WHO as an answer to the perennial problem of manpower shortage and as an affirmation of non-Western national identities.

China provided an example of effective health care in an undeveloped country which borrowed some Western techniques but which in its grass-roots origins stood outside WHO's model of health care development. It was an example which contradicted most of the assumptions of Western medical paternalism: an effective health care system which served one-fifth of the global population without Western-style physicians. Through the example of China the persistent problems which WHO had conceptualised as 1) how to solve manpower shortages, i.e. how to provide more health care workers trained in Western techniques and to Western professional standards, and 2) how to 'create an infrastructure', i.e. how to establish and sustain Western-style health centres in lands of incredible poverty, were eventually to be dissolved in favour of a new WHO ideology, that methods of health care must not be imposed on the people but must come *from* the people, and that, as in China, such methods were inseparable from politics at large. The new WHO ideology, borrowed from China, was to be encapsulated in the Alma Ata declaration and the rhetoric of 'primary health care'.

The Soviet initiative to reinvent WHO

It was the Soviet Union, however, which expanded on China's example to remake WHO's *raison d'être*, and thereby to score a small Cold War victory. Cold War hostilities had appeared in an extreme form shortly after the founding of WHO, when the Soviet Union and its satellites withdrew in 1950, only to rejoin in 1957. Through the 1960s the Soviets were readier than the United States to inject Cold War messages into the WHO arena. They had taken aim at the former colonial powers with various memoranda and in the late 1960s they had introduced resolutions into WHO deploring the 'epidemiological situation' in Vietnam.

By 1975 the Soviet Union had seized the initiative in sustaining the momentum for change at WHO. It was the Soviet Union that turned the half-hearted proposals for change, first manifest in the Executive

Board's 1971 study of 'Methods of Promoting Basic Health Services', into a call, in 1975, for an international health conference on primary health care whose rhetoric would become central to WHO ideology. In 1976 the Assembly passed a major resolution on promoting primary health care, and a year later passed its resolution encouraging the use and development of traditional medical practices. Alma Ata followed in 1978. In retracing the early steps on WHO's road to Alma Ata we see that Soviet leadership was crucial.

At the World Health Assembly which met in 1975, one of WHO's two general committees discussed the report of the Director General on the promotion of national health services. Two proposed resolutions had been offered in response to the report. The first was an anodyne expression of thanks to the Director General for his report, offered by an *ad hoc* group of the Executive Board. The second was far stronger; it began by reaffirming the 'impossibility of accepting any longer a position in which the overwhelming majority of the population in many countries lacks the opportunity to exercise its inalienable right to the protection and improvement of its health'.[55] It went on to recommend the convening of an international conference devoted to the topic of primary care. This proposal had been put forward by countries of the Communist Bloc: Cuba, Czechoslovakia, Mongolia and the USSR.

The response to the Soviet initiative was intriguing, for it did not divide clearly, as might have been expected, along lines demarcating developed and undeveloped countries. At least as important a divider was the question of professional medical privilege. The US delegate, product of a medical establishment consistently hostile to governmental involvement with health care, favoured the first proposal. He complained that:

> The title of the agenda item was confusing; the point at issue was primary health care – i.e. that component of the existing system that was required to extend services to the majority, in their own localities, in an acceptable manner, and at a cost that the country could afford – not the promotion of *national health services, organizations, or systems.* [Emphasis added]

He concluded 'therefore, ... the draft resolution proposed by the Soviet delegation, though it was in itself correct and good, did not concern the subject under discussion'. Yet the promotion of some sort of national health service, organisation or system, as a means of providing primary health care, had been precisely the point of the discussion.

The US delegate's reaction epitomised the professional medical outlook which had so long dominated WHO, and the frank words of numerous other delegates underlined that truth. The Norwegian delegate warned that:

> at a time when certain groups with a strong antiprofessional bias in a number of countries were tending to oversimplify the problem of health care and to deny the need for special medical competence ... any WHO document ... should strike a proper balance [regarding the relationship of primary care to specialized services]

The delegate from Egypt declared that:

> Primary Health Care in all countries was based on the services of the *doctor* [emphasis added] who, as the most highly qualified member of the health care team, should be responsible for the directing of health units with the help of nurses, auxiliaries and paramedical personnel who could take over from him only under exceptional circumstances.

The United States, Norway, Egypt and five other countries came out for the toothless proposal, which did not include a call for an international conference, against the Soviet one.

Opposing medical interests, the Belgian delegate claimed that '[t]he most difficult task undoubtedly would be to persuade doctors trained along necessary lines to agree to the necessary changes'. The delegate from Cameroon lamented that 'Powerful vested interests opposed any change ... much resistance was encountered among medical and health personnel to any suggestion of creating new cadres with medical functions between those of physicians and nurses.'

In the end, the Executive Board agreed to allow a working group consisting of the chairman of the *ad hoc* group and the delegates from the USSR, Cuba, Czechoslovakia and Mongolia – the sponsors of the second proposal – to work out a new proposal. The new proposal was quite similar to the original Soviet one, and it retained the call for an international conference. The proposed resolution was carried.

In January 1976 the Executive Board acted on the resolution. The Soviets continued to lead in the matter. Halfdan Mahler, three years into his service as Director General, was hesitant. Mahler was 'not convinced that the time was opportune ... action should be directed to the regional, sub-regional, and national levels and pursued with clear knowledge and awareness of the problems and present solutions of individual countries'.[56] The Soviet board member, Dr Venediktov, pressed on immediately; he was 'surprised ... [and] failed to understand how the desirability of holding the conference could now be questioned'.

While the other members listened, very probably quite surprised themselves, Venediktov went on to describe bluntly the ideological interests behind the policy.

> It was not enough to send another group of experts to a few countries and produce another book ... It had been stated in a book on *Health and Developing Countries*, published by the Rockefeller Foundation some years before, that the authors had been unable to visit a number of countries, including the Soviet Union and China; that book had failed to bring out the spirit of Primary Health Care.

He stressed the USSR's desire to sponsor the conference: 'The Soviet Government was prepared to show participants what had been done in that connexion in its country over the past 50 years.' Venediktov moved quickly to close off the possibility of invitations from other countries to hold the conference, though he was unsuccessful in doing so.

The US board member could agree only falteringly, and in his last remark he complained, probably without even understanding the manoeuvre which he had just witnessed, that 'there was a tendency to view the program as a kind of competitive ideological effort. He trusted that, in future, it would be seen rather as a means of progress toward health for all.'

A new ideology for WHO

Primary health care and 'Health for all by the year 2000' were in fact the result of a competitive ideological effort, though they represented more of an ideological than a substantive change. The Chinese example had undermined the assumptions of Western medical paternalism, and the Soviets had turned the Chinese lesson into a new ideology of health. The changes in WHO activities, however, were less striking. The only major change in the flow of WHO funds was a cut in administrative expenses, in favour of increased funding for technical co-operation (to rise from 51 per cent in 1977 to 60 per cent in 1981).[57] WHO documents have consistently criticised the 'domination of the health planning process by members of the medical profession',[58] yet WHO still grants as many fellowships as it ever has, proportionately, for medical education.[59]

At all events, in the late 1970s WHO began to promote the training of health workers with basic skills, and that has been perhaps the most concrete change in its fieldwork. An important element of the policy has been traditional medicines and health workers, a subject on which WHO has sponsored numerous seminars and conferences. The imagery of war on disease, physicians-the-world-over, disappeared from WHO's publications in favour of the low-key community health worker.

If budgets and fieldwork did not change drastically, the new WHO ideology did provide a rationale for different battles. The leadership of

Halfdan Mahler was critical in this regard. If Mahler had hesitated in the earliest stages of the making of Primary Health Care policy, he had staked his career and perhaps the WHO itself on even more radical stands by the late 1970s.[60] In 1977 he spearheaded a drive to produce a list of essential drugs to help the developing nations order their health budgets, a move which provoked extreme hostility among drug interests touting the virtues of the free market. By 1981 the chairman of a major US drug company was telling his colleagues at a trade meeting that:

> An innovative minority conceives the world's technology, raises most of the world's food and produces most of the world's goods. This minority is being challenged by a hostile majority ... [We must] put intense pressure on the UN – and on its specialized agencies – to give realistic instead of unrealistic advice to developing countries. For this year and next, 70% of WHO's budget will be paid by 13 industrialized countries. Certainly this entitles the industrialized world to stand up to WHO. We must have the will to do so.[61]

In general WHO's declared enemies have changed from mosquitoes to actors all too human, whether 'imperial' medical interests or multinational corporations.[62] To wage its new wars, the declaration of Alma Ata has served as its ideological touchstone. The Alma Ata goal of 'Health for all by the year 2000' has become a WHO mantra. The organisation's latest *Report on the World Health Situation* was renamed around the new mission: *Evaluation of the Strategy for Health for All by the Year 2000: Seventh Report of the World Health Situation*. By the 1970s WHO had abandoned the war on disease, and through the challenge of the socialist giants it discarded its assumptions of the natural beneficence of Western professional medicine in favour of a more politicised rhetoric of health.

Notes

I would like to express my deep thanks to the Rotary Foundation, from whom I received a scholarship which allowed me to study for a year at the University of Cambridge, and to Dr Andrew Cunningham, whose guidance was essential throughout this project.

1 *First World Health Assembly, 1948*, WHO Official Records 13: 32.
2 *The Work of WHO for 1976–77*, WHO Official Records 243: ix.
3 *Primary Health Care: Report of the International Conference on Primary Health Care*, Geneva: WHO, 1978: 3.
4 *Second World Health Assembly, 1949*, WHO Official Records 21: 80.
5 *First World Health Assembly, 1948*: 34.
6 *Second World Health Assembly, 1949*: 80.
7 *Second World Health Assembly, 1949*: 84.
8 *Fourth World Health Assembly, 1951*, WHO Official Records 35: 111.
9 *Third World Health Assembly, 1950*, WHO Official Records 28: 107.
10 *Fifth World Health Assembly, 1952*, WHO Official Records 42: 92–3.

11 *The Work of WHO for 1951*, WHO Official Records 38: 1.
12 *Third World Health Assembly, 1950*: 112.
13 *The First Ten Years of the World Health Association*, Geneva: WHO, 1958: 373.
14 *First Report on the World Health Situation, for 1954–56*, WHO Official Records, 94: 10.
15 *The First Ten Years*: 375.
16 Principal enemies included malaria, tuberculosis, venereal diseases, treponematoses, viral diseases, zoonoses.
17 It must be noted here that none of these early efforts, including the first years of the malaria programme described later, were directed towards Africa, because of a perception of the sheer magnitude of the problem there.
18 *Annual Report of the Director General for 1948*, WHO Official Records 16: 7.
19 See Gordon Harrison, *Mosquitoes, Malaria, and Man: a History of the Hostilities since 1880*, London: John Murray, 1978: 222–58.
20 *Proposed Regular Programme and Budget*, WHO Official Records 89: 1960.
21 Harrison, *Mosquitoes*: 257.
22 C. F. Brockington, *World Health*, Edinburgh: Churchill Livingstone, 1975: 179.
23 *Ibid.*: 179. Emphasis in original.
24 *Handbook of Resolutions and Decisions of the World Health Assembly and the Executive Board I, 1948–72*, Geneva: WHO, 1973: 7–8.
25 *Handbook of Resolutions and Decisions*, 8.
26 As reprinted in 'United Nations', *Encyclopaedia Britannica* XXIX, London: Encyclopaedia Britannica, 1992: 147.
27 *Fifteenth World Health Assembly, 1962*, WHO Official Records 119: 84–97.
28 *Twentieth World Health Assembly, 1967*, WHO Official Records 161: 148.
29 There were, of course, exceptions to this rule. In the field of agricultural economics René Dumont was an example of at least one European who had forcefully warned, among others, former pupils of his who had become officials in new African states against the wholesale adoption of European practices. See his *False Start in Africa*, London: Earthscan, 1988.
30 *Primary Health Care*: 3.
31 Part II of this study is an elaboration of a fact pointed out by Kenneth Warren: the Chinese and Soviet background to Alma-Ata. The Soviets were purportedly so astonished by the success of the Chinese barefoot doctor system that 'according to a retired UNICEF official, the USSR was moved to demonstrate its own forms of Primary Health Care' by hosting an international conference. Kenneth Warren, 'The Alma-Ata declaration: health for all by the year 2000?' in *1990 Britannica Book of the Year*, London: Encyclopaedia Britannica, 1990: 26.
32 *Twentieth World Health Assembly, 1967*, WHO Official Records 160–1: 399.
33 *Twenty-first World Health Assembly, 1968*, WHO Official Records, 168–9: 218.
34 Mao Zedong, '26 June Directive', reprinted in Ruth and Victor Sidel, *The Health of China*, London: Zed Press, 1982: 4.
35 AnElissa Lucas, *Chinese Medical Modernization*, New York: Praeger, 1982: 136.
36 Victor Sidel, 'The barefoot doctors of the People's Republic of China', *New England Journal of Medicine*, 15 June 1972: 1294–5.
37 See *A Barefoot Doctor's Manual*, Philadelphia, Pa: Running Press, 1977.
38 Sidel, 'The barefoot doctors': 1295.
39 Sidel and Sidel, *The Health of China*, 39.
40 Revolutionary Committee of the Shanghai First Medical College, as quoted in Sidel, 'The barefoot doctors': 1294. It is astounding that, despite Sidel's reference to the political origins of the barefoot doctor system, he was quite confident that Chinese practices offered America 'a number of lessons', presumably transferable without the Cultural Revolution. He described the barefoot doctors as a factory manager might proudly describe his floor hands: they had high 'job satisfaction' and a commitment to 'service'.
41 As reprinted in Sidel, 'The barefoot doctors': 1298.
42 Sidel and Sidel, *The Health of China*: 7.

43 *Twenty-sixth World Health Assembly, 1973*, WHO Official Records 210: 143–4.

44 In fact China was not the first developing country to speak of revolutionary politics and health care. In 1968 the delegate from the Congo, announcing his country's plans to train more auxiliary health workers, had declared that the 'time has come when our younger generation must realize that they must go and join the masses to fight side by side with them and understand their problems'. *Twenty-first World Health Assembly, 1968*, WHO Official Records 168: 218. It was to take a success on the scale of China's for such claims to be taken seriously.

45 *Twenty-sixth World Health Assembly, 1973*: 172.

46 *Twenty-sixth World Health Assembly, 1973*: 215.

47 *Twenty-sixth World Health Assembly, 1973*: 248.

48 *Alternative Approaches to Meeting Basic Health Needs in Developing Countries: a Joint UNICEF/WHO Study*, Geneva: WHO, 1975: 7.

49 *Ibid.*: 49.

50 *Ibid.*: 96.

51 *Twentieth World Health Assembly, 1967*, WHO Official Records 161: 321.

52 *Twenty-second World Health Assembly, 1969*, WHO Official Records 177: 337.

53 *Twenty-eighth World Health Assembly, 1975*, WHO Official Records 227: 534.

54 *Thirteenth World Health Assembly, 1977*, WHO Official Records 241: 466. Support for the resolution was strong but not unanimous. The delegate from Fiji 'did not wish to be associated in any way with those who took advantage of human ignorance' (p. 467).

55 This and the following quotations are taken from *Twenty-eighth World Health Assembly, 1975*: 528–43.

56 This and the following quotations are taken from *Fifty-seventh Session of the Executive Board, January 1976*, WHO Official Records 232: 184–92.

57 *The Work of WHO for 1976–77*, WHO Official Records 243.

58 *Sixth Report on the World Health Situation for 1973–77*, Geneva: WHO, 1980: 2–3.

59 Since its foundation WHO has granted fellowships for three types of studies: (1) Health Organisation and Services, (2) Communicable Diseases, and (3) Clinical Medicine, Basic Medical Sciences, and Medical and Allied Education. Since the 1960s the ratio of fellowships distributed in those categories has consistently been about 3:1:1.

60 See M. Muller, *The Health of Nations: a North–South Investigation*, London: Faber, 1982, and Milton Silverman, Philip R. Lee and Mia Lydecker, *Prescriptions for Death: the Drugging of the Third World*, London: University of California Press, 1982, for harshly critical accounts of multinational pharmaceutical corporation activities in the developing world. Both studies portray WHO and Director General Mahler in a very positive light.

61 As quoted in Muller, *Health of Nations*: 179.

62 WHO gained prestige with its successful challenge in the early 1980s of Nestlé Corporation's marketing of infant formula in the developing world. International organisation specialists have considered the episode one of the few important successes in the implementation of an international code. 'WHO and UNICEF played crucial roles … as grantor of legitimacy, creator of consciousness, center of debate'. Catherine Sikkink, 'Codes of conduct for transnational corporations: the case of the WHO/UNICEF code', *International Organization* 40, 4 (1986): 840.

CHAPTER TWO

AIDS from Africa: Western science or racist mythology?

Rosalind J. Harrison-Chirimuuta

There is little argument that science has contributed greatly to our understanding of the external world, so much so that knowledge acquired by scientific means is considered more likely to be true than other forms of knowledge. This holds for medicine as for other branches of science, and the practical application of medical science has given rise to therapies of unquestioned benefit. One of the great achievements of medical science was the discovery of micro-organisms and the recognition of their role in a large number of different infectious diseases. The provision of clean water and sanitation, disinfection and sterilisation during surgery, immunisation and antibiotics – all are based on an understanding of the behaviour of micro-organisms. Yet from the successes of last century we come, at the end of this century, to a challenge that has so far defeated the best that medical science has to offer. The US government alone is spending about a billion dollars a year researching the Acquired Immune Deficiency Syndrome,[1] but there is still no cure, no proven effective treatment, no vaccine, nor even agreement as to how the Human Immunodeficiency Virus destroys the immune system. Is this because AIDS is just a more difficult problem than medical science has dealt with before, but with persistence will be conquered, or could there be something fundamentally wrong with the scientific investigation of the illness? In this chapter I endeavour to examine the AIDS science that claims that AIDS originated in Africa and the possibly racist underpinnings of this science. I discuss the alternative possibility of a laboratory origin of HIV. Finally, I look at the political and economic aspects of AIDS research in particular and science in general that may have encouraged or promoted the belief that AIDS originated in Africa.

The first step in the construction of AIDS science was the recognition of a new phenomenon: the epidemic of fatal, wasting disease in previously healthy homosexual US men, first reported in 1981.[2] Unexplained wasting diseases had occurred in the past and had been reported in the medical literature, but were sporadic, not epidemic.[3] The next stage of the scientific response was the elaboration of a hypothesis that could be subjected to investigation and challenge. The initial hypothesis proposed that AIDS was due to toxins, particularly nitrites, which were popular with homosexual men as a sexual stimulant. The toxin hypothesis soon fell into disfavour when similar illnesses were described in intravenous drug users and haemophiliacs. Infectious agents such as the hepatitis B virus transmitted via blood to blood and sexual contact disproportionately affected these groups of patients, and a second hypothesis, that AIDS was caused by an unknown infectious agent, was proposed and widely accepted. The search for the infectious agent was intense and the result was the Human Immunodeficiency Virus, HIV (initially called HTLV III). Inductivism, naive or otherwise, certainly had no place in AIDS science, as the hypothesis long preceded the evidence. That HIV is the sole cause of AIDS was quickly accepted as theory if not fact by the great majority of scientists engaged in research into AIDS. Dissenting views and alternative hypotheses have remained on the heretical fringes of AIDS science and have been paid little attention in mainstream scientific conferences and publications.[4]

The phenomenon of a new infectious disease inevitably raised the question of its source. The possibility that this could lie within the United States, where the epidemic began, was never entertained by scientists or general public. But when, in 1982, Haitians were diagnosed with AIDS, the as yet unidentified infectious agent was immediately assumed to come from that country.[5] A Haitian origin soon fell into disfavour, at least in part because no evidence could be found that AIDS existed in Haiti prior to its appearance in the United States,[6] and was soon superseded by the African hypothesis, with or without the rider that the virus had stopped over in Haiti *en route* to the United States. The African origin of AIDS was immediately accepted in the West with minimal critical assessment, and there was significant debate only on the issues of whether the reservoir of HIV was in a remote tribe of Africans or in African monkeys, and at what point it was spread from Africa to the West.

Although Western scientists accepted the African origin without difficulty, many Africans were unconvinced and argued that the fundamental concepts of the AIDS from Africa hypothesis resided in racial theory and not in science. For example, Yinka Adeyemi, the science and health correspondent of the Nigerian Weekly *Concord*, wrote in July 1985:

> To the average European researcher in virus cancers, the notion that the Acquired Immune Deficiency Syndrome (AIDS) had its origin in Africa is now a scientific fact ... Yet, arguments by such scientists whose minds are made up about the African connection are replete with fundamental loopholes and illogicalities that render them not plausible ...
>
> A common notion which cuts through the reasoning of most Western scientists is that a visit should be made to Africa before any researcher concludes whether a disease is new. For instance, De Cock wrote that Ebola virus, Marburg virus and Lassa fever were all initially thought to be new diseases when they first surfaced 'but all of them turned out to have been endemic in Africa'.
>
> There are even more offensive notions ... Gallo, who first identified the AIDS-causing virus in man, said at the Dakar conference: 'Viruses closely related to HTLV, but distinct from it, have been isolated from Old World monkeys. This and other facts led us to propose that the ancestral origin of HTLV is in Africa.'
>
> Comments such as this immediately raise problems because of the socio-historical implications. To the ordinary man, Gallo will be understood as saying that: 'We (European scientists) conclude that AIDS originated from Africa because we found AIDS virus in monkeys, and Africans are closer to monkeys.'[7]

Later the same year, at a symposium on AIDS and Africa held in Brussels, there were heated arguments between Western medical scientists claiming an African monkey origin for HIV and African scientists and government officials who rejected such a hypothesis as unproved.[8] They questioned why such a rare evolutionary event should have been confined so long to Zaire, and Dr David Desiré Benoni of Gabon asked, 'Why do they not look for a monkey in the US? AIDS started there and could equally well have been brought to Zaire by wealthy homosexuals.'[9] African doctors at this meeting also said that HIV tests were unreliable in their patients and gave a high rate of false positivity.

Unsurprisingly the charge of racism was rejected by Western scientists and the following quotation, from three leading British AIDS researchers, was a typical response:

> In the case of some early studies in Africa, techniques were used that had not been sufficiently well validated for African sera, given the prevalent hypergammaglobulinaemia and a notorious tendency to 'stickiness' and false positive reactions in antiglobulin assays. The observations derived from these studies have led to some confusion and have also tended to damage the credibility of foreign scientists working in Africa – especially among local leaders. Additional problems have been created when investigators have spent a short time collecting sera and basic data in a developing country, often with little guidance from local investigators, and then published the data without reference to the original context.

> This has tended to produce scientific data that has not been adequately placed in an anthropological perspective. Even worse, it has led to denial and resentment, jeopardising essential and potentially fruitful collaboration between investigators in the developed and developing world in a study of an issue of mutual concern. This has been particularly damaging when the pursuit has apparently been the origin of AIDS and HIV, an essentially academic question, however interesting. Such investigations have often been taken to imply blame on the region that appears to be the source. Although they were certainly never intended to impugn any community in this way, it is not difficult to see how such perceptions arose.[10]

It is difficult to untangle the confusion of ideas here. What on earth are data placed in an anthropological perspective? But whilst there is acknowledgement that the behaviour and practices of AIDS researchers may have left something to be desired, there is no acknowledgement that Africans have questioned the scientific basis of the 'AIDS from Africa' hypothesis. Although the views of Western scientists have prevailed over the last decade, the 'fundamental loopholes and illogicalities' have not been removed by force of argument or scientific evidence. I will, therefore, attempt to delineate the essentials of AIDS science and racial ideology pertinent to this debate.

If HIV or indeed some other as yet unidentified micro-organism is the cause of AIDS there are a limited number of possibilities as to its origin: a human population that has harboured the virus for many years and from whom the virus has spread in recent years, an animal reservoir of the virus or a mutation of an existing human or animal virus. The first possibility, a human reservoir of HIV, the 'isolated tribe' or 'village disease', was presented in detailed form in 1984:

> This report proposes that the infectious agent causing AIDS ... is endemic and unrecognised in parts of sub-Saharan Africa, from where it recently disseminated into external populations ...
>
> In rural Africa diagnosis is often inexact. Fever is readily attributed to malaria without confirmation, and pneumonia is often assumed to be pneumococcal or tuberculous ... In such a situation immunodeficiency would go unrecognised.
>
> Useful analogies can be drawn between the sudden appearance of AIDS and the recent recognition of some African viral haemorrhagic fevers ... [Marburg, Ebola and Lassa].
>
> As Kaposi's sarcoma was a feature in about one-third of reported cases of AIDS, it would seem mandatory to look for AIDS where Kaposi's sarcoma has its highest incidence in the world, equatorial Africa ...
>
> The incubation period of AIDS is thought to be one or more years. The first American cases are likely to have become infected in the early to

> mid 1970's, a time when tourism from the United States to Africa was developing as a result of heightened cultural interest ...[11]

There are serious weaknesses in the medical aspects of this hypothesis. For example, it is quite inappropriate to draw parallels between the haemorrhagic fevers and AIDS, as the former have no carrier state in humans and can be transmitted from human to human only during the acute illness. Outbreaks therefore occur in limited geographical locations and the infected person either dies or recovers completely. It is the historical inaccuracies, though, that are more spectacular. For centuries before the Portuguese sailed around the Cape powerful West African kingdoms conducted trade across the Sahara to the Mediterranean,[12] and every year thousands of West Africans undertook the pilgrimage to Mecca.[13] On the East African seaboard there were city states that flourished on trade between the central and southern African kingdoms, such as Monamatapa in Zimbabwe, and Asia as far as the Ming dynasty China.[14] With the advent of the Portuguese began 400 years of the African slave trade, during which millions of Africans were transported to the New World and Europe, and African women were regularly raped from the time of capture.[15] Following the demise of the slave trade came the scramble for Africa, when almost the entire continent was colonised by the European powers. If AIDS was the cause of a tumour as common as Kaposi's sarcoma in equatorial Africa the disease would have spread to the rest of the world hundreds if not thousands of years earlier. The idea that tourists from the United States in the mid 1970s were the means by which AIDS reached America was breathtakingly naive. Nonetheless attempts were made to find an 'isolated tribe' harbouring HIV, without success, and the quest for an African origin increasingly focused on African monkeys.[16]

Reading the scientific literature about a simian (monkey) origin for the human immunodeficiency virus can be a confusing business. It is easy to gain the impression that simian retroviruses can readily infect humans, but evidence for this is absent. The Simian Immunodeficiency Viruses that have been isolated from monkeys are, like all other retroviruses, species-specific, i.e. in nature no monkey retrovirus can infect a human or indeed a different species of monkey, and there is no monkey reservoir of the human immunodeficiency virus.[17] Only laboratory chimpanzees have been reported to be successfully infected with HIV, but they do not become ill.[18] Thus a simian origin for HIV requires two chance events, a mutation of a monkey virus into a virus that could infect a human, and blood-to-blood contact between the monkey with the mutant virus and a human. Even between humans AIDS is not very efficiently transmitted via limited blood-to-blood contact, much less so than hepatitis B, as is evidenced by the minimal risk of becoming seropositive from needle stick injuries between medical personnel and patients.[19] AIDS researchers have claimed that Africans inject themselves with monkey blood or give their children dead monkeys as toys, claims that Africans have rejected as preposterous, and even for the minority of Africans who hunt and eat monkeys the prospect of human infection with even a mutant strain of SIV is very remote.[20] A far more efficient potential route for the transmission of simian viruses to humans occurred not in Africa but in Europe during the 1920s. Thousands of European men underwent an operation that was believed to slow the ageing process and bring about 'rejuvenation'.[21] The technique was pioneered by Dr Serge Voronoff, a Russian working in Paris, and involved the transplantation of testicles from living chimpanzees, monkeys and other simian species directly onto the testicle of the human recipient. The procedure was so popular that the detective writer Dorothy Sayers included it in the plot of *The Unpleasantness at the Bellona Club*. However spurious the benefits of the operation, there were no reported ill effects, and there was no subsequent epidemic of AIDS.

The improbability of transmission of a mutant retrovirus from monkeys to humans has not deterred AIDS scientists from wild speculations. Claims that a Simian Immunodeficiency Virus (SIV) isolated from laboratory Macaque monkeys had been isolated from wild African green monkeys and was similar to a virus isolated from West African prostitutes were disproved when the virus was found to be a laboratory contaminant.[22] Undeterred, scientists have estimated that SIV mutated into HIV in the last few decades, their conclusion based on estimates of the rate of mutation of the viruses and their degree of genetic dissimilarity.[23] Even if such an improbable event did occur, given the colonial ties and trading links between Africa and Europe, the virus would have caused an epidemic in Europe at the same time as or before the epidemic in the United States. Yet all the documented evidence points to an epidemic beginning in America and from there spreading to Europe.[24] Arguments that Haitians acquired the infection in Zaire and took it back to Haiti, where it was acquired by American tourists, are also quite implausible, as the European presence in Zaire was large and the Haitian presence minimal. Whatever the logic, Western fascination with African 'isolated tribes' and their sexual practices continued unabated, and drew the following response from a Ghanaian scientist:

> Some people have decided that the origin of AIDS will be forever associated with Africa, hence such unscientific statements as 'there is now

> little doubt human AIDS began in Africa'. Their evidence is that 'not only is the disease widespread in Central Africa but only in Africa are there monkey species naturally infected with lentiviruses related to human immunodeficiency virus'. An African might have written similarly of syphilis in Europe in the Middle Ages: 'There is little doubt that syphilis began in Europe. Not only is the disease widely spread there, but only in Europe it seems are people naturally susceptible to the disease'. At that time there was not a single case of syphilis reported from black Africa, even though there were sailors going to and returning from Africa to Europe, thanks to acquired immunity against syphilis because of widespread Yaws. We all know now that syphilis did not begin in Europe.
>
> If members of the Idjwi tribe had practices that would constitute an efficient means of trans-species transmission and could be responsible for the emergence of simian immunodeficiency virus (SIV) infections of man and thus AIDS, why have they only now developed AIDS? Perhaps A. Karpas (*Nature* **348**, 578: 1990) would have us believe that they had acquired an immunity to AIDS until they suddenly lost it in 1959. Sexual practices in East Zaire, in a small circumscribed tribe, led to a suggestion that SIV could have given rise to HIV-2 infection of man in West Africa thousands of miles away. How elastic is Karpas's imagination?[25]

Other arguments in support of an African hypothesis have been presented that are peripheral to the origin of HIV. These arguments can be considered in three categories, and I will deal with each in turn. Firstly there have been a number of cases of AIDS-like illnesses reported in Africans or people who have been to Africa that antedated the AIDS epidemic in the United States; second are the reports of positivity to AIDS tests in African blood taken decades before the AIDS epidemic in America and Europe; and thirdly there is the sheer scale of the AIDS epidemic in Africa – AIDS must have been in Africa longer than elsewhere for it to have affected so many people.

With regard to the early AIDS-like cases, these can be considered evidence of an African origin of AIDS only if they were genuine cases of AIDS and if such cases occurred only in Africa. In reality sporadic AIDS-like cases have been reported in the medical literature for many years but, with few exceptions, only those with an African connection have been highlighted.[26] Two of these cases were investigated further and were found to be spurious. The Danish surgeon who worked in Zaire and died in 1977 has been given a great deal of attention in medical and popular literature, but a sample of her blood that had been preserved was found to be HIV negative, although this fact has been mentioned only in private correspondence and not in the medical literature.[27] The other, a Manchester seaman who sailed to many continents, including Africa, and died in 1959 has been regarded as the first documented case of HIV infection. Samples of his tissue were preserved and were reported as containing HIV, but when further tests were carried out in a different laboratory the original findings were disputed.[28]

The next issue, that of positive tests from stored African serum, has been alluded to in the quotations from the British scientists above. No blood test can be considered perfectly reliable, and all tests will have a greater or lesser percentage of false positive and negative results. In the case of patients who have more than average amounts of circulating antibodies in response to other infections, the chances of them giving a false positive reaction are higher. This is undoubtedly the case with people continually exposed to malarial infection and other parasitic and infectious diseases – the notorious tendency to 'stickiness'.[29] Evidence that false positivity was a major problem in both stored serum samples and samples taken for population studies of HIV in Africa was available from the mid 1980s but has been largely ignored.[30] Claims that early tests were unreliable but that those used now can be trusted are also untenable. Research published in 1994 found that antibodies to Mycobacterium antigens, i.e. antibodies produced by patients with tuberculosis and leprosy, give a positive test for HIV.[31] Long before this research was published African physicians appreciated the difficulty of attributing meaning to a positive HIV test in a patient with tuberculosis. Dr Konotey-Ahulu, a Ghanaian physician, wrote in 1987:

> I asked what advice the doctors [in Congo-Brazzaville, a predominantly Roman Catholic country] gave to a married man with tuberculosis who was found to be seropositive and they said: 'Nothing.' The patient was not even told he might have AIDS because the doctors, quite rightly, said that they had nothing else to go on but seropositivity for human immunodeficiency virus as assessed by ELISA and pulmonary tuberculosis ... and in any case 'the man has improved on anti-tuberculous therapy and the wife is still seronegative'.[32]

Yet, despite all the evidence that tests for HIV are unreliable, a single positive blood test taken from an unknown African and stored in a freezer for a quarter of a century is frequently quoted as evidence that AIDS originated in Zaire.[33]

On the grounds that the health services of most African countries cannot afford the diagnostic tests for AIDS the World Health Organisation has different criteria for defining AIDS in Africa, based on signs and symptoms only, from the rest of the world.[34] This case definition includes patients who have prolonged cough, fever and weight loss, the classic presenting symptoms and signs of tuberculosis. If the tuberculosis is confirmed but, resources permitting, the patient is found to be HIV positive, it is assumed that tuberculosis has developed because the patient is infected with HIV. It is then quite conceivable, when resources are limited, that treatment will be withheld on the grounds that the patient will die anyway. It is fortunate that at least some African physicians have relied on their clinical judgement rather than the conclusions of Western AIDS researchers. The implications of both clinical criteria and diagnostic tests that fail to distinguish between HIV and treatable diseases common in Africa extend beyond personal and family tragedy. Both are used, separately or together, to estimate the extent of the HIV epidemic in Africa and will lead to exaggeration.

There are other reasons to dispute the scale of the African AIDS epidemic. In the West a progression has been reported from HIV infection to AIDS of around 5 to 7 per cent per annum.[35] This ratio is a function of the rate of progression from infection to manifest disease. If the huge number of reported seropositive Africans are seropositive for the same reasons as their counterparts in the West they should be developing AIDS and dying at a comparable rate and the continent should be witnessing a death rate far in excess of that which is occurring. Seropositive Africans do have a higher death rate than non-seropositive Africans,[36] but that would be the case even if the majority of the seropositives were false positives but suffering from chronic malaria, tuberculosis or other diseases that could give rise to a false positive response. A further difficulty with the African epidemic is the equal or near equal sex incidence of seropositivity found in population studies, which, it is claimed, is due to the heterosexual transmission of HIV in Africa.[37] Studies in the West have shown repeatedly that HIV positivity is far more likely to be transmitted from semen donor to semen recipient (whether the latter is male or female) than the reverse, and there is no reason why this should be different in Africa.[38] If heterosexual intercourse is the major means of transmission of HIV in Africa, HIV seropositivity and AIDS would disproportionately affect women. An equal sex ratio implies not sexual transmission but the converse, non-sexual transmission, and one obvious explanation would be that the large majority of seropositives in Africa are false positives due to malaria, tuberculosis and other infections that affect men and women equally.

If the evidence of an African origin is contradictory or insubstantial, are there any more credible alternatives? One possibility that has been paid scant attention in the vast scientific literature about HIV and AIDS is an artificial origin of a mutant virus. This neglect would seem rather surprising, as the risk of mutant viruses emerging from laboratories has been widely debated for many years. For example, in 1966 Professor and Nobelist Sir MacFarlane Burnet, a leading microbiologist, wrote:

> I remember vividly the beginnings of molecular biology. For me it began when Schlesinger showed in 1934 that a bacterial virus contained thymonucleic acid – we call it DNA now ... For thirty years I have watched this structure develop around the central bacterium-phage theme, bringing in as needed contributions from the chemistry of nucleic acids and proteins, from the genetics of higher organisms, and the pharmacology of antibiotics. It has been a magnificent achievement, to be ranked with the elucidation of subatomic structure as one of the two major triumphs of twentieth-century experimental science. It seems almost indecent to hint that, so far as the advance of medicine is concerned, molecular biology may be an evil thing ...
>
> The human implications of what is going on in this sophisticated universe of tissue-cultured cells, bacteria, and the viruses which can be grown at the expense of one or other are at best dubious, at worst frankly terrifying ... Amongst many billions of essentially independent units, mutations will range widely, particularly under the impact of chosen mutagenic agents. Almost always, cultural conditions can be so manipulated that any mutant of interest, whether of a mammalian cell line, a bacterium, or a virus can be caused to outgrow the other forms and can be isolated in pure culture or its equivalent. Theoretically, anything within the physical possibility of mutation can be obtained by current techniques from cell line, bacterium or virus, and can be isolated in unlimited quantity. It is interesting to contemplate the possibilities for human good or evil in the mutations thus obtained ... For the foreseeable future the only function of viruses is to destroy higher forms of life ...
>
> The latest development has been the recognition that, in some way, a portion of the genetic material of a virus can be incorporated into the genome of the infected cell and induce changes in the behaviour of the cell ... Potentially, viruses could be evolved in biological laboratories to insert episomes into a variety of cells to produce a variety of effects. There would always be the reservation, however, that to provide the appropriate conditions for selective survival the effect of the episome must be easily recognisable under laboratory conditions. At present the only two readily observable effects are death or malignant transformation. Practical applications of molecular biology to cancer research might also be sinister – they are not likely to be helpful.
>
> ... Medicine must make use of all the sciences, but it must also recognise the limitations that the progress of evolution and the nature of man place on their utilisation.[39]

Professor Burnet was not an isolated voice. In the early 1970s several molecular biologists also expressed concern at the risks of molecular biology, and published a book, *Biohazards in Biological Research*.[40] In February 1975, at Asilomar in California, an international conference of 150 molecular biologists agreed a policy of self-regulation that included 'appropriate safeguards, principally biological and physical barriers adequate to contain the newly created organisms, [should be] employed' and 'certain experiments ... ought not to be done with presently available containment facilities'. In the following years the debate entered the body politic, and by 1976 the US National Institutes of Health released guidelines for research into recombinant DNA molecules, and the following year the Federal Interagency Committee on Recombinant DNA Research issued an interim report on *Suggested Elements for Legislation* that was subsequently enacted by the US government.[41]

Whether or not HIV is a mutant laboratory virus, there is at least one documented cross-species transmission of a virus that has been attributed to the development of mutant forms of the virus in the laboratory. Between 1978 and 1980 a new disease appeared in dogs in widely separated geographical locations which was found to be due to a parvovirus related to parvoviruses infecting cats and mink. During the first half of this century Feline Panleukopenia Virus (FPV) had repeatedly given rise to huge epidemics in various parts of the world, but this parvovirus had never infected dogs, and all attempts to infect dogs experimentally had failed. It has been proposed that strains of FPV and the Mink Enteritis Virus (MEV) were deliberately or accidentally adapted to growth in canine cells in the laboratory. Passage of the feline virus in canine cells may have been undertaken to attenuate the virus to make it suitable for a feline vaccine, or the virus may have accidentally contaminated canine cell cultures. Attenuated FPV given to cats as a vaccine may then have infected the canine population.[42]

It is virtually impossible for any molecular biologist researching AIDS in the early 1980s to be unaware of the debate about the risks of molecular biology and the subsequent legislation regulating their activities. Even before the AIDS epidemic, retroviruses were the subject of intense research activity because of their ability to turn RNA into DNA, and their possible role in causing cancer. Hundreds of thousands of African green monkeys and other species have been exported from Africa to research laboratories in Europe and America, where they have been subjected to experimental infections and their tissues have been used in cell culture. If HIV is a mutant monkey virus, it is surely more probable that it came from a laboratory than from monkey with naturally mutated virus biting man somewhere in darkest Africa. That the latter hypothesis and not the former has been pursued suggests that factors other than science have been guiding the activities of AIDS researchers. If one factor was fear of being accused of causing the AIDS epidemic, the other was a conscious or unconscious acceptance of racial ideology.

If there are parallels between racist ideology as it applies to Africa and Africans, and the tenets of the 'AIDS from Africa' hypothesis, what are the essential racist beliefs, and how may they have influenced AIDS researchers? It can be generally agreed, I trust, that the world view of any individual is acquired from the society in which she or he is raised, and that these perceptions and values are often unconscious, at least until challenged. It can also be agreed, I hope, that racist beliefs are the result of a historical process and are not innate to the human condition. This, certainly, was the view of Morgan Godwyn, one of the first Europeans to analyse racism as a class ideology. He was the grandson of a bishop and the son of a canon, who went to Virginia, then to Barbados, as a minister of religion. In 1680 he published a book, *The Negro's & Indians Advocate,* the essential thesis of which is contained in the following passage:

> [A] disingenuous and unmanly *Position* hath been formed: and privately (*and as it were in the dark*) handed to and again [i.e. to and fro], which is this, That the *Negro's*, though in their Figure they carry some resemblances to Manhood, yet are indeed *no Men* ... If *Atheism and Irreligion* were the true Parents who gave it Life, surely *Sloth and Avarice* have been no unhandy Instruments and Assistants to midwife it into the World, and to Foster and Nurse it up. Under whose Protection getting abroad, it hath acquired sufficient strength and reputation to support itself; being now able not only to maintain its ground, but to bid defiance to all its *Opposers*; who in truth are found to be but very *few*, and those scarcely *considerable.* The issue whereof is, That as in the *Negroe's all pretence to Religion* is cut off, so their *Owners* are hereby set at Liberty and freed from those importunate Scruples, which Conscience and better Advice might at any time happen to inject their unsteadie Minds.[43]

Godwyn is arguing very clearly that racism, at least as applied to Africans, was a product of the greed of the planters and slave merchants, which they used to justify their actions in their own eyes as well as in those of the rest of society. Initially they spread their views in a furtive manner but later gained sufficient confidence to speak openly, and ultimately their views gained general acceptance.

There is ample historical evidence for Godwyn's arguments. One of the earliest historical records of contact between Europeans and Sub-Saharan Africans can be found in the Portuguese royal archives. In 1482 Diego Cão sailed down the West African coast and discovered the estuary of a river so great that its silt-laden waters discoloured the ocean miles from the shore. On a subsequent journey Cão sailed up the estuary, landed near Matadi of today and there met some of the people of the country. Although, of course, there was no common language the Portuguese understood that they were in the territory of a powerful ruler whose capital was distant from the coast. Cão left four Franciscan monks to see if they could contact the king and took hostages back to Portugal. There they were well received by the king, clothed, converted to Christianity and encouraged to act as future interpreters. In 1487 they were sent back to the Congo with Cão's third expedition, and Cão himself, together with a retinue of fellow countrymen and the Congolese interpreters, was invited to visit the ruler of the land, the Mweni-Congo, at his capital of Mbanza in the hills behind the coast. There the Europeans found this African ruler seated on a royal stool of ivory, surrounded by his counsellors and his men-at-arms. The meeting was a great success. Within a few years of this visit to Mbanza the 'royal brothers' of Portugal and the Congo were writing letters to each other that were couched in terms of complete equality of status. Twenty-two of the Mweni-Congo's letters (he was baptised King Affonso) are preserved in the royal archives of Portugal. Written between 1512 and 1540 by various secretaries, the most important of whom, baptised as João Texeira, was evidently Congolese, they show a good command of the Portuguese language and bear on a wide variety of topics. Relations were also established between Mbanza and the Vatican, and a son of the Mweni-Congo was educated in a Portuguese seminary and appointed in Rome as bishop of his country.

In the early years of Portuguese contact slave trading was undertaken on a small scale. The practice of one African monarch turning over a number of his captives to another who was his ally was common in Iron Age Africa and was far from rare in medieval Europe. Indeed, European merchants and sea captains were still selling European slaves to the markets of North Africa. But as the overseas slave trade increased chaos descended on the Mweni-Congo's kingdom. Repeatedly the Mweni-Congo asked his Portuguese 'brother' to provide him with a ship, or the means of making one, but the Portuguese were determined to retain their maritime monopoly, and ultimately the Mweni-Congo sought to bring the slave trade to an end. In a strongly worded letter to John III the Mweni-Congo wrote:

> We cannot reckon how great the damage is, since the above-mentioned merchants daily seize our subjects, sons of the land and sons of our noblemen and vassals of our relatives: Thieves and men of evil conscience take them because they wish to possess the things and wares of this Kingdom ... They grab them and cause them to be sold ... and so great, Sir, is their corruption and licentiousness that our country is being

> utterly depopulated ... [We] need from [your] Kingdoms no other than priests and people to teach in schools, and no other goods but wine and flour for the holy sacrament: that is why we beg Your Highness to help and assist us in this matter, commanding your factors that they should send here neither merchants nor wares, because it is *our will that in these kingdoms [of Congo] there should not be any trade in slaves nor market for slaves.*[44]

Needless to say, such pleas were entirely ignored.

Such was the change in European perceptions of Africa over the subsequent 400 years of the slave trade that it was possible for Joseph Conrad to write of much the same place and people:

> The reaches opened before us and closed behind, as if the forest had stepped leisurely across the water to bar the way for our return. We penetrated deeper and deeper into the heart of darkness ... We were wanderers on prehistoric earth, on an earth that wore the aspect of an unknown planet. We could have fancied ourselves the first of men taking possession of an accursed inheritance, to be subdued at the cost of profound anguish and of excessive toil. But suddenly, as we struggled round a bend, there would be a glimpse of rush walls, of peaked grass-roofs, a burst of yells, a whirl of black limbs, a mass of hands clapping, of feet stamping, of bodies swaying, of eyes rolling, under the droop of heavy and motionless foliage. The steamer toiled along slowly on the edge of a black and incomprehensible frenzy. The prehistoric man was cursing us, praying to us, welcoming us – who could tell? We were cut off from the comprehension of our surroundings; we glided past the phantoms, wondering and secretly appalled, as sane men would be before an enthusiastic outbreak in a madhouse. We could not understand because we were too far and could not remember, because we were travelling in the night of first ages, of those ages that are gone, leaving hardly a sign – and no memories ...
>
> The earth seemed unearthly. We are accustomed to look upon the shackled form of a conquered monster, but there – there you could look at a thing monstrous and free. It was unearthly, and the men were – No, they were not inhuman. Well, you know, that was the worst of it – this suspicion of their not being inhuman. It would come slowly to one. They howled and leaped, and spun, and made horrid faces; but what thrilled you was just the thought of their wild humanity – like yours – the thought of your remote kinship with this wild and passionate uproar. Ugly. Yes, it was ugly enough; but if you were man enough you would admit to yourself that there was in you just the faintest trace of a response to the terrible frankness of that noise, a dim suspicion of there being a meaning in it which you – you so remote from the night of first ages – could comprehend. And why not? The mind of man is capable of anything – because everything is in it, all the past as well as all the future ...

> And between whiles I had to look after the savage who was fireman. He was an improved specimen; he could fire up a vertical boiler. He was there below me, and, upon my word, to look at him was as edifying as seeing a dog in a parody of breeches and a feather hat, walking on his hind-legs. A few months of training had done wonders for that really fine chap. He squinted at the steam-gauge with an evident effort of intrepidity – and he had filed teeth, too, the poor devil, and the wool of his pate shaved into queer patterns, and three ornamental scars on each of his cheeks. He ought to have been clapping his hands and stamping his feet on the bank, instead of which he was hard at work, a thrall to strange witchcraft, full of improving knowledge. He was useful because he had been instructed; and what he knew was this – that should the water in that transparent thing disappear, the evil spirit inside the boiler would get angry through the greatness of his thirst, and take a terrible vengeance. So he sweated and fired up and watched the glass fearfully (with an impromptu charm, made of rags, tied to his arm, and a piece of polished bone, as big as a watch, stuck flatways through his lower lip), while the wooded banks slipped past us slowly, the short noise was left behind, the interminable miles of silence – and we crept on, towards Kurtz.[45]

Heart of Darkness is a novel, but Conrad had worked in the Congo and was presenting an albeit dramatised version of the European conception of 'darkest Africa'. His fictional account followed many others that claimed to be factual or even scientific. For example, David Hume, the great British empiricist, wrote in 1748:

> I am apt to suspect the negroes, and in general all the other species of men (for there are four or five different kinds) to be naturally inferior to the whites. There never was a civilised nation of any other complexion than white, not even any individual eminent either in action or speculation. No ingenious manufacture amongst them, no arts, no sciences ... Such a uniform and constant difference could not happen, in so many countries and ages, if nature had not made an original distinction betwixt these breeds of men. Not to mention our colonies, there are NEGROE slaves dispersed all over Europe, of which none ever discovered any symptoms of ingenuity: tho' low people, without ingenuity, will start up amongst us, and distinguish themselves in every profession. In JAMAICA indeed they talk of one negroe as a man of parts and learning; but 'tis likely he is admired for very slender accomplishments, like a parrot, who speaks a few words plainly.[46]

One of the most prolific exponents of this line of reasoning was Edward Long, the son of a Jamaica planter. In his three-volume history *History of Jamaica* we find another of the central themes of racist ideology:

> When we reflect on ... their dissimilarity to the rest of mankind, must we not conclude, that they are a different species of the same *genus*? ...

> Nor do [orang-utans] seem at all inferior to the intellectual faculties to many of the Negroe race; with some of whom, it is credible that they have the most intimate connexion and consanguinity. The amorous intercourse between them may be frequent ... and it is certain, that both races agree perfectly well in lasciviousness of disposition.[47]

And Thomas Atwood, chief judge of Dominica and later of the Bahamas, stated:

> Negroes are in general much addicted to drunkenness, thievery, incontinency [i.e. promiscuity] and idleness ... Idleness is so very predominant in negroes, and their dislike of labour is so great, that it is very difficult to make them work; sometimes it is necessary to have recourse to measures that appear cruel, in order to oblige them to labour.[48]

Racism 'being now able not only to maintain its ground, but to bid defiance to all its *Opposers*' profoundly influenced many of the leading European intellectuals and writers of the last three centuries: John Hunter, the father of British surgery, Carl Linnaeus, the Swedish botanist, and Charles Bonnet, the Swiss naturalist, are but a few who contributed to the pseudo-science of racism; Charlotte Brontë, William Thackeray and many others reflected in their literary work the racism prevailing in the society around them.

As Europe began to come to terms with the Nazi holocaust, racism lost much of its intellectual respectability, a process hastened by independence in the colonies and the black civil rights movement in the United States. But whilst the expression of racism may be less acceptable, the underlying racist beliefs, particularly those pertaining to Africa and Africans, remain integrated into the European and North American world view. Thus in the scientific literature on AIDS and Africa all the racist themes can be found underpinning arguments for which scientific evidence is contradictory or absent. Africans are primitive people living in isolated tribes cut off from civilisation, so could have harboured diseases for centuries before they spread to the rest of the world. They are evolutionarily closer to monkeys, and thus could more readily acquire monkey diseases, perhaps by having sexual relations with monkeys or at least involving them in their sexual practices. They are sexually unrestrained, and a sexually transmitted disease would therefore spread more rapidly among them than among any other people. Their intelligence is limited and they cannot understand the complexity of a disease such as AIDS; their objections to being attributed with its source are harmful to themselves and do not need to be taken seriously. We are all the products of our culture, and it is unlikely that the Western scientists who accepted the 'AIDS from Africa' thesis so uncritically were aware of the source of their views.

This may be understandable, but their failure even to consider, let alone debate, the objections raised by Africans is surely quite unacceptable. It is also bad science.

If the intrinsic scientific merits of the 'AIDS from Africa' hypothesis are insufficient to justify its retention, and it is being sustained by a combination of desire to distract attention from a laboratory origin and racist beliefs about Africans, what is the historical context in which this has taken place? It is appropriate to begin with the development of biological warfare during the Second World War, when all the major combatants tested such weapons – in the case of the Germans and Japanese, on a large number of human subjects. After the war the Americans, in close collaboration with the British, allocated substantial resources to develop these weapons. So important did they regard biological warfare that they gave Japanese scientists who had regularly sacrificed human prisoners during experiments immunity from prosecution for war crimes in exchange for the information so gathered. For two decades from the early 1950s more than 200 experiments were conducted in the United States alone. 'Harmless' bacteria were released on military and civilian targets, including whole cities. In other experiments pathogenic bacteria were tested on animals on rafts off the Bahamas, the carcasses of the animals being burned at sea. The scientists conducting these experiments were based at the US military base at Camp Detrick, later renamed Fort Detrick, in Maryland, and in Britain at the Microbiological Research Establishment at Porton Down. The diseases considered most promising in the 1950s were anthrax, brucellosis, tularaemia, psittacosis and Q fever, caused by bacteria, and viral haemorrhagic fevers such as Rocky Mountain spotted fever and Rift Valley fever.[49]

Unlike bacteria, viruses survive and multiply only within cells, and laboratory experimentation with viruses became very much easier when 'immortal' cell lines were developed during the 1950s. The determination of the molecular structure of DNA by Watson and Crick in 1953 opened up the possibility of manipulation of the genetic structure of micro-organisms, and the possibilities were not lost on those engaged in biological warfare research. As early as 1962 forty scientists were employed at the US biological warfare laboratories on full-time genetics research, and when Professor MacFarlane Burnet wrote of the dangers of molecular biology in 1966 he would undoubtedly have been aware that his fellow scientists were using such knowledge for military purposes. By 1969 the US Department of Defense sought funding to manufacture a new biological agent, presenting the following testimony to the House Appropriations Committee:

> Within the next 5 to 10 years, it would probably be possible to make a new infective micro-organism which could differ in certain important respects from any known disease-causing organisms. Most important of these is that it might be refractory to the immunological and therapeutic processes upon which we depend to maintain our relative freedom from disease.[50]

It is important to realise that, whatever the intentions of scientists, molecular biology research was and remains imprecise, and the results are therefore unpredictable. The first immortal cell line was taken from the cervical cancer of a young American woman who died in 1951, and was called HeLa after the first two letters of her first and last names. This cell line was passed to laboratories throughout the world and grew so well that in the late 1960s it was discovered that many laboratory cell lines thought to have been immortalised by laboratory techniques were contaminations by HeLa cells, and many experiments were discredited. Viral contamination of cell cultures has also been persistently problematic. A notable example was a 'new' human retrovirus called HL23 which was cultured from human leukaemia cells. This 'new' virus was subsequently found to be two 'old' contaminating monkey viruses.[51] The debacle of the African green monkey virus hailed as the precursor of HIV but found to be a laboratory contaminant was a similar and far from unusual event.

Public disquiet about the dangers of biological warfare found political expression in 1968 when, at the Standing Eighteen Nation Disarmament Committee in Geneva, the British proposed that the disarmament of biological weapons should be negotiated separately from that of chemical weapons and introduced a draft Biological Weapons Convention which would commit all signatory states to renouncing the weapons for all time. The United States and the Soviet Union initially greeted the proposal with little enthusiasm, but under mounting domestic pressure President Nixon supported it. The Soviet Union abandoned its opposition, and in 1972 the two countries signed a treaty that they would 'never in any circumstances develop, produce, stockpile, or otherwise acquire or retain' any biological weapons. The US government was left with a research establishment at Fort Detrick capable of producing almost every known human pathogen and millions of infected mosquitoes, fleas, ticks and flies to deliver them to target populations. In a consummately political move, President Nixon ordered a large part of this establishment to be transferred to the National Cancer Institute, and Litton Biotechnic, a division of Litton Industries, was privately contracted to run the operation.[52] No longer useful for waging war on communism, the army's DNA and genetic engineering programmes were co-ordinated into anti-cancer research and molecular biology programmes for President Nixon's ill-fated War on Cancer, which officially began with the signing of the National Cancer Act on 23 December 1971. Officials were hopeful that a cancer cure would be discovered in time for America's bicentennial birthday celebrations in 1976. Working on the premiss that viruses caused cancer, numerous experiments were conducted inoculating viruses, with and without prior alteration of their genetic structure, in cell cultures or laboratory animals not normally infected by the virus. By 1976 there was still no proven association between human cancer and virus infection nor any prospect of effective treatment. The Director of the National Cancer Programme was forced to resign, and future efforts were directed towards researching possible environmental factors responsible for cancer.[53]

For obvious reasons scientists engaged in biological warfare research do not publish their findings in scientific journals, and the extent of overlap between biological warfare research and cancer research is not public knowledge. It is well known that some of the leading scientists who failed to find a cure for cancer were later credited with the discovery of HIV and became the 'godfathers' of AIDS research. If the origin of the AIDS epidemic could be traced even circumstantially to laboratory experiments for biological warfare or cancer research, the trail could end with these leading AIDS experts. It is hard to believe it is a coincidence that these same scientists have been the most ardent proponents of an African monkey origin for HIV.

There is little doubt, either, that biological warfare research did not cease in 1972, but continued either within the terms of the disarmament treaty or covertly outside them. For no good scientific reason AIDS researchers have associated the Ebola epidemic in Zaire in 1976 with the origin of AIDS. In the film *And the Band Played On*, based on the book by Randy Shilts, a team from the World Health Organization investigated and attempted to control the epidemic. This was untrue. The medical team were members of the US military who received support from the South African government, and the same military team was also studying Lassa fever in West Africa.[54]

AIDS science has at its heart a small number of assumptions, and at first glance it may seem difficult to understand why there is so little debate or even diversity of opinion among the many scientists participating in this complex research activity. Part of the explanation lies with normal scientific practice. Each field of science, or at least of mature science, has a core of theories, described by Lakotas as the 'hard core' of research programmes, or, in a somewhat different conceptual framework, by Kuhn as paradigms.[55] Scientists working in the field are unlikely to challenge the existing paradigm, in part because of training and discipline, which can constitute a form of internal censorship, and in part from external peer pressure. The latter can be of a very direct nature, as scientific careers can progress only if funds can be obtained for research projects and the results of research are published in learned journals. Leading scientists in the field normally have influence over the allocation of funds in their field of research and, by the process of peer review and editorial control, over publication in scientific journals.

Yet even 'normal' science does not function independently of its social, economic and political context. The days of the independent scientist conducting experiments in the study at home are long gone, and the political and economic priorities of government and industry now largely determine the allocation of funds. And, as scientists bring into their work their own particular cultural baggage, so too the results of their work are expected to conform with the prevailing cultural norms or vested interests. From the beginning of the epidemic the political aspects of AIDS have been exceptionally prominent. The conflict over who first isolated HIV was resolved not in scientific meetings or publications but in the White House, where the French scientist Luc Montaigner and the American Robert Gallo were officially recognised as 'co-discoverers' of HIV, and the extremely lucrative royalties from blood tests for HIV were divided accordingly.[56] Such is the murkiness of AIDS science that Montaigner is now regarded as the sole discoverer, and Gallo has been found guilty of scientific misconduct.[57] But, as I have endeavoured to argue above, the high-profile political endorsement of scientists like Gallo may be motivated by more than money. The manner in which science is organised and funded in the late twentieth century makes it possible for a small group of scientists very well connected with the political, military and industrial establishments to dominate their area of research, and in so doing, to promote the interests of their sponsors rather than seek scientific truth.

Science is but one means of acquiring knowledge and understanding of the world around us and, like all human endeavours, it contains our partial understandings and individual and collective prejudices. However, the central aim of science is to find theories that best explain available knowledge, and if the scientific process deviates from that aim, failure is likely, if not inevitable. If AIDS is caused by a virus that did not come from Africa but from a laboratory it would be foolish to expect success from scientists who may have deliberately or accidentally created the virus and who wish to divert attention from their past activities. The very failure of AIDS science, though, may be grounds for optimism, for flawed hypotheses cannot survive for ever and sooner or later the obvious must be confronted. For those already suffering from AIDS it will, unfortunately, be far too late.

Notes

1 P. H. Duesberg, 'AIDS acquired by drug consumption and other noncontagious risk factors', *Pharmacology and Therapeutics* 55 (1992): 201–77.
2 M. S. Gottlieb, H. M. Shanker, P. T. Fan, A. Saxon, J. D. Weisman and I. Polanski, 'Pneumocystis pneumonia – Los Angeles', *Morbidity and Mortality Weekly Report* 30 (21 1981): 250–1.
3 W. Sterry, M. Marmor, A. Konrads and G. K. Steigleder, 'Kaposi's sarcoma, aplastic pancytopaenia, and multiple infections in a homosexual (Cologne, 1976)', *Lancet*, 23 April 1983: 924; see also H. P. Katner and G. A. Pankey, 'Evidence for a Euro-American origin of Human Immunodeficiency Virus (HIV)', *Journal of the National Medical Association* 79 (10 1987): 1068–72; G. Williams, T. B. Stretton and J. C. Leonard, 'Cytomegalic inclusion disease and *Pneumocystis carinni* infection in an adult', *Lancet* (ii 1960): 951–5.
4 The alternative hypothesis to HIV as the cause of AIDS could be summarised briefly as follows. (1) HIV is a harmless passenger virus and AIDS is caused by non-infectious factors such as drugs (Duesberg). (2) HIV is a necessary but not the sole cause of AIDS (Root-Bernstein). (3) HIV does not exist, and what are described as viruses are non-infectious virus-like particles (Pappadopoulos *et al.*).
5 'Opportunistic infections and Kaposi's sarcoma among Haitians in the United States', *Morbidity and Mortality Weekly Report* 31 (1982): 353–4, 360–1; J. Viera, E. Frank, T. J. Spira and S. H. Landesman, 'Acquired immune deficiency syndrome in Haitians', *New England Journal of Medicine* 308 (3 1983): 125–9.
6 K. M. De Cock, 'AIDS: an old disease from Africa?' *British Medical Journal* 289 (4 August 1984): 306–8.
7 Y. Adeyemi, 'The origin of AIDS', *Concorde Weekly*, 11 July 1985: 46.
8 F. Misser, 'Trying to break the African connection', *New African* (220 1986): 13–14.
9 'Scientists attack AIDS slur on Africa', *New Scientist*, 28 November 1985: 15.
10 A. J. Pinching, R. A. Weiss and D. Miller, 'AIDS and HIV infection: the wider perspective', *British Medical Bulletin* 44 (1 1988): 58.
11 De Kock, 'An old disease?'
12 B. Davidson, *Old Africa Rediscovered*, London: Gollancz, 1959.
13 C. H. Robinson, *Hausaland, or, Fifteen Hundred Miles through Central Soudan*, London: Sampson Low, 1900.
14 P. S. Garlake, *Great Zimbabwe*, London: Thames & Hudson, 1973.
15 B. Davidson, *The African Slave Trade*, Boston and Toronto: Little Brown, 1980.
16 'Evidence for origin is weak', *New Scientist*, 15 October 1987: 27; P. J. Kanki, J. Alroy and M. Essex, 'Isolation of a T-lymphotrophic retrovirus related to HTLV-III/LAV from wild-caught African green monkeys', *Science* 230 (22 November 1985): 951–4.
17 M. Fukawawa, T. Miura, A. Hasegawa, S. Morikawa, H. Tsujimoto, M. Keizaburo, T, Kitamura and M. Hayami, 'Sequence of simian immunodeficiency virus from African green monkey, a new member of the HIV/SIV group', *Nature* 333 (2 June 1988): 457–61.
18 D. C. Gajduser, H. L. Amyx, C. J. Gibbs, D. M. Asher, R. T. Yanagihara, P. Rodgers-Johnson, P. W. Brown *et al.*, 'Transmission experiments with human T-lymphotropic retroviruses and human AIDS tissue', *Lancet*, 23 June 1984: 1415–16.
19 G. H. Freidland, B. R. Saltzman, M. F. Rogers, P. A. Kahl, M. L. Lesser, M. M. Mayers and R. S. Klein, 'Lack of transmission of HTLV-III/LAV infection to household contacts of patients with AIDS or AIDS-related complex with oral Candidiasis', *New England Journal of Medicine* 314 (6 1989): 344–9; P. Jones and P. Hamilton, 'HTLV-III antibodies in haematology staff', *Lancet*, 26 January 1985: 217.
20 F. Noireau, 'HIV transmission from monkey to man', *Lancet*, 27 June 1987: 1498–9;

J. Green and D. Miller, *AIDS: the Story of a Disease*, London: Grafton Books, 1986: 66; 'HIV origin "a continuing mystery": green monkey theory disputed', *Skin and Allergy News* 19 (1 1988): 28–9.

21 D. Hamilton, *The Monkey Gland Affair*, London: Chatto & Windus, 1986.

22 H. Kornfield, N. Reidel, G. A. Viglianti, V. Hirsch and J. Mullins, 'Cloning of HTLV-4 and its relation to simian and human immunodeficiency viruses'. *Nature* 326 (9 April 1987): 610; C. Mulder, 'A case of mistaken non-identity', *Nature* 331 (18 February 1988): 562; C. Mulder, 'Human AIDS virus not from monkeys', *Nature* 333 (2 June 1988): 396; S. Connor, 'Laboratory mix-up solves AIDS mystery', *New Scientist*, 25 February 1988: 32.

23 M. McClure, 'Where did the AIDS virus come from?' *New Scientist*, 30 June 1990: 54–7.

24 J. E. Osborn, 'The AIDS epidemic: multidisciplinary trouble', *New England Journal of Medicine* 314 (12 1986): 779–82; M. Melbye, R. J. Biggar, P. Ebbesen, M. G. Sarngadharan, S. H. Wiess, R. C. Gallo and W. A. Blattner, 'Seroepidemiology of HTLV-III antibody in Danish homosexual men: prevalence, transmission, and disease outcome', *British Medical Journal* 289 (8 September 1984): 573.

25 S. K. Owusu, 'Origin and spread of AIDS', *Nature* 350 (1988): 184.

26 H. P. Katner and G. A. Pankey, 'Evidence for a Euro-American origin of human immunodeficiency virus', *Journal of the National Medical Association* 79 (1987): 1068–72.

27 I. C. Bygbjerg, 'AIDS in a Danish surgeon (Zaire, 1976)', *Lancet*, 23 April 1983: 925; letter from Dr Bygbjerg to Dr Grote, 18 April 1988.

28 G. Corbitt, A. S. Bailey and G. Williams, 'HIV infection in Manchester, 1959', *Lancet* 336 July 1990: 51; 'Researchers in US dispute first case of AIDS', *British Medical Journal* 310 (15 April 1995): 957.

29 R. J. Biggar, 'Possible non-specific associations between malaria and HTLV-III/LAV', *New England Journal of Medicine* 315 (7 1986): 457–8.

30 G. Hunsmann, J. Schneider, I. Wendler and A. F. Fleming, 'HTLV positivity in Africans', *Lancet*, 26 October 1985: 952–3; I. Wendler, J. Schneider, B. Gras, A. F. Fleming, G. Hunsmann and H. Schmitz, 'Seroepidemiology of human immunodeficiency virus in Africa', *British Medical Journal* 293 (27 September 1986): 782–5.

31 O. Kashala, R. Marlink, M. Ilunga, M. Diese, B. Gormus, K. Xu, P. Mukeba, K. Kasongo and M. Essex, 'Infection with Human Immunodeficiency Virus Type 1 (HIV-1) and Human T Cell Lymphotrophic Viruses among leprosy patients and contacts: correlation between HIV-1 cross-reactivity and antibodies to lipoarabinomannan', *Journal of Infectious Diseases* 169 (1994): 296–304.

32 F. I. D. Konotey-Ahulu, 'Clinical epidemiology, not seroepidemiology, is the answer to Africa's AIDS problem', *British Medical Journal* 294 (20 June 1987): 1593–4.

33 A. J. Nahmias, J. Weiss, X. Yao, P. Kanki, M. Essex *et al.*, 'Evidence for human infection with an HTLV III/LAV-like virus in Central Africa, 1959', *Lancet*, 31 May 1986: 1279–80.

34 *Weekly Epidemiological Record* (10 1986): 71.

35 R. M. Anderson and R. M. May, 'Epidemiological parameters of HIV transmission', *Nature* 333 (9 June 1988): 514–22.

36 D. W. Mulder, A. J. Nunn, A. Kamali, J. Nakiyingi, H.-U. Wagner and J. F. Kengeya-Kayondo, 'Two-year HIV-1-associated mortality in a Ugandan rural population', *Lancet* 343 (23 April 1994): 1021–3.

37 R. J. Biggar, M. Melbye, L. Kestens *et al.*, 'Seroepidemiology of HTLV-III in a remote population of eastern Zaire', *British Medical Journal* 290 (16 March 1985): 808–10; R. M. Anderson, R. M. May, M. C. Boily, G. P. Carnett and J. T. Rowley, 'The spread of HIV-1 in Africa: sexual contact patterns and the predicted demographic impact of AIDS', *Nature* 352 (15 August 1991): 581–9.

38 W. L. Heyward and J. W. Curran, 'The epidemiology of AIDS in the US', *Scientific American*, October 1988: 52–9; E. D. Acheson, 'AIDS: a challenge for the public health', *Lancet*, 22 March 1986: 662–5.

39 F. M. Burnet, 'Men or molecules? A tilt at molecular biology', *Lancet*, 1 January

1966: 37–9.
40 A. Hellman, M. N. Oxman and R. Pollack (eds), *Biohazards in biological research*, Cold Spring Harbour, N.Y.: Cold Spring Harbour Laboratory, 1973.
41 C. Grobstein, *A Double Image of the Double Helix: the Recombinant DNA Debate*, San Francisco: Freeman, 1979.
42 G. Siegl, 'Canine parvovirus: origin and significance of a "new" pathogen', in K. I. Berns (ed.), *The Parvoviruses*, New York and London: Plenum Press, 1984.
43 Quoted in P. Fryer, *Staying Power: the History of Black People in Britain*, London and Sydney: Pluto Press, 1987: 148. Emphasis in the original.
44 This account can be found in B. Davidson, *The African Slave Trade*, Boston, Mass. and Toronto: Little Brown, 1980, part 4.
45 J. Conrad, *Heart of Darkness*, Harmondsworth: Penguin Books, 1989.
46 Quoted in Fryer, *Staying Power:* 152.
47 *Ibid.*: 159.
48 *Ibid.*: 164.
49 R. Harris and J. Paxman, *A Higher Form of Killing: the Secret Story of Gas and Germ Warfare*. London: Chatto & Windus, 1982.
50 *Ibid.*
51 A. Cantwell, *AIDS and the Doctors of Death*, Los Angeles: Aires Rising Press, 1988.
52 Harris and Paxman, *A Higher Form.*
53 Cantwell, *Doctors of Death.*
54 Personal communication from a participant in the Ebola control programme.
55 I. Lakatos, *The Methodology of Scientific Research Programmes*. Cambridge University Press, 1978; T. S. Kuhn, *The Structure of Scientific Revolutions*, University of Chicago Press, 1970.
56 'AIDS truce brings history to a halt', *New Scientist*, 9 April 1987: 21; 'Settlement on AIDS finally reached between US and Pasteur', *Nature* 326 (9 April 1987) 533.
57 'Inside the Gallo probe', *Science* 248, 22 June 1990: 1494–507; 'HSS: Gallo guilty of misconduct', *Science* 259, 8 January 1993: 1168–70.

CHAPTER THREE

Elders and experts: contesting veterinary knowledge in a pastoral community

Richard Waller and Kathy Homewood

A meeting supposedly once occurred between a group of Maasai elders and a colonial veterinary officer who was attempting to explain the benefits of stock improvement schemes. After listening in silence the Maasai countered with a generous offer: 'Send some of your young men to live with us and we will teach them to keep cattle properly.' Whether apocryphal or not, the vignette captures something of the ambiguity of an encounter between two systems of knowledge, one based on Western scientific principles of investigative and curative medicine and directed towards market production and the ultimate eradication of disease, the other based on inherited knowledge drawn from local observation and experience and directed towards the reproduction and survival of both herd and household. The advocates of each system distrusted the other. The argument continues today essentially unchanged, despite the far greater powers of intervention now assumed by state, development aid and veterinary authorities.

In the last decade the history of Western medicine in non-Western settings has been re-examined. It has moved from the simple confrontational triumphalism of *Man against Tsetse*[1] or *Tropical Victory*[2] to a much more nuanced understanding of the factors involved in medical intervention.[3] These include not only complex and changing natural and socio-political environments but also shifts and developments in Western science and in its perception of, and relation to other therapeutic systems. There is growing appreciation of the wider context of power relations in colonial societies.[4] Recent studies have acknowledged that combating disease provided an opportunity for social control as well as a demonstration of the superiority of Western civilisation and a way of measuring the success of colonial rule. 'Natives' as well as 'germs' might have been the target. Moreover, pathogens, like 'the actinic rays of the sun', could stand metonymously for the alien and hostile environment with which colonisers had to contend.[5] Disease acquired a descriptive power, and its spread from 'native' to 'settler' seemed to be both a consequence of and a metaphor for unregulated culture contact. Thus the imposition of Western medical knowledge and practice, sometimes by force and usually without consultation, calmed imperial fears and served a number of imperial purposes.[6]

Western medical practitioners in the tropics did more than cure the ills of imperialists and their subjects. As exponents of an alien and supposedly superior system of knowledge they sought to reshape the bodies and minds of their patients, and to claim a universal validity for their particular construction of health and disease. Algerians in the mid-nineteenth century, for example, would have to learn 'a new way of being sick' in order that French medicine might reach them. This meant viewing themselves and their bodies in a different relation to the natural and social environment.[7] A century later, Western vets complain that African pastoralists define diseases according to different taxonomies and often aggregate and disaggregate symptoms 'wrongly'.[8] They too must learn what disease 'is', and perceive their environment differently. Herd owners have also had to be brought to see their animals not as a totality, an integral part of the household and its reproduction, but as individual items of property with a realisable market value.[9] This perceptual shift, like the individuation of the human body, has created a field in which science can operate to improve, rather than merely to control. Now, as then, these shifts take place within a field of unequal power relations between state and pastoralists, to which differential access to veterinary resources contributes substantially.

During and after the colonial period, Western medical practitioners received government support in their attempts to redefine disease and its treatment, not only because disease, whether in humans or in animals, was a threat and because medical aid was seen as an important means to 'win the confidence' of the colonised,[10] but also because the collation of data and the creation of knowledge which scientific investigation involved were a crucial part of the wider imperial project. But experts did not always agree among themselves. The field of tropical medicine is littered with the debris of old jealousies and disputes. The celebrated clash between the London and Liverpool Schools at the turn of the century reveals that the medical profession was divided not only over issues of scientific theory and procedure but also about the proper role and objectives of medicine in the tropical colonies.[11] Similar divisions existed in veterinary science.[12] The Kenya and Tanganyika governments pursued different, and not always compatible, policies with regard to livestock and its improvement.[13] Within the veterinary service in Kenya there were disputes between research-oriented and field-oriented officers and between 'interventionist' and 'isolationist' schools of thought. Both accepted, almost axiomatically, that African herds were the focus of disease, but the former believed that it was both possible and essential to combat stock diseases by active intervention within the Reserves, while the latter argued that, since disease could not be effectively eradicated in African herds, veterinary resources should be directed to the needs of white commercial stock owners and African areas sealed off by quarantine barriers.[14] Science in the colonies often spoke in private with many and discordant voices, even if it appeared monolithic and authoritative to its lay public, and there was always more at stake professionally than simply the study and cure of disease.[15]

Colonial officials, however, did not always appreciate scientific intervention in the business of governing. The administration in Kenyan Maasailand, for instance, while urging and welcoming the appointment of district Veterinary Officers, was concerned about the impact on the local community. District administrators complained bitterly about the imposition of quarantine, which, they argued, was often imposed needlessly and without consultation and, by disrupting the stock trade, made Maasai development impossible.[16] Distrust sprang in part from the field administrators' reluctance to accept experts with a rival claim to authority in 'their' districts,[17] but it was also rooted in a different and highly localised set of ruling priorities which contradicted the universalising tendencies of colonial science. Until the 1940s vets and agriculturalists, with a few influential exceptions, were the servants rather than the masters of local policy. As disputes over Kenyan veterinary policy demonstrate, the discourse of expert technical opinion was subject to challenge and denial – although also to affirmation – in the interests of local governance. Moreover, the Veterinary Department frequently found its ostensibly 'neutral' scientific authority being used to further political ends. In its practical expression, no less than in its theoretical assumptions, colonial veterinary science was shaped by and implicated in power relations.[18]

Colonial medical history is still too often written, implicitly at least, from the colonisers' perspective. Although we are beginning to learn in some detail how power infuses colonial (and postcolonial) medical practice and how cultural assumptions shape and have shaped the construction of scientific knowledge and method, we know far less about how this enterprise was viewed and understood by its colonial subjects. Their voices only rarely made themselves heard.[19] Often we are left to infer thought from mute action. And Africans often literally 'voted with their feet', thus confirming the view of their would-be benefactors that they were incapable of understanding the benefits of scientific medicine.[20]

Less has been written specifically on the development and application of Western veterinary medicine in Africa – surprisingly, perhaps, in view of the impact on African historiography of John Ford's work on the history of trypanosomiasis.[21] Yet veterinary medicine was very much a 'tool of empire'.[22] At the time of conquest, pack animals as well as people had to be protected from disease. Later the health, growth and commercial exploitation of the 'national herd' have been central to the development of the colonial and postcolonial economy.[23] Where land ownership and herd ownership were unequally split between white settlers and African pastoralists, as they were in Kenya and Rhodesia, stock diseases acquired political and symbolic importance, and quarantine barriers demarcated racial space.[24] More recently the policy of expanding and intensifying livestock production has continued to direct veterinary resources into the commercial sector, focusing on well-capitalised ranching enterprises and on grade cattle in high-potential mixed farming areas rather than on pastoralist producers on extensive rangelands. Veterinary medicine is now an important tool of development, and veterinarians have become the guardians of substantial national resources and class interests.[25]

Understanding of the colonial context of veterinary medicine and of the wider issues of knowledge, power and perception involved has lagged behind the sophistication of modern studies of the human 'body politic' and its ills. Ford's work on the ecology of disease has been taken up and developed within the frame of colonial historiography,[26] but colonial veterinary intervention is still explained largely in terms of colonial practice: as a potent form of extra-economic market control and a way of safeguarding local capital accumulation.[27] There is little acknowledgement that actual practice might be derived as much from veterinary theory applied in a colonial situation as from the particular political and economic imperatives of the state. Struggles between vets and herd owners are presented simply in terms of control over animals and markets, and Africans are usually cast as victims and evaders. Rarely are they – or vets themselves, for that matter – allowed to speak for different systems of knowledge and experience.[28]

In this chapter we seek in a preliminary way to suggest how the debate on veterinary medicine may be taken beyond the study of the political and economic effects of stock control and into the area of the historical sociology of knowledge, drawing on the growing literature on medicine and society for our comparisons. Taking the opening scene as our text, we focus on the interaction between vets and the

Maasai of Kenya and Tanzania during and after the colonial period. We consider Maasai and Western veterinary thought and practice as the products of two different systems of knowledge, sometimes converging or interlocking but often at odds over fundamental issues. We also draw attention to the fact that strategies based on the different systems of knowledge lead to different biological/ecological outcomes, and we suggest that modern epidemiological events should still be interpreted in the light of conflicts between state policy and pastoralist strategy.

While issues of knowledge had much wider reference than simply the health of the herds, it was inevitable that, within an administration always driven by pragmatic considerations of cost, disease and its control would be the prime focus of veterinary concern and the point on which elders and experts most often found themselves opposed. Accordingly, in order to provide a frame for discussion, we take four contrasting diseases as our main case studies.[29]

East Coast Fever (ECF) was endemic to parts of Maasailand before the era of colonial rule, although it was first recorded for Kenya in 1904.[30] It has since spread and is now one of the most serious cattle diseases in East Africa. ECF is a tick-borne protozoan disease which causes high mortality in susceptible animals which have not been able to acquire or maintain immunity through exposure to disease challenge as calves. Because it is vector-borne, ECF may be considered as an 'ecosystemic' disease involving land as well as the herd.[31] As such, ECF carried political and symbolic overtones in the colonial period. Areas where the disease was endemic were revealingly described in colonial writing as 'dirty', in contrast to those where ticks could not thrive or from which the disease had been eradicated, which were 'clean'. Pastures could, it was believed, be 'cleansed' or kept 'clean' by the regular dipping of stock to kill infective ticks. The line between 'clean' and 'dirty' was clearly and legally marked on the landscape by fences, roadside dips and quarantine stations, although the difficulties and expense of control posed by a patchwork of endemically stable (otherwise 'dirty') and unstable (otherwise 'clean') areas were obvious.[32] Unless they were tested and certified immune to ECF, a cumbersome procedure involving quarantine in a 'temperature boma', transport oxen and cattle from 'dirty' areas could not move into or through 'clean' ones – especially if it involved crossing the line from African Reserves to (white) settled areas – as they might introduce the disease to susceptible herds and uninfected tick populations. Recent research has, however, disproved the belief, on which much of the veterinary rationale for the policy of control depended, that immune stock cannot infect ticks. It was not appreciated until the 1970s that there was a carrier state in which animals, while showing no clinical symptoms themselves, could, nonetheless, transmit the protozoon to feeding ticks which then infected other, susceptible, animals.[33] The search for security in fences and dips was thus an illusion created by the conjunction between incomplete scientific understanding and an urge to impose order and distance.

Little veterinary attention, beyond survey work, was paid to the control of the disease within Maasailand itself until late in the colonial period, but the fact that the Reserve contained both endemic and non-endemic areas was important in shaping the patterns of local stock exchange and marketing.[34] At the end of the colonial period, and in the first decades of independence, serious attempts were made to control the vector population through regular and sometimes compulsory cattle dipping with acaricides in both Kenya and Tanzania. In the 1960s a major dip construction programme began, but the growing number of susceptible exotic and cross-bred animals, the rapid emergence of acaricide resistance in ticks, the mounting costs and declining efficiency of dipping, and the lack of effective ways of dealing with carriers and disease reservoirs, have all conspired to exacerbate the impact of ECF on an increasingly vulnerable stock population.[35]

Trypanosomiasis too is a long-established vector-borne disease caused by a parasitic protozoon. In this case the vector is a tsetse fly, which, like different species of tick, has particular habitat requirements. Because other forms of the trypanosome cause sleeping sickness in humans and because the fly and its freight spread with visible and appalling rapidity throughout large parts of Eastern and Central Africa in the first decades of colonial rule, trypanosomiasis commanded scientific and colonial attention and quickly came to symbolise the struggle of Man against Nature. About two-thirds of Tanzania (much of it high-potential land) and a quarter of Kenya are now infested. Indigenous cattle breeds have varying degrees of resistance and, with mild disease challenge, commonly develop sub-clinical infections which may not become apparent until the animal is under stress, but exotics are at much greater risk.

As with ECF, the control of the vector within the ecosystem offered the first and obvious line of attack. Ambitious and ultimately unrealisable socio-ecological engineering projects were undertaken in an attempt to separate the fly from its human and animal hosts and to destroy its woodland breeding grounds. These schemes involved clearing large areas of bush, eliminating wildlife populations and resettling huge numbers of people and their livestock. Their interventionist style caught both the public and the scientific imagination, but the results, proportional to the effort involved, were disappointing.[36] Late colonial and postcolonial governments have attempted a double strategy of control: reducing the vectors and tackling the pathogen with drugs – but with equally limited results.

Maasailand escaped much of this activity, even though the fly was present and spreading. Human trypanosomiasis was rare and thus did not threaten labour supplies or peasant production; settlement and land use were sparse. Loss of access to grazing land was probably a more significant result of tsetse encroachment in Maasailand than direct loss of stock. Attention in any case was focused elsewhere, in western Tanganyika or in the Belgian Congo, where scientific reputations and empires were being built.[37] However, when the fly threatened to cross boundaries into the European settled areas, a programme of eradication and land reclamation was set in motion which did, for a while, push tsetse back from parts of western Maasailand.[38] Much of southern Maasailand was also invaded, but limited tsetse eradication measures in the 1940s tended to benefit cultivators rather than pastoralists. While Tanzania has continued the same strategy of barrier clearance to control the vector, Kenya in the 1950s and 1960s developed trypanocidal drugs for both prophylaxis and therapy – to which resistance has now emerged.[39]

Vector-borne diseases in general perhaps appealed to the colonial imagination because their conquest involved more than the microscope and the syringe. It stressed prevention as well as cure and presented scientists as heroic figures leading an army of experts against a tangible foe. The fight against tsetse in particular evoked images of an African landscape being transformed and ordered by Western science and technology in the pursuit not merely of microbes but of a greater social and civilising purpose.[40] As we indicate below, however, alternative therapeutic systems may perhaps offer a surer and less costly, if also less spectacular, means of control.

By contrast, neither Contagious Bovine Pleuro Pneumonia (CBPP) nor rinderpest is a vector-borne disease, and neither was originally present in East Africa. CBPP reached Maasailand from the south in the early 1880s. Its impact was severe, but dwarfed in memory by that of the great rinderpest pandemic ten years later which struck and virtually destroyed the Maasai herds in the early months of 1891.[41] After their initial onslaught both diseases recurred at intervals and became endemic in the Maasai herds.

CBPP is a mycoplasma disease which spreads by droplet infection from breathing in the nasal discharge of infected animals within the herd. Although acute cases may die within two weeks, of fever and respiratory distress, other animals recover either completely or as 'lungers', apparently healthy animals which may still carry and transmit the disease to others. The presence of carriers together with the long incubation period of up to six months means that the disease may spread undetected through a herd or remain dormant for long periods. It also prompted one of the most unpopular of veterinary interventions, the inspection of herds and the slaughter, often without compensation, of all suspect animals – a measure with consequences to the owners potentially more serious than the disease itself.[42] Rinderpest is a viral infection which can be transmitted through contact in a similar way and which causes high levels of mortality in non-immune cattle and in some species of wild animals. At first its extreme virulence ensured that outbreaks of the disease burnt themselves out, but as rinderpest established itself it developed a milder strain from which animals could develop some immunity.[43]

Rinderpest and CBPP thus differed from the vector-borne diseases in their relation to the wider ecology of stock management. They were essentially contagious diseases of the herd which presented colonial governments with different perceptions of danger and problems of control. The threat of vector-borne diseases was conceptualised in terms of space; that of contagious diseases in terms of contact, the invasion in this case being that of diseased animals themselves rather than of their parasites. The concept of contagion, together with the existence of carriers which appeared safe but were in fact deadly, made such diseases suitable as a veterinary justification for the essentially political act of removing or restricting the grazing of African-owned animals in the vicinity of settler areas.[44] It also prompted the first attempts to cure, rather than merely isolate, epidemics in Maasai herds.[45] Rather than attempting to alter the disease environment, veterinary authorities have sought a 'magic bullet' approach to eradication through inoculation and slaughter, with varying success. Rinderpest has been virtually eliminated by mass vaccination campaigns in the 1960s and 1970s but CBPP remains a major hazard.[46]

Having introduced the major cattle diseases of Maasailand, we turn to the general comparison of Western and Maasai concepts of disease and treatment. Maasai veterinary praxis is based on three underlying assumptions about the construction of knowledge, about the nature and role of disease and about the value of the herds it threatened.

Maasai have traditionally looked on stock disease as something that can be identified and understood through a process of deduction based on empirical observation. Practical knowledge and skill in dealing with the herds, gained through learning and experience, have an overriding authority and value. Some herd owners are acknowledged to be expert managers and diagnosticians whose advice is widely sought. There is nothing particularly arcane about their knowledge. It can be acquired by anyone diligent and observant enough and is passed on to a favoured or particularly promising son. By contrast, the knowledge brought by Western vets did seem arcane and was apparently acquired less by experience than by the mastery of scientific theories and techniques. It was often difficult for elders and vets to recognise each other as equally but differently expert. Even the means of validation were different: in the one case through the survival of the herd; in the other by diploma and professional appointment. Attempts on the part of government to bridge the conceptual gap and to teach the basics of 'improved' herd management through the establishment of practical training schemes at the Ngong Veterinary Centre and the inclusion of 'animal husbandry' in the Maasai school curriculum largely failed either to spread enlightenment in the Reserve or to overcome the elders' scepticism. If anything, this initiative in communication merely reinforced local stereotypes: that Maasai were unteachable, and that government had little of value to teach.[47]

Maasai had particular ideas about the place that disease occupied in their world. Whereas Western science saw 'health' as normal – indeed, defined it as the normal state – and disease by contrast as abnormal, requiring medical intervention to return the body to normality, Maasai regarded disease as a natural, inevitable but potentially stable part of the environment. Their world was not divided spatially or conceptually between disease and health. Intervention might be required to curb undue loss, but disease could not simply be eradicated. Nor was a disease-free state necessarily desirable. Maasai were aware of the vulnerability of animals without acquired immunity, and used movement and controlled exposure to endemic disease as a way of protecting herds against epidemic outbreaks. Models of herd size and composition recognised the fact of unpredictable mortality and allowed for it by increasing numbers and maximising breeding potential.[48] Management and therapeutic techniques, therefore, were predicated on the constant presence of disease and tended to work with rather than against the ecological grain.

Colonial veterinary policy, by contrast, moved increasingly in the opposite direction. Both their professional training and the demands of the economy led vets to work towards the creation of an environment from which disease would gradually be excluded by scientific means. In Kenya especially, the trajectory of the stock industry itself encouraged this thinking, starting with a small settler enclave of high-value and often exotic stock which required constant protection, and moving outwards to create ever larger areas in which commercial stock rearing could be safely carried on – and diminishing areas in which disease remained largely unchecked. Priority was given to control, of movement as much as of disease itself, and to the development and protection of capital assets. In Tanganyika, too, controlled zones were created and extended – one, indeed, along the interterritorial border cutting Maasailand in half – though here the emphasis was less selective, with veterinary services more equally, if sparsely, distributed. Quarantine regulations symbolised Western attitudes to disease and preventive medicine in East Africa. Indeed, it was in the imposition of quarantine restrictions that veterinary medicine in the service of the state had its most obvious and serious impact on the African stock economy. By defining and confining areas of disease, quarantine created safe spaces maintained by a system of scientific surveillance, of which the district Veterinary Officer and his staff of scouts were the local agents. Quarantine barriers could also be erected to block the spread of epidemics. They often cut arbitrarily across the lines of stock movement and trade, turning vets into policemen, and they created two landscapes: one remade and guarded apprehensively by Western science and veterinary medicine, the other left to 'Nature' and 'unimproved' pastoralism.[49]

Contrasting views of disease sprang in part from different theories of causation and underpinned different therapies. For Western medical science, cause lay in the invasion and colonisation of the body by unseen (except by science) and alien agents of mortality which might in principle be observed, identified and then destroyed, often with the help of other, benign, agents – antibodies, in the revealing term. It followed that therapy would be conceived of in invasive terms, whether the penetration of the patient's body by drugs or the inscription of quarantine lines on the land. Maasai, lacking the scientists' belief in and insight into the microbial other world, did not regard disease as the sign of an alien presence. On the contrary, disease, once observed, appeared to operate within a familiar and predictable frame of cause and effect. As Merker noted, Maasai did not regard disease as necessarily having supernatural causes or implications.[50] Diseases were diagnosed by their characteristic external symptoms and effects. Rinderpest, for example, quickly became known as *olodua* (gall bladder/bile) from the way in which the disease could be recognised.[51] In the case of foot-and-mouth, the symptomatic skin lesions – and not the viral infection itself – constitute the disease. Generally, each disease is assigned a specific identifying cause which may then be prevented, avoided or dealt with. Malignant catarrhal fever (MCF), for example, is attributed to grazing on pastures fouled by calving wildebeeste, and such areas are accordingly avoided.[52] Thus Maasai veterinary practice is based on knowledge of a complex system of external symptomology and causation which served both to identify disease and to guide therapy.[53] This was quite different from colonial veterinary medicine, based on a scientific methodology which located cause in an unseen world of pathogens and separated cause and symptom in its classificatory system.[54] As East African veterinary officers became more confident of their ability to isolate and identify pathogens, first in the laboratory and then in the field, they lost interest in Maasai views of disease, its causation, prevention and treatment. While indigenous and colonial conclusions sometimes coincided in practice, as with MCF, the very different systems of thought from which they came made dialogue between elders and experts difficult. Western vets often found Maasai explanations 'unscientific', even bizarre, while Maasai dismissed veterinary explanations as irrelevant to their concerns.[55]

Elders and experts disagreed over the nature and cause of disease; they were also divided over the value of the herds they both sought to protect. Differences here lay close to the root of conflict over the politics and economics of pastoralism which divided Maasai from their rulers throughout the colonial period and beyond. Maasai saw the herd as a totality in itself, the support and guarantee of the continuation of social reproduction: not merely as a capital asset and the aggregate of individual animals, as vets were trained to see it. Disease, then, threatened social disaster, not just the loss of valuable markets or capital investment. The Maasai social and totalising perception of disease and the herd often conflicted with the primarily economic and individualising view mandated by government.

Colonial veterinary authorities worked within a framework of economic policy which gave primacy to the market value of stock and which directed them towards the protection of valuable animals and the general improvement of stock quality, defined in market terms. While aware in a general way of the subsistence and social value of herds in pastoral areas, vets, like administrators, tended to see the accumulation of stock as something archaic and irrational that acted as a brake on development but would in time be superseded by a more enlightened attitude to stock wealth. Bigger herds would then be replaced by better beasts as the object of accumulation. As veterinary goals in the Reserves moved beyond the mere suppression and policing of disease, vets came to redefine their role in African areas as that of educating opinion and creating the conditions under which scientific asset management would be both possible and profitable to pastoralists.[56]

Practical experience of range conditions in Maasailand, however, suggested that this veterinary utopia was unlikely to be realised.[57] Drought and disease continued to take a regular toll of the herds, and improvement schemes from the late 1930s onwards, largely paid for by the Maasai themselves from compulsory stock sales, could not compensate for earlier losses of grazing and water resources. Prudent stock owners, therefore, made cautious and highly selective use of what Western veterinary science had to offer, based on an assessment of how it might contribute to the continuation of subsistence pastoralism and the survival of the herds, and of whether its rationale accorded with their own knowledge and experience.[58] Maasai resisted reducing the herds. Colonial medicine could neither command the rain nor forbid epidemics nor compensate for the harm to family and community fortunes that the sudden decimation of the herd would do. Numbers still counted. And they were sceptical of the value of exotic breeds which, while perhaps increasing productivity, were all too vulnerable to ambient disease and poor range conditions. Grade (cross-bred) cattle, however, obtained from settler farms and stock traders, were easily incorporated into the herds, since their viability and value were proven by experience.[59]

In principle, Maasai were not averse to the idea of treatment, but they could not understand how vets hoped to cure simply by invading the body or cordoning off the land into protected spaces, while apparently neglecting either to address the overt manifestations of disease or to make use of the environmental constraints within which it operated. Foot-and-mouth, for example, was seen as a form of lesion which could be externally treated by cautery: it did not require quarantine, which the Maasai refused to apply. Similarly, while Maasai understood the importance of immunity, and themselves practised forms of immunisation, their attitude towards early veterinary inoculation campaigns was influenced by the fact that the techniques appeared to contradict logic and experience.[60] Herd owners were initially highly sceptical of the value of artificially infecting an otherwise healthy adult animal directly with disease. Whereas calves infected with ECF and mild rinderpest might recover and then be immune to further attack, adult animals infected usually succumbed. Their scepticism was increased and justified by the dangerously unstable behaviour of the early inoculations – which seemed to kill as often as they cured.[61] Later, herd owners were willing to pay for some immunisations, though not for others. Selectivity here was not, however, determined primarily by cost. It was guided partly by experience but also by the relative contribution it might make to the survival and subsistence value of the herd as a whole. Treatment against anthrax, for example, was sought when cases occurred in the herds. Anthrax, unlike other diseases, turned cattle into their opposite: not just dead meat but deadly meat. By contrast, treatment for foot-and-mouth was ignored, since the disease had little obvious effect on the well-being of the herd. Similarly, while Maasai reluctantly submitted to CBPP inoculations, they resisted testing for carriers, since that might lead to their slaughter and the dead loss of an animal which would otherwise have contributed, if only its hide.

There was another concern. Practice based on a different kind of knowledge had wider social implications beyond the management of the herds. It required Maasai to re-evaluate their concepts of land, wealth and obligation as well as their ideas about disease and the bovine body. By 1950 communities were becoming accustomed to grazing divisions, water control and cash payment for 'the needle', while some richer and 'progressive' owners were dipping their cattle and enclosing pasture. In the long run, as some had already foreseen, these changes would create a different order in which access to land and resources would be limited and individualised and in which wealth would come from outside, no longer accumulated within the community through experience, prudence and good fortune.[62] Some elders might then become experts themselves, and dominate others.

Maasai responses, given the very different premises on which they were based, were inevitably construed as backward, apathetic and even obstructive by hard-pressed vets and administrators, and this construction fitted well with the experts' image of stubbornly conservative elders.[63] Yet, in scrutinising and selecting rather than fully embracing veterinary aid, and in continuing to accept limited loss in order to safeguard the herd and to defend the value of their own system of medical knowledge by 'passive resistance', Maasai were following the harsh logic required to maintain subsistence pastoralism under increasingly adverse conditions. To do otherwise would have meant making a conceptual and practical shift which was as potentially dangerous and divisive as it was difficult.

The last part of our chapter deals directly with the practical outcome of disputes over knowledge and authority, for different systems of veterinary knowledge informed different and competing strategies of stock management in postcolonial as well as colonial times. Although the governments of Kenya and Tanzania have pursued somewhat different policies, the outcome for their pastoral populations has been very similar.[64]

We may begin by outlining briefly how Maasai stock owners have attempted to deal with disease and how this has conflicted with state policy. Chief among indigenous strategies has been the use of space and movement to control or avoid outbreaks. An early response to rinderpest was to attempt to outrun it, leaving sick cattle on the way. Later, Maasai were willing to co-operate with veterinary authorities in isolating infected herds away from contact with others.[65] Such a use of space implied, of course, that there was space to be used. It became difficult to find once the Maasai were confined within legally defined Reserves in both Kenya and Tanganyika. Maasai complained of restrictions on movement throughout the colonial period.[66] It was probably in part the realisation that there was increasingly nowhere to run that encouraged Maasai to accept inoculation as an alternative to avoidance once it became freely available and demonstrably effective. In so doing, of course, they were beginning to reshape their therapeutic system to conform to veterinary ideas about intervention, protection and control.

An important corollary of the use of space was the selective use and management of pasture. Maasai herd owners were well acquainted with the different types of pasture to be found on their land. Indeed, an important aspect of 'possessing the land' was learning its ecology. They were able to use the knowledge to maintain the health of the herds by rotating them seasonally through different types of pasture. In this respect their practice was in advance of that of the white pastoralists who replaced them in parts of the Rift Valley, as some contemporary critics of the dispossession of the Maasai pointed out.[67] Maasai were also aware of the connection between some diseases and the insects that carried them, and of how this vector relationship fitted into, and was affected by, the wider ecosystem. Just as they observed that malaria was common in mosquito-ridden areas and therefore moved into such places only when mosquito challenge was low during the dry season, so they connected trypanosomiasis with the bite of the tsetse fly and either avoided areas of tsetse bush or took cattle through them only between sunset and sunrise when the fly is dormant and the risk least.[68] Again, this required space and freedom of movement. The creation and enforcement of colonial boundaries militated against the careful use of natural checks within the ecosystem and forced Maasai on to the defensive with regard to disease. In the case of trypanosomiasis, flexible use of the rangeland mosaic can maintain partial immunity and endemic stability but that presupposes access to a wide range of pastures and the ability to move freely between them. In Ngorongoro, Potkanski has noted a Maasai model of ECF which involves the differential management of immune (highland) and non-immune (lowland) animals so as to maintain endemicity.[69] Closer settlement has reduced this flexibility, and drought especially forces owners to take their animals into 'diseased' areas to find pasture – sometimes death. Pastoralists will face similar – if not worse – choices in the future as their grazing areas dwindle further and their movement patterns are disrupted under the pressure of development and wildlife conservation.[70]

Lack of space and restricted movement risk more than immediate stock losses, however. Both Waller and Giblin have drawn attention to the relationship over time between shifts in grazing patterns, vegetation change and the spread of disease vectors. Controlled grazing kept the latter in check and was always a crucial ingredient of management strategies.[71] Yet Maasai modes of land use and management have conflicted not only with past veterinary orthodoxies but also with recent Western perceptions of landscape and its value.[72] Grass burning and close grazing by a succession of different animals has been an effective method of cleaning pasture of ticks and other parasites[73] and of preventing the spread of tsetse bush, but it has been castigated by outsiders as ecologically 'destructive'.[74] Pastoral land use has been conventionally but erroneously regarded as inimical to the interests of conservation and economic development alike.[75] Pastoralists have been regularly accused of 'ruining' their land by overgrazing and poor management – a convenient argument for denying them access to pasture land which has been repeated over some sixty years of colonial and postcolonial overrule.[76] Given the Western focus on eradication and the power differential involved in relations between elders and experts, it is not surprising that dipping, symbolically, has usually prevailed over burning. The result has been, ironically, a real if gradual deterioration in pasture resources, caused not by Maasai land use but by its interdiction.

There have, however, always been dissidents. Among the most perceptive was Hornby, the Chief Veterinary Officer of Tanganyika in the mid 1930s. Hornby initially took a consistently more open-minded view of indigenous management techniques, including close grazing and burning, than many of his colleagues, especially in Kenya, who were still locked into familiar but unexamined arguments about the connections between over-stocking, over-grazing and erosion.[77] More recently, grazing management has been an area in which the opinions of experts and elders have begun belatedly to converge. Some of the former now give a cautious but still sceptical reception to methods of disease and pasture control, including naturally acquired immunity, derived from 'indigenous' knowledge.[78] Indeed, current scientific thought on ECF is both a vindication of and a compromise with indigenous systems of control.[79] Yet new strategies based on this understanding are doomed because they run counter to every other trend in land use and tenure and because they presuppose a reassessment of the national livestock industry, perhaps accepting lower productivity for less expenditure and risk.[80]

States are driven by economics, not epistemology, and the linkage that we have observed between the creation of veterinary knowledge, veterinary practice and colonial capitalism has been strengthened in the postcolonial world. East African governments are wholly committed to the development and protection of valuable capital assets and, therefore, reluctant to drop now-familiar strategies despite the weight of empirical evidence against them. Quarantine and prophylactic measures are geared to the needs of a developing export market, not those of subsistence pastoralism and the local market. Foot-and-mouth policy is a clear case in point. The European Union bans the import of meat from affected areas. Kenya's meat exports are important both to government and to highly capitalised commercial producers. Government has, therefore, concentrated on creating disease-free zones protected by an outer ring of compulsory vaccination. Highly disruptive quarantines are imposed on local pastoral producers in Maasailand and elsewhere in order to block the movement of infected animals.[81] The parallel with colonial thinking and practice is clear. Given East Africa's involvement in the international economy, the very idea of a fundamental change in the object and focus of veterinary care might appear to threaten national development. At the same time, experts are themselves part of the larger power structure of scientific and professional authority, and their position might also be threatened by a re-evaluation of the basis of knowledge.[82] Such concerns keep governments and experts alike prisoners of the illusion of scientific intervention.

Elders and experts, the latter again backed by the state, are still largely failing to understand one another. Yet the future looks increasingly ominous for both. The inequalities of power which enabled one system of knowledge to dominate the other remain, and they have had the further and continuing effect of marginalising local pastoralists both politically and economically. Pastoralists can no longer live entirely in the world of their own experience, but they have small access to the resources of the world of Western expertise. Thus they hang suspended between the two systems. The degree of discrimination which they were once able to exercise is steadily diminishing, and much of their knowledge has been invalidated by developments beyond their control. Although some Maasai have learnt to view their animals as capital assets, it has been to the detriment of the community as a whole. Commercial ranching by an emergent pastoral bourgeoisie has encouraged the privatisation and sale of grazing land and the dividing up of formerly shared resources.[83] Ironically, this has increased the vulnerability of both commercial producers, who have entered the domain of Western prophylaxis, and subsistence pastoralists, who remain largely outside but whose resource base is being further eroded by commercial expansion.

The ideology of colonial veterinary science may have triumphed, but at a high cost. While Western veterinary practitioners have largely succeeded in subordinating or silencing their rivals and critics they have not been equally successful in their fight against disease. Three of our four case-study diseases remain a serious threat to the livestock industry; and even the fourth, rinderpest, illustrates some of the dangers of success. Because the disease has been eradicated, a growing stock population is now at risk of reinfection in epidemic form, since it has neither exposure to disease nor artificial immunity. Experts have succeeded only too well over the last half-century in creating an artificial and highly unstable environment in which the health of the herds, now conceived of as absence of disease, has become critically dependent on access to prophylactic drugs and on expensive technical intervention. But this is hardly the veterinary utopia they once envisaged, and it is arguable that governments have neither the resources nor the close structures of control and consent to maintain this precarious state, as the case of ECF shows. Under pressure, veterinary orthodoxies are being re-examined and perhaps a paradigm shift may occur. But, if it does, it will not necessarily mean that the elders' offer to teach has been accepted. Experts will appropriate and reshape indigenous knowledge and, in a sense, change places with elders who have now learnt to see things differently.

Notes

1 J. J. McKelvey, *Man against Tsetse: Struggle for Africa* (Ithaca, N.Y.: Cornell University Press, 1973).

2 M. Gelfand, *Tropical Victory: an Account of the Influence of Medicine on the History of Southern Rhodesia* (Cape Town: Juta Press, 1953).

3 Several historians have commented on the use of military metaphor in medical writing. The same may be said of veterinary propaganda with its talk of 'campaigns' and its use of the visual imagery of the needle and the syringe. See, for example, comments in T. Ranger and P. Slack (eds), *Epidemics and Ideas* (Cambridge University Press, 1992): 14.

4 N. Gallagher, *Medicine and Power in Tunisia, 1780–1900* (Cambridge University Press, 1983); S. Marks and N. Anderson, 'Typhus and social control: South Africa, 1917–50', in R. MacLeod and M. Lewis (eds), *Disease, Medicine and Empire* (London: Routledge, 1988): 257–83.

5 D. Kennedy, 'The perils of the midday sun: climatic anxieties in the colonial tropics', in J. M. MacKenzie (ed.), *Imperialism and the Natural World* (Manchester University Press, 1990): 118–40.

6 D. Arnold (ed.), *Imperial Medicine and Indigenous Societies* (Manchester University Press, 1988); R. MacLeod and M. Lewis (eds), *Disease, Medicine and Empire* (London: Routledge, 1988).

7 A. Marcovich, 'French colonial medicine and colonial rule: Algeria and Indochina', in MacLeod and Lewis, *Disease, Medicine and Empire*: 103–17 at p. 106.

8 C. M. McCorkle and E. Mathias-Mundy, 'Ethnoveterinary medicine in Africa', *Africa*, 62 (1992): 59–93, quoting others.

9 The trope used to discuss this in the colonial literature is another apocryphal story

in which an African herd owner 'explains' to a colonial interlocutor that cattle, like banknotes, are worth the same whatever their physical condition. In fact few, if any, herd owners thought this way, as one Narok District Commissioner discovered to his cost in the 1940s, but the story, like the encounter between elders and expert, dramatises and simultaneously trivialises difference. Versions of both the banknote story and the death of DC Grant can be found in N. Farson, *Last Chance in Africa* (London: Gollancz, 1949). Stock owners who were persuaded to adopt a more 'progressive' view were differently and appropriately presented – see, e.g., photographs of 'The Rev. Daudi Mokinyo ... on his ranch'; and 'A better farmer's wife offers salt to her better cow ...' in E. Huxley, *A New Earth* (London: Chatto & Windus, 1960).

10 Marcovich, 'French colonial medicine'; Gelfand, *Man against Tsetse.*

11 M. Worboys, 'Manson, Ross and colonial medical policy: tropical medicine in London and Liverpool, 1899–1914', in MacLeod and Lewis, *Disease, Medicine and Empire*: 21–37; J. M. MacKenzie, 'Experts and amateurs: tsetse, Nagana and sleeping sickness in East and Central Africa', in MacKenzie, *Imperialism and the Natural World*: 187–212.

12 See, for example, M. Worboys, 'Germ theories of disease and British veterinary medicine, 1860–90', *Medical History* 35 (1991): 308–27; P. F. Cranefield, *Science and Empire: East Coast Fever in Rhodesia and the Transvaal* (Cambridge University Press, 1991).

13 Differences sharply summarised in: 'Masai Question', memo. by Cameron, 11 June 1926, encl. in Dundas to Amery, 1 July 1926, Public Record Office (PRO) CO 691/86/6202; Evidence of H. Brassey-Edwards (Chief Veterinary Officer, Kenya), 31 May and 28 March 1933, and 'Some Aspects of the Veterinary Situation in Kenya, affecting Cattle Trade and Livestock Movement', memo. by McCall (Chief Veterinary Officer, Tanganyika), n.d., printed in Kenya Land Commission (KLC), Evidence and Memoranda, 3 vols. London: HMSO, 1934: 3103–13, 3168–74.

14 The dispute over the direction and focus of veterinary activity in Kenya came to a head in the early 1920s in the conflict between the new Director of Agriculture, Holm, and Montgomery, formerly the Veterinary Pathologist, over the acceptance and implementation of the recommendations of the 1920 Veterinary Conference which advocated increased intervention and investment in African pastoral areas. The 'isolationists', backed by settler opinion, won, despite the fact that Montgomery had the support of the Chief Veterinary Officer and the Chief Native Commissioner and the confidence of the Colonial Office in London. Although a separate budget for African areas was finally agreed, no major development initiatives were undertaken, and in 1930 Montgomery, by then Colonial Office Veterinary Adviser, voiced the general disquiet in London about the lack of pastoral development in Kenya, claiming that the disease situation in the African reserves was as bad if not worse than it had been twenty years earlier. See I. R. G. Spencer, 'Pastoralism and colonial policy in Kenya', in R. I. Rotberg (ed.), *Imperialism, Colonialism and Hunger* (Lexington: Lexington Books, 1983); memo. by R. E. Montgomery, n.d. (1917), in Economic Commission, *Evidence* (Nairobi, 1919): 210–17; report and memo. by Stordy, November 1919, encl. in Amery to Smith, 9 December 1919, Malawi National Archives (MNA) S1/46/20; *Report of a Conference of the Veterinary Departments of Kenya Colony, Uganda Protectorate and Tanganyika Territory – Summary* (Nairobi, 1920; Montgomery minute on Grigg to Passfield, 15 September 1930, Passfield to Byrne, 9 July 1931, in CO 533/403/7.

15 Among other issues were severe budgetary constraints on research and concern about professional status. Despite persistent demands for autonomy, and the recommendations of the Lovatt Committee, set up in 1927 to consider the upgrading of colonial veterinary services, the Veterinary Service in Kenya remained a subdepartment under the overall control of the Director of Agriculture until 1937. See Agricultural Department Annual Report, 1920/21; Grigg to Passfield, 25 February 1930, Director of Agriculture to Colonial Secretary, 22 October 1929, memo. by Kenya Veterinary Medical Association, n.d., and minutes on file, all in CO 533/391/3; note by Stockdale (Colonial Office Agricultural Adviser), 9 June 1931, in file 16259/30, CO 533/401/12. The Chief Veterinary Research Officer, Daubney, a man with a background in laboratory research, then became the first director (and from 1939 also director of the long-awaited East African Veterinary Research Institute) in succession to the long-serving Chief Veterinary Officer, Brassey-Edwards, whose earlier career, like that of his predecessors, had been spent as a veterinary officer in the field (see Parkinson minute, 26 June 1929, on file 15724/29, CO 533 389/2, and Daubney biography in D. W. Throup, *Economic and Social Origins of Mau Mau* (London: James Currey, 1987): 265–6). For financial constraints see, e.g., Stockdale note above and papers in file 17124/31: Kabete Laboratory, CO 533/406/15. Autonomy for the Veterinary Department eventually brought increased research and development funding and a significant shift in government perceptions of the service and its role. Greater specialisation and professionalisation are also evident in the *East African Agricultural Journal*, which reappeared in 1935, after a lapse of more than twenty years, as a journal of scientific record with serious veterinary coverage.

16 R. D. Waller, 'Uneconomic growth: the Maasai stock economy, 1919–29', unpublished conference paper, Cambridge, 1975; R. Tignor, *The Colonial Transformation of Kenya* (Princeton University Press, 1976); Spencer, 'Pastoralism and colonial policy in Kenya'.

17 B. Berman, *Control and Crisis in Colonial Kenya* (London: James Currey, 1990).

18 See, e.g., correspondance cited in note 15 above and in file 15724/29: Appointment of Chief Veterinary Officer, Kenya, CO 533/389/2 (Brassey-Edwards's promotion was opposed in Kenya on the grounds of his insensitivity to settler concerns) and the Leroki case (fn. 44 below). See also MacKenzie, 'Experts and amateurs'. The relationship changed with the 'second colonial invasion' (of the technocrats) after the Second World War. See D. A. Low and J. M. Lonsdale, 'Introduction: towards the new order, 1945–63', *History of East Africa* III (Oxford: Clarendon, 1976): 12–14.

19 In the colonial literature, sceptical or negative African responses to Western medicine are often caricatured as foolish, ignorant and even comic, or are presented as one side of a contest between 'superstition' and 'science'. See M. Vaughan, *Curing their Ills* (Cambridge: Polity Press, 1991; Stanford University Press, 1991). While such stereotypes may be seen as part of a larger contemporary attempt to subordinate or suppress local systems of knowledge, even as extensive and recent a study of the impact of colonial medicine as Lyons's (see note 20 below) has curiously little to say about the indigenous social and intellectual context of healing. Moreover, as Pool has indicated, attempts to achieve a more 'emic' perspective have often involved the reinterpretation of local discourse within the more familiar categories of Western biomedicine, which in turn has led to a reductionist convergence between Western and indigenous medical systems. See R. Pool, 'On the creation and dissolution of ethnomedical systems in the medical ethnography of Africa', *Africa* 64 (1994): 1–19. Study of the incorporation of symbols of Western medicine in other discourses of power, including dance, witchcraft eradication and popular protest, may, however, open some promising avenues of research.

20 A. Beck, 'Medicine and society in Tanganyika, 1890–1930: a historical enquiry', *Trans. of the American Philosophical Society* 67 (3 1977); M. Lyons, *A Colonial Disease: a Social History of Sleeping Sickness in Northern Zaire, 1900–40* (Cambridge University Press, 1992).

21 Ford, *The Role of Trypanosomiasis in African Ecology* (Oxford University Press, 1971).

22 D. R. Headrick, *Tools of Empire: Technology and European Imperialism in the Nineteenth Century* (New York: Oxford University Press, 1981).

23 S. Sandford, *Management of Pastoral Development in the Third World* (Chichester: Wiley, 1983); C. Kerven, *Customary Commerce* (London: Overseas Development Institute, 1992); P. L. Raikes, *Livestock Policy and Development in East Africa* (Uppsala: Scandinavian Institute of African Studies, 1981).

24 P. Mosley, *The Settler Economies: Studies in the Economic History of Kenya and Southern Rhodesia, 1900–63* (Cambridge University Press, 1983).

25 Raikes, *Livestock Policy*; Sandford, *Management of Pastoral Development*.

26 Especially by J. L. Giblin. See his 'East Coast Fever in socio-historical context: a case study from Tanzania', *International Journal of African Historical Studies* 23 (1990): 401–21; 'Trypanosomiasis control in African history: an evaded issue?', *Journal of African History* 31 (1990): 59–80: *The Politics of Environmental Control in North-eastern Tanzania* (Philadelphia, Pa.: University of Pennsylvania Press, 1992).

27 R. M. A. Van Zwanenberg, with A. King, *An Economic History of Kenya and Uganda, 1800–1970* (London: Macmillan, 1975); G. Kitching, *Class and Economic Change in Kenya* (New Haven, Conn.: Yale University Press, 1980); Kerven, *Customary Commerce*.

28 There is no equivalent in veterinary history as yet for, e.g., Vaughan's studies of the politics and poetics of colonial health policies or for the work on indigenous therapeutic systems. See Vaughan, *Curing their Ills*; S. Feierman, 'Struggles for control: the social roots of health and healing in modern Africa', *African Studies Review* 28 (1985): 73–147; S. Feierman and J. Janzen (eds), *The Social Base of Health and Healing in Africa* (Berkeley, Cal.: University of California Press, 1992). Studies by Peires and Ranger, e.g., are partial exceptions, but they deal with the prophetic apprehension of medical and veterinary catastrophe rather than with more mundane therapeutic practice. See J. B. Peires, *The Dead will Arise* (Johannesburg: Ravan Press, 1989); T. Ranger, 'Plagues of Beasts and Men: Prophetic Responses to Epidemic in Eastern and Southern Africa', in T. Ranger and P. Slack (eds) *Epidemics and Ideas* (Cambridge University Press, 1992): 241–68. The growing literature on what has been called 'veterinary anthropology' (McCorkle and Mathias Mundy, 'Ethnoveterinary medicine in Africa'), while giving African herd owners status and a voice, is still written from within the paradigm of Western medical science, even in the way in which it defines a specific field of indigenous medical systems. See Pool, 'On the creation and dissolution of ethnomedical systems'. It also lacks historical depth and specificity and avoids analysing the issue of power in the constitution of knowledge.

29 General descriptions of these diseases and their aetiologies are to be found in R. T. B. Hall, *Diseases and Parasites of Livestock in the Tropics* (London: Longman, 1997); D. J. Pratt and M. D. Gwynne (eds), *Rangeland Management and Ecology in East Africa* (London: Hodder & Stoughton, 1977); G. M. Mugera (ed.), *Diseases of Cattle in Tropical Africa* (Nairobi: Kenya Literature Bureau, 1979); R. Norval, B. Perry and A. Young, *The Epidemiology of Theileriosis in Africa* (London: Academic Press, 1992); Ford, *The Role of Trypanosomiasis*. The authors are also grateful to Philip Wheatley for compiling a much more detailed reference bibliography.

30 In 1911 it was confirmed, despite its different epidemiology, as being the same disease that was raging in epidemic form in southern Africa. See P. F. Cranefield, *Science and Empire: East Coast Fever in Rhodesia and the Transvaal* (Cambridge University Press, 1991); R. D. Waller, 'The lords of East Africa: the Maasai in the mid nineteenth century (*c.*1840–80)', Ph.D. thesis, Cambridge, 1979; Norval, Perry and Young, *The Epidemiology of Theileriosis*.

31 Giblin, 'East Coast Fever'.

32 Over 200 miles of fencing, paid for by government funds, had already been erected in Kenya before 1914 in an attempt to control ECF, but the passing of a Cattle Cleansing Ordinance to make dipping compulsory had to wait until after the First World War. However, despite re-enactments, neither dipping nor fencing rules were enforced until the 1940s because white farmers could not meet the cost – correspondence and memos. encl. in Sadler to Elgin, 26 October 1907 and 8 September 1908, CO 533/32 and /47; Grigg to Passfield, 23 January and 14 February 1930, CO 533/396/10 and /397/5; Byrne to Passfield, 10 June 1931, CO 533/396/10; Agricultural Department *Annual Reports*, 1909/10, 1920/21, 1929–30, 1950; M. I. Keating, 'Tick control by chemical ixodicides in Kenya: a review, 1912 to 1981', *Tropical Animal Health and Production* 15 (1983): 1–6.

33 Norval, Perry and Young, *Epidemiology of Theileriosis*.

34 R. D. Waller, 'Interaction and identity on the periphery: the trans-Mara Maasai', *International Journal of African Historical Studies* 17 (1984): 243–84. See also E. A.

Lewis, *Investigations into the Tick Problem in the Masai Reserve* (Nairobi: Department of Agriculture, 1934). A total of three dips had been provided for the Maasai, two of which were near Nairobi, after the establishment of the reserve in 1913, but, not surprisingly, they were avoided – Masai Province, *Annual Report*, 1920/21, Kenya National Archives (KNA) PC/SP 1/2/2. A dipping scheme and the establishment of a branch veterinary laboratory were also proposed, but the idea disappeared with the spending cuts of the early 1920s.

35 Raikes, *Livestock Policy*; D. P. Kariuki, 'Current state of theileriosis in Kenya, 1989', in A. Young, J. Mutugi and A. Maritim (eds) *Progress towards the Control of East Coast Fever (Theileriosis) in Kenya* (Nairobi: Kenya Agricultural Research Institute, 1990): 17–26.

36 C. F. M. Swynnerton, 'The tsetse flies of East Africa', *Trans. Royal Entomological Society of London* 84 (1936); Ford, *The Role of Trypanosomiasis*; Lyons, *A Colonial Disease*; MacKenzie, 'Experts and amateurs'.

37 Professional correspondence cited in Cranefield, *Science and Empire*, Lyons, *A Colonial Disease*, and the official papers dealing with Swynnerton's rapidly escalating projects in Tanganyika make the connections between project funding and professional status very clear. See encl. in Scott to Thomas, 30 September 1924, CO 691/72. See also Ford, *The Role of Trypanosomiasis*.

38 R. D. Waller, 'Tsetse fly in western Narok, Kenya', *Journal of African History* 31 (1990): 81–101; R. Lamprey and R. D. Waller, 'The Loita-Mara region in historical times: patterns of subsistence, settlement and ecological change', in P. Robertshaw (ed.), *Early Pastoralists of South-western Kenya* (Nairobi: British Institute in Eastern Africa, 1990): 16–35.

39 Raikes, *Livestock Policy*; H. E. Jahnke, *Tsetse Flies and Livestock Development in East Africa* (Munich: Weltforum Verlag, 1976).

40 British colonial propaganda placed vets beside nutritionists, agronomists, water engineers and other scientific experts in its portrayal of post-war development initiatives in Africa. See, e.g., W. R. Moore, 'Britain tackles the East African bush', *National Geographical Magazine* 97 (1950): 311–52, p. 314 and photographs. As an example of vector as villain, the early Disney cartoon film on malaria shown to village audiences in the Central African Federation in the 1950s can hardly be bettered – copy in MNA. The link between high technology and tsetse continues in, e.g., the use of remote sensing techniques. See D. J. Rogers and S. E. Randolph 'Mortality rates and population density of tsetse flies correlated with satellite imagery', *Nature* 351 (1991): 739–41.

41 R. D. Waller, 'Emutai: crisis and response in Maasailand, 1883–1902', in D. H. Johnson and D. M. Anderson (eds), *The Ecology of Survival* (Boulder, Colo.: Westview Press, 1988): 73–112.

42 In view of its political repercussions the colonial authorities in Kenya, unlike the present government, decided not to apply the most drastic method of CBPP control to African herds, contenting itself with the slaughter of visibly affected animals and preventive quarantines and inoculations in contact cases. See (Kenya) Agricultural Department *Annual Reports*, 1920/21, 1921, 1936; Tignor, *The Colonial Transformation*.

43 The 'gastro-enteritis' from which Maasai stock on Laikipia were reportedly suffering before the Move of 1912 may have been one such milder strain, as the Maasai themselves believed. See Laikipia District, *Annual Report*, 1910/11, KNA:DC/LKA 1/1.

44 A striking case concerns the attempted removal of the Maa-speaking Samburu from the Leroki plateau in the 1920s to make way for an extension of white ranching from Laikipia partly on the grounds that CBPP and rinderpest might spread uncontrollably from African herds to the European-settled areas. See Spencer, 'Pastoralism and colonial policy in Kenya'; G. Simpson, 'Land and Murder in Colonial Kenya: the Leroghi Land Dispute and the Powys Murder Case', unpublished paper, 1995.

45 Sandford, *Management of Pastoral Development*; Tignor, *The Colonial Transformation*.

46 CBPP vaccination remains problematic in its duration and effectiveness, and quarantine is still evaded by stock owners who fear slaughter without compensation. See R. J. Sweet, *A Development Plan for the Pastoral Sector of Isiolo District* (Isiolo Livestock Development Project document, Kenya Government Arid and Semi-arid Lands Project, 1991); Mugera, *Diseases of Cattle*.

47 'Bringing practical education to the people', *East African Standard*, 27 August 1926; A. G. Doherty, *Veterinary Education of Natives* (Nairobi: Agricultural Department, 1929); Agricultural Department *Annual Reports*, 1924, 1927; Masai Province, *Annual Reports*, 1928, 1929, 1937, PC/SP 1/2/2; *Report of the Agriculture Commission* (Nairobi, 1929): 32; correspondence in file KNA:DC/Ngong 1/17/3: Ngong Veterinary Training Centre; Tignor, *The Colonial Transformation*. Although some Maasai took advantage of the opportunity of vocational training and subsequently found employment as vet scouts or as stockmen on settler farms, few seem to have put what they learned into practice in the cattle camps – where the distance between pastoral reality and veterinary theory was at its greatest.

48 G. Dahl and A. Hjort, *Having Herds* (Stockholm, University of Stockholm, Department of Social Anthropology, 1976); Waller, 'The lords of East Africa'.

49 For disruptions see complaints about the inter-territorial border in Masai Province, *Annual Reports*, 1921, 1925, 1927, PC/SP 1/2/1. For the grand strategy of containment see, e.g., East African Governors' Conference, *Conference on Rinderpest: Report* (Nairobi, 1938) and *id.*, *Report of Proceedings of the Second Conference on Rinderpest* (Nairobi, 1939).

50 M. Merker, *Die Masai* (Berlin: Reimer, 1910): 179. There is little indication, *pace* Ranger ('Plagues of beasts and men'), that Maasai prophecies and traditions about the coming of rinderpest saw the epizootic as a punishment or judgement or as a physical sign of moral collapse; or that their responses were couched in terms of social renewal. Indeed, contemporary accounts, though awe-inspired, are highly pragmatic, more concerned with the social and economic effects of loss than with moral causes. See Waller, 'Emutai'. Descriptions of the first Maasai encounters with CBPP convey an intention to investigate and observe the new phenomenon as much as a sense of powerlessness and despair. See J. Thompson, *Through Masailand* (London: Sampson Low, 1885): 204–10. The possibility arises that a moral dimension has been supplied by outsiders.

51 Merker, *Die Masai*.

52 MCF is not, in fact, transmitted through contact with wildebeeste placenta but via droplet infection from newborn wildebeeste calves, which can develop a mild form of the disease at birth. After calving, the wildebeeste herds migrate and the calves recover. Maasai belief and action, based on the observation of apparent causal effect, nonetheless achieves the object of removing susceptible cattle from a source of infection. See Mugera, *Diseases of Cattle*; K. Homewood and W. A. Rodgers, *Maasailand Ecology: Pastoral Development and Wildlife Conservation in Ngorongoro, Tanzania* (Cambridge University Press, 1991).

53 This does not, however, preclude the 'pluralistic' use of protective and curative charms and medicines, especially when other means have failed.

54 The difference emerges clearly if a comparison is drawn between Merker's account of Maasai stock diseases, which was gathered from informants around the turn of the century and was evidently arranged according to their descriptive system, and modern veterinary handbooks for East Africa, which are arranged according to very different taxonomic principles. See Merker, *Die Masai*; Mugera, *Diseases of Cattle*.

55 In one example of miscommunication Trans-Mara Maasai witnesses to the Kenya Land Commission asserted that the fly had expanded its range, brought by elephants which had increased owing to the disappearance of 'Dorobo' hunters. The observation was ignored as fanciful but Maasai were aware that hunters alter the bush habitat by their use of fire and also kill bushbuck and pig, among the tsetse's favourite hosts (KLC, 1934: 1203; Lamprey and Waller, 'The Loita–Mara region in historical times'). Giblin gives another example of a differently constructed sequence of causation among the Parakuyu Maasai. See his *The Politics of Environmental Control*,

p. 174. In this context it is worth noting the survival of 'magico-religious' as a residual descriptive category in the modern technical literature. In a survey of 'magic, religion and ethnoveterinary medicine', for example, McCorkle and Mathias-Mundy urge researchers to take 'the supernatural' seriously for 'diplomatic' reasons, though the authors also acknowledge the possibility that apparent evocations of the supernatural may, in fact, 'embody practical veterinary and management acumen'. (See their 'Ethnoveterinary medicine in Africa' 135–7; but contrast Pool, 'On the creation and dissolution of ethnomedical systems': 16–17).

56 For the evolution of veterinary attitudes, compare memos by Brassey-Edwards and Mulligan and Troughton, printed in KLC, 1934: 3114–18, 3138–41, with *The Improvement of the Native Cattle of Kenya*, Kabete: Veterinary Department, 1948.

57 Basic material for this and the following paragraph is taken from Masai Provincial and District Annual Reports, and from Agricultural and later Veterinary Department Reports.

58 They were able to do this partly because they and their herds were on the periphery of the colonial state. Stock owners closer to the centres of development had far less choice. See Throup, *Economic and Social Origins of Mau Mau.*

59 G. R. Sandford, *An Administrative and Political History of the Masai Reserve* (London: Waterlow, 1919); W. McG. Ross, *Kenya from Within: a Short Political History* (London: Allen & Unwin, 1927). Maasai had always circulated breeding stock through raiding and trading. Obtaining grade cattle from farms was an extension of this, since the stock concerned were usually Boran crosses, with which Maasai were familiar. However, concern about the viability of exotic stock was still being expressed by elders in the 1980s. The first imported government stud bull in Maasai land died, appropriately, of rinderpest – and perhaps loneliness. See Masai Province, *Annual Report*, 1917/18, PC/SP 1/2/2.

60 In the case of CBPP a form of variolation was sometimes used, analogous to a similar technique for smallpox, in which matter taken from a diseased animal was rubbed or bound into an incision made in the nose or tail of a healthy animal (Merker, *Die Masai*: 170). This procedure, however, seemed visually and conceptually quite different from colonial immunisation, which involved several injections of live vaccine brought in from outside, often with fatal results (Mugera, *Diseases of Cattle*).

61 The first rinderpest immunisation, for example, was by 'double inoculation', described later as 'costly, clumsy, heart-breaking and dangerous'. It involved injecting the pathogen and then the antibody in turn, simultaneously inducing and curing the disease and leaving the animal, if it survived, with lifelong immunity, but the reaction could be severe. Later, inactive and attenuated virus preparations were developed, culminating in the Kabete Attenuated Goat (KAG) vaccine of the 1940s. See *Conference on Rinderpest: Report*: 3–4; 'Notes on Animal Diseases', IV (rinderpest) and XV (CBPP), *East African Agricultural Jnl* 5 (1939/40) and 8 (1942/43); Tignor, *The Colonial Transformation.*

62 R. D. Waller, 'Re-making Maasailand: pastoral land and land use after the Maasai moves, 1914–1950', unpublished paper, 1994.

63 See Sandford, *An Administrative and Political History of the Maasai Reserve*, p. 111, for typical comments on Maasai as 'lazy and listless' stock owners. Twenty-five years later, sentiments were similar though touched by a spirit of optimism – e.g. Masai Province, *Annual Report*, 1945, PC/SP/1/2/3.

64 K. Homewood, 'Development and the ecology of Maasai food and nutrition', *Ecology of Food and Nutrition* 29 (1992): 61–81; K. Homewood, 'Development, demarcation and ecological outcomes in Maasailand', *Africa* 65 (1995): 331–50.

65 Waller, 'Emutai'.

66 Waller, 'Re-making Maasailand'.

67 Ross, *Kenya from Within*; M. P. K. Sorrenson, *The Origins of European Settlement in Kenya* (Nairobi: Oxford University Press, 1968). 'Nakuruitis' provides a particularly illustrative case. This 'disease' was diagnosed among settler herds in the Lake Nakuru area. It required a full-scale investigation sponsored by a special sub-com-

mittee of the government Committee of Civil Research in London before it was established that the 'disease' was caused by mineral, especially cobalt, deficiency in the pasture, and that cattle could not graze there for long periods without supplements – something Maasai herd owners had always known and had tried to convey to sympathetic white listeners. See CO 533/376/13.

68 Waller, 'The lords of East Africa'; *id.*, 'Tsetse fly in western Narok'. According to Merker (*Die Masai*: 179–80), Maasai believed that mosquitoes injected poison with their bite which then caused fever. He was careful to note that his information about malaria dated from the mid 1890s, at a time when German colonial doctors in the territory were still uncertain about its transmission and control. See Beck, 'Medicine and society': 14–15. Maasai may not, however, have initially made the connection between ticks and ECF. Merker's list correctly names and indicates the disease (*ol tigana*) but links it to the eating of a poisonous plant. However, it is clear from elsewhere in his account that Maasai in the 1900s knew that tick bites could cause disease (relapsing fever) in humans.

69 T. Potkanski, *Property Concepts, Herding Patterns and Management of Natural Resources among the Ngorongoro and Salei Maasai of Tanzania* (London: IIED, 1994).

70 K. Homewood and W. A. Rodgers, *Maasailand Ecology: Pastoral Development and Wildlife Conservation in Ngorongoro, Tanzania* (Cambridge University Press, 1991); Homewood, 'Development and the ecology of Maasai food and nutrition'; *id.*, 'Development, demarcation and ecological outcomes in Maasailand'.

71 Waller, 'The lords of East Africa'; Waller, 'Tsetse fly in western Narok'; J. L. Giblin, 'East Coast Fever'; *id.*, *The Politics of Environmental Control.*

72 'Conservationism' may now be a serious threat to pastoralism. This sentimental creed is a particularly worrying example of the current Western 'primitivism'; which seeks to appropriate what is left of other cultures and to shape them in its own image. See N. Thomas, *Colonialism's Culture* (Cambridge: Polity Press, 1994; Princeton University Press, 1994); Spear and Waller, *Being Maasai.* Activists are making determined attempts to recreate an idealised or mythical pre-colonial Eden by pressing governments to drive pastoralists off their land in order to 'restore' ecological harmony (and, incidentally, to provide a playground for capital). Their arguments against pastoral land use are an odd, and reductionist, mixture of old colonial ideas of conservation and echoes of the historical arguments of 'Merrie Africa[nists]' like Kjekshus who have popularised the misleading notion that colonial capitalism was, in itself, an ecological catastrophe. See H. Kjekshus, *Ecology Control and Economic Development in East Africa* (London: Heinemann, 1977). Whereas we subject Western scientific paradigms to critical scrutiny, we accept that veterinary medicine has brought benefits as well as problems, and we do not subscribe to a construction of 'Nature' so fundamentally at odds with the one we are describing. Indeed, we note a strange similarity in the encounters between elders and both experts and conservationists. Totalising and essentialist statements about pastoralists come very close in sentiment to earlier notions of 'contagious' and 'ignorant' natives. See J. Knowles and D. Collett, 'Nature as myth, symbol and action: notes towards a historical understanding of development and conservation in Kenyan Maasailand', *Africa* 59 (1989): 433–60; D. Brockington and K. Homewood 'Received wisdom, science and pastoralists', in M. Leach and R. Mearns (eds), *The Lie of the Land: Challenging Received Wisdom in African Environmental Change and Policy* (London: James Currey, 1995).

73 When ticks feed on a resistant animal with circulating antibodies they lose their capacity to infect.

74 M. Birley, 'Resource management in Sukumaland, Tanzania', *Africa* 52 (1982): 1–30; R. W. Sutherst, 'Ectoparasites and herbivore nutrition', in J. B. Hacker and J. H. Ternouth (eds), *The Nutrition of Herbivores* (Sydney: Academic Press, 1987).

75 K. Arhem, *Pastoral Man and the Garden of Eden* (Uppsala: Scandinavian Institute of African Studies, 1985); R. Bell, 'Conservation with a human face: conflict and reconciliation in African land use planning', in D. Anderson and R. Grove (eds), *Con-*

servation in Africa (Cambridge University Press, 1987): 79–101; E. Fratkin, *Surviving Drought and Development: Ariaal Pastoralists of Northern Kenya* (Boulder, Colo.: Westview Press, 1991).

76 The sentiments expressed in the majority opinion of the East Africa Commission of 1925 and those reported for the Ngorongoro Crater wildlife conservation debate fifty years later are remarkably similar in their opposition to the 'wastefulness' and 'destructiveness' of pastoral land use, despite the difference in time and context. See *Report of the East Africa Commission*, April 1925, Cmd 2387; Homewood and Rodgers, *Maasailand Ecology*.

77 However, after he became Director of Tsetse Research, Hornby appears to have moved over to the majority opinion. See *Interim Report of a Committee appointed to Advise as to ... the Problem of Overstocking ...*, Nairobi, 1941; H. E. Hornby, 'Overstocking in Tanganyika Territory', *East African Agricultural Journal* 1 (1935/36): 355–66; D. M. Anderson, 'Depression, dust bowl, demography and drought: the colonial state and soil conservation in East Africa during the 1930s', *African Affairs* 83 (1984): 321–45.

78 For example, Norval, Perry and Young, *The Epidemiology of Theileriosis*: 307, 335.

79 The importance of naturally acquired immunities had been recognised since the 1920s but not seriously pursued.

80 Kariuki, 'Current state of theileriosis'.

81 Raikes, *Livestock Policy and Development*.

82 'Expert' status is still conferred by Western academies, even if located in Nairobi or Addis Ababa. Moreover, the international pharmaceutical industry itself has a powerful vested interest in the maintenance of the scientific *status quo*. See B. Williams, C. Campbell and R. Williams, 'Broken houses: science and development in the African savanna', *Agriculture and Human Values*, 1995, in press.

83 H. Hedlund, 'Contradictions in the peripheralisation of a pastoral society: the Maasai', *Review of African Political Economy* 15/16 (1979): 15–34; D. J. Campbell, 'Land as ours, land as mine: economic, political and ecological marginalisation in Kajiado District', in T. Spear and R. D. Waller (eds), *Being Maasai* (London: James Currey, 1993): 258–72.

CHAPTER FOUR

Dances with doctors: Navajo encounters with the Indian Health Service

Stephen J. Kunitz and Jerrold E. Levy

The recent experience of American Indians with European medicine differs from that of many other non-European peoples because Indians are a submerged minority, having been engulfed demographically by waves of European immigrants. Unlike the indigenous peoples of many other temperate regions who were similarly engulfed, however, increasingly in this century Indians in the western United States have been the recipients of free health services provided by the federal government. Unlike the native peoples of Australia, Canada and New Zealand, for instance, who simply by virtue of their rights as citizens are the beneficiaries of national health care schemes, American Indians are the beneficiaries of a health care system which is devoted solely to their care and provides them with a full range of public and personal services, particularly if they reside on reservations as members of federally recognised tribes. This makes their situation unique among native peoples, and unique among minority groups in the United States as well.[1]

In this chapter we first describe the development of this system over the course of most of the present century. We sketch briefly the evolution of federal policy with respect to Indian health services. The point we should like to make is that, as in other areas of Indian policy, there has been continuous debate between assimilationists and pluralists over what should be the government's stance with respect to Indians. Increasingly in recent decades Indians have been participants in the debate, but for the most part at the national level of policymaking Indians have been the subjects of policy, not the creators. It is primarily at the regional and local level that Indian responses and influence are felt, but it is federal policy that creates the context for the regional and local exercise of such influence.

Thus in the second part of the chapter we consider in detail the changing relationship between Indian people and providers of care at the individual and tribal level, paying particular attention to the experience of Navajo Indians, the largest American Indian tribe, numbering over 200,000 people living on a reservation of 24,000 square miles.

I. Federal health services for Indians

Federal appropriations

A useful way to get a broad overview of the expansion of the growth of services is to consider the pattern of federal appropriations for Indian health services over the course of the twentieth century.[2] In Figure 4.1 we have displayed the appropriations in current and constant (1993) dollars for each year from 1911 to 1993. The level of appropriations for Indian health services was very low for the first several decades of this century, in 1911 $40,000. Substantial increases were first made in the late 1920s, but the period of real growth began shortly after World War Two, when appropriations increased at a faster rate than did federal outlays in general.[3] The rate of increase remained higher until the late 1970s, when it slowed to the rate for all federal outlays, where it has remained.

In constant dollars the amount of money *per capita* for Indian beneficiaries has increased substantially since World War Two, as Table 4.1 indicates, although it is still lower than the amount spent on the health care of other citizens. The most dramatic increases occurred between the mid 1950s and mid 1970s, after which the rate slowed. This was the result of several years of high inflation in the late 1970s. Real growth resumed in the early 1980s, but at a slower rate than in previous periods.

Federal recognition

The data apply only to members of federally recognised tribes, most of which are found in the western United States, where conquest came later than in the east, and where treaties were made with Congress, not with the original thirteen colonies. Many of the treaties signed by Indian tribes included a commitment on the part of Congress to provide health care as well as education, agricultural implements, and other goods and services,[4] but many other treaties, such as the Navajos' treaty in 1868, contained no such provision. The provision of health care does not derive only from treaty rights, however, but also from the federal government's role as trustee.[5] Thus members of federally recognised tribes receive health benefits whether such benefits are mentioned in their treaty or not, and whether they live on a treaty

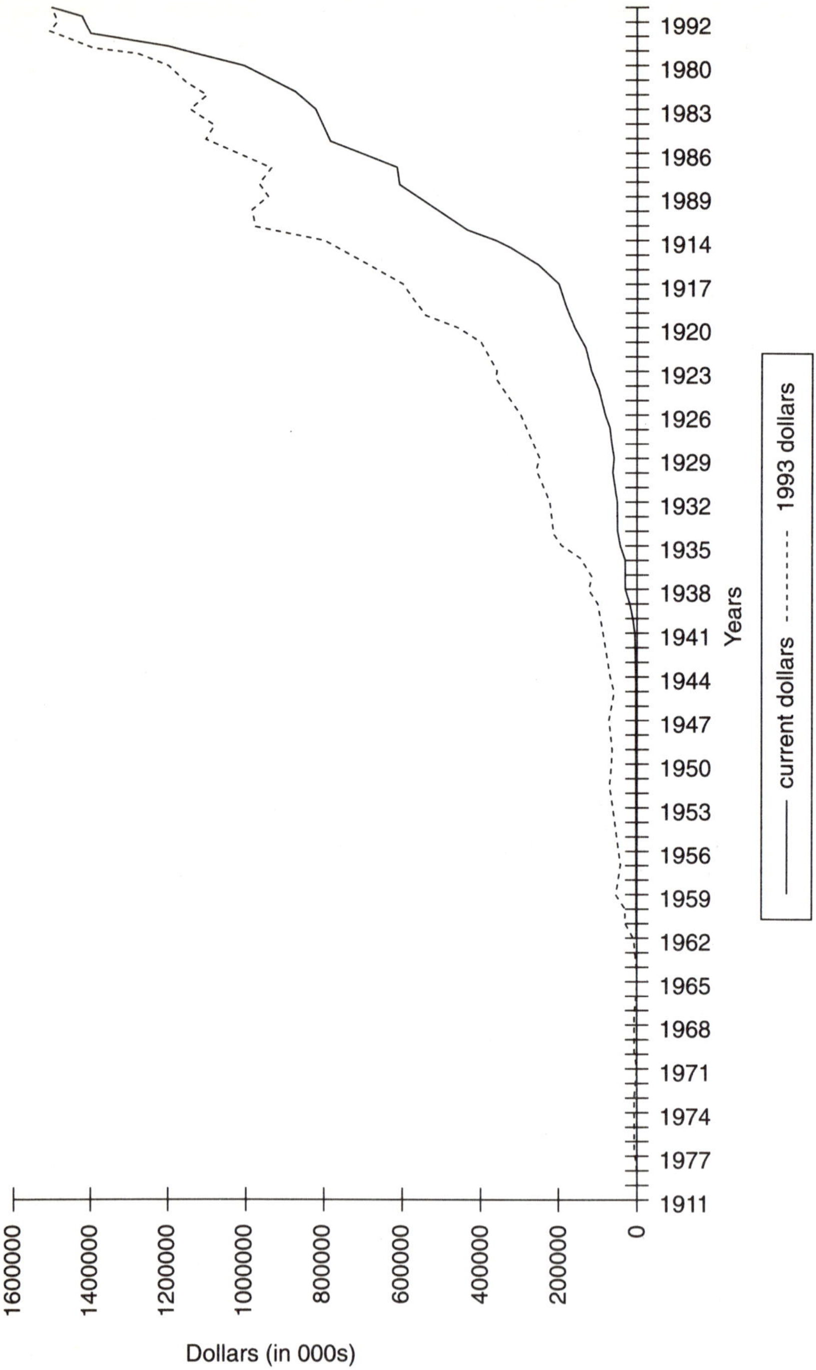

Figure 4.1 Annual appropriations for Indian health services

or executive order reservation, or, since the passage of legislation in the mid 1970s, whether they live on a reservation at all.

Table 4.1 *Per capita appropriations for Indian health services, 1955–92*

Year	*Per capita appropriations (1993 $)*[a]	*Average annual rate of change (%)*
1995[b]	396	
		6·4
1965[c]	755	
		3·5
1975[d]	1,080	
		0·3
1985[e]	1,115	
		1·8
1992[e]	1,270	

Sources

[a] Division of Resource Management (Finance), Indian Health Service, Rockville, Md.

[b] *Health Service for American Indians*, Public Health Service Publication No. 531, US Department of Health, Education and Welfare, Public Health Service, Office of Surgeon General, Division of Public Health Methods, Washington, D.C.: US Government Printing Office.

[c] *Indian Health Highlights*, US Department of Health, Education and Welfare, Public Health Service, Bureau of Medical Services, Division of Indian Health, Office of Program Planning and Evaluation, Rockville, Md, June 1966.

[d] *Selected Vital Statistics for Indian Health Service Areas and Service Units, 1972 to 1977*, DHEW Publication No. (HSA) 79–1005, US Department of Health, Education and Welfare, Public Health Service, Health Services Administration, Indian Health Service, Division of Resource Coordination, Office of Program Statistics, Rockville, Md, 1979.

[e] *Trends in Indian Health 1991*, US Department of Health and Human Services, Public Health Service, Indian Health Service, Office of Planning, Evaluation and Legislation, Division of Program Statistics. Rockville, Md, 1991.

Health care of a minimal sort had been provided to Indians by military physicians in the early nineteenth century, when Indian affairs were administered by the War Department. In 1849 the Bureau of Indian Affairs was transferred to the Department of the Interior, and health services of a sort continued to be provided. The health of Indians became of increasing concern to the bureau throughout the latter half of the nineteenth century, prompted in part by a recognition that the number of Indians was declining.[6] Moreover, by the late nineteenth century, policy had shifted and, instead of Indians being treated as separate nations by the federal government, assimilation now became the goal.[7] This could work only if education were provided, and improved health was understood to be an essential ingredient. In fact Indian children sent to boarding schools had extremely high death rates, making the provision of health care in those settings particularly pressing.

The Meriam Report and the New Deal

The first several decades of this century saw the entry of professionals and experts into government at all levels. In Indian affairs the first instance was the so-called Meriam Report,[8] carried out at the request of the Commissioner of Indian Affairs during the Coolidge administration.[9] The report was damning in its assessment of the implementation of Indian policy and recommended the creation of a much more highly professionalised service, not only in medicine and public health but in education, economics, agriculture and administration.

Moreover, once a more highly professional staff had been recruited, Meriam recommended that administration should be decentralised. Because local conditions differed, it was important that agency superintendents should have the flexibility to deal with them directly rather than simply carrying out orders from the central office in Washington. Underlying the report was the assumption that, under the direction of efficient and humane professionals, within three generations Indians would be assimilated into the larger society and the federal government's obligation would be ended.[10]

When the Hoover administration took office in 1928 the new Secretary of the Interior, Ray Lyman Wilbur, and his Commissioners of Indian Affairs acted on the recommendations of the Meriam Report. Among other things, they reorganised 'the bureau into five divisions: health, education, agricultural extension, forestry, and irrigation. Each division had a technical or professional director to insure a more direct relationship between the reservation superintendents and Washington.'[11] Wilbur shared with Meriam the belief that improved administration and services would ultimately lead to Indians' assimilation into American life.[12] Indeed, it was this belief that rationalised increased funding for Indian services, for once Indians had been raised to the same educational and health standards as the rest of the population the government's responsibilities would have been discharged and support could be withdrawn. It is this policy which accounts for the increased appropriations for Indian health services beginning in the late 1920s.

The goal of assimilation was one that was most emphatically

rejected by John Collier, Commissioner of Indian Affairs during the New Deal administration of Franklin D. Roosevelt. He had a long history as a social reformer in New York City and California before becoming involved with Indian issues in the 1920s. His life and career have been the subject of several studies, and only a few points need be made here.[13] First, like his predecessors, he shared the faith of social reformers in value-free research, and it was during his long reign as Commissioner that the Bureau of Indian Affairs supported several major ethnographic studies and field surveys.

Second, also like other reformers, his plans often ran into opposition from parties whose interests were threatened. In Collier's case this included many western politicians and businessmen, many field-level employees of the bureau itself, and some Indian tribes. He was never able to overcome all this opposition, although he won some impressive victories.

Third, although he believed in the importance of community control and decentralisation, he was often authoritarian in practice, notably in the case of the implementation of the Indian Reorganisation Act over the objections of many Indians, and of livestock reduction over the objections of many Indian stockmen. Under his administration there occurred the same growth of government bureaucracies that characterised the New Deal more generally. On the other hand, the kind of professionalisation and decentralisation that had been recommended by the Meriam Report was implemented.[14] Despite the changes, a survey in the mid 1930s found that a high volume of services was being provided to a population suffering from high rates of morbidity by staff who were underpaid, overworked and based in inadequate facilities.[15]

Finally, the coming of World War Two largely eviscerated many of the programmes Collier had developed in the 1930s: road and irrigation system construction, the Indian Civilian Conservation Corps, and attempts to build an adequate health service.[16] Moreover, his advocacy of Indians' control of their land and resources, and of cultural pluralism in opposition to the more widespread notions of assimilation, had continued to antagonise vested interests, who recommended in 1943 that the Bureau of Indian Affairs should be dismantled and its functions distributed to other agencies as a way of freeing Indians from dependence. It was not until the Eisenhower administration in the 1950s that these recommendations were acted on, however.

Thus from the 1920s to the 1940s partially successful attempts were made to professionalise the Bureau of Indian Affairs bureaucracy. Moreover, whether people believed in assimilation or tribal sovereignty, all agreed that improvements in health and education were crucial to Indians' well-being. This continued to be an important point of agreement.[17]

Termination

During the Eisenhower years, with the return of the Republicans to the White House, the forces that had favoured dismantling the Bureau of Indian Affairs and the reservation system emerged with added strength and succeeded in terminating the federal recognition of several tribes. One step toward dismantling the Bureau of Indian Affairs was to remove health care from its jurisdiction. The original plan called for counties and states in which reservations were located to assume responsibility for health care. Local governments resisted, however, arguing that the added financial burden would be too heavy for them to carry. The second option was to transfer the Indian Health Service to the US Public Health Service. This was accomplished in 1955. The arguments in favour of the transfer were similar to those Meriam and Wilbur and other assimilationists had used in the past: that, in order for assimilation to work, health had to be improved, and the only way to do that was to make it the responsibility of a professional, highly skilled and dedicated corps that would be able to recruit health care personnel more successfully than the bureau had, and that would be able to be more successful in obtaining funds from Congress.[18] The organisation that was established was staffed by physicians, nurses, pharmacists, sanitarians and other health professionals, many of whom were commissioned officers in the Public Health Service – along with the army, navy, and air force one of the four uniformed services. It was highly structured bureaucracy with a chain of command stretching from remote field clinics to general hospitals, regional area offices, and headquarters in Washington.[19] It was successful in obtaining an increase in funds, as Figure 4.1 shows. Thus the paradox emerged again: though weakening the Bureau of Indian Affairs bureaucracy the assimilationists had created and begun the process of institutionalising an entirely new bureaucracy that continued to flourish until only recently.

Self-determination

With the return of a Democratic administration in 1960 the policy of termination was halted. Most crucial for our story, the civil rights movement, which originated with African-Americans in cities, had important consequences for Indians on rural reservations. The Kennedy and Johnson administrations created new processes for providing federal money to poor people. Instead of following traditional routes through state and municipal bureaucracies, new community organisations were created which were to receive direct grants, thus buying the allegiance of the dispossessed for the Democrats. Some Indian tribal governments were designated Community Action Program Boards and received funding for programmes such as legal aid and ancillary health services.[20] In addition, the passage of the 'new careers' amendment to the Economic Opportunity Act meant that both the Bureau of Indian Affairs and the Indian Health Service began to hire many more local Indians than they had previously in para-professional positions such as teachers' aides, veterinarians' aides, community health representatives, and mental health and substance abuse workers. Finally, the phrase 'maximum feasible participation' of the poor in the programmes affecting them, which was a crucial part of the Economic Opportunity Act, was interpreted to mean that there should be 'community control' of agencies providing services. The result in the Indian Health Service was that local service units have ultimately achieved a great deal of independence from the area office. The point of all this was several-fold: to reduce unemployment; to create new careers, mainly in human services, for those newly hired; to make agencies more responsive to the demands and needs of their client populations; and, in the cities, to buy peace.

The growing political acceptance of community control, originating in the civil rights movement of the 1960s, was transformed by Republican administrations in the 1970s and 1980s into 'self-determination'. It has often been argued that Democrats favour the creation of a large federal government and that Republicans wish to reduce the federal government and devolve responsibility for various government activities to state and local governments, or have government play no role at all. During the Reagan administration in the 1980s this was called the 'New Federalism', but devolution had begun earlier, under the Nixon and Ford administrations in the late 1960s and early 1970s with passage of the Indian Self-determination and Educational Assistance Act (PL 93-638). The new law created mechanisms whereby tribes could contract with the Secretaries of the Interior and of Health, Education and Welfare to develop new services or assume control over services previously provided by the federal government. These were for the most part health, education and welfare programmes, the management of natural resources remaining under the control of the Department of the Interior.[21]

A year later the Indian Health Care Improvement Act (PL 94-437) was passed. Its purpose was not simply to build new facilities but to create new and needed services and attract more Indians into health-related occupations. Combined with a federal policy of Indian preference in hiring, this has meant increasing employment for Indians not simply in tribal bureaucracies but in the federal bureaucracies serving Indians as well. Moreover, as more Indians were attracted to the health professions through scholarship assistance they have assumed increasingly responsible positions within the two federal agencies.

The 'New Federalism' of the Reagan years was consistent with previous Republican legislation, but funding levels decreased for many programmes. This was true of the support for the Bureau of Indian Affairs, which between 1974 and 1988 first increased over three years and then decreased such that by 1988 the level of funding was only $5 million more than it had been (in 1974 dollars) in 1974: an increase from $411 million to $416 million.[22] Over the same period the Indian Health Service Direct Program outlays increased (in 1974 dollars) from $217 million to $398 million. Moreover, '[B]etween 1976 and 1988, full-time permanent positions in the Bureau of Indian Affairs *declined* by one-third (33.0 percent), while full-time permanent positions in the Indian Health Service *increased* by more than one-third (40.1 percent).'[23]

Whether the bureau's recent history can be said to enhance true self-determination by Indian tribes is a matter of debate.[24] What is important in the present context is that until recently appropriations for health programmes have continued to increase at the same time as Indian education and employment in the health sector have also continued to increase. Funding for Indian health services increased dramatically in the 1970s, although the rate of increase remained virtually constant from the late 1970s and inflation eroded some of the benefits of the increase in current dollars in the late 1970s and early 1980s.[25] Nonetheless, by the early 1990s *per capita* spending was still substantially less than health expenditures for other US citizens.

This brief introduction to the history of Indian policy in general and Indian health care policy in particular is intended to demonstrate that until recently, whether federal policy favoured assimilation on the one hand or tribal sovereignty and cultural pluralism on the other, the end result in respect of funding of services has been continuous increase. Similarly, over the past two or three decades both assimilationists and pluralists have supported the decentralisation of services and responsibilities to area offices and to service units answering to tribal governments and community health boards. In the following section we examine more closely some of these processes on the Navajo Reservation, and in the final section we explore a range of responses on the part of Navajos to these changes.

II. A brief history of the Navajos

The Navajos are Athapaskan-speakers related to the Apaches who seem to have entered the American Southwest near what is now north-western New Mexico some time in the fifteenth and sixteenth centuries. Initially hunters and gatherers, they adopted agriculture and many cultural traits from the Pueblos, with whom they had numerous contacts, especially between 1690 and 1770, when they hosted Pueblo refugees from the Spanish reconquest of the area subsequent to the Pueblo revolt of 1680. After the Spanish had introduced livestock to the region the Navajos increasingly took to pastoral pursuits, until, by 1850, they obtained over half their sustenance from stock raising. Raids by the Ute Indians to the north, increased warfare with the Spaniards and the search for new grazing led them to spread south-west from their original homeland in the San Juan River drainage, and by the nineteenth century they were as far west as the Colorado and Little Colorado rivers in what is now Arizona.[26]

In the first half of the nineteenth century Navajos engaged in raiding for livestock and slaves. Ultimately their depredations became such that troops were sent after them. In 1864, 8,000 gave themselves up and spent the next four years at the Bosque Redondo in eastern New Mexico. It is estimated that perhaps as many as 2,000 Navajos avoided captivity. In 1868 the Navajos returned to a treaty reservation which straddled what is now the New Mexico–Arizona border. Soon they spilled over the boundaries of the original reservation and moved westward to lands they had occupied before their incarceration. Their reservation was expanded by executive order several times over the next sixty years until by the mid 1930s it had attained its present size of about 24,000 square miles.

Upon their return to the reservation Navajos were issued with livestock, food and farm implements and were encouraged by government agents to become self-sufficient. Their stock increased rapidly just at a time when the Southwest was entering an epicycle of erosion. The combination of heavy grazing and altered weather patterns caused sufficient concern about destruction of the range that in the 1930s, during John Collier's reign as Commissioner, livestock reduction was carried out. The story has often been told.[27] Suffice it to say that livestock reduction completely disrupted the traditional stratification and subsistence systems. To partially compensate for this, the Indian Civilian Conservation Corps was used to provide jobs, but it was the coming of World War Two that provided most employment, as many Navajo men entered the armed forces and many other men as well as women went to work in war industries off the reservation. The money they sent back created something of a boom on the reservation, but their return after the cessation of hostilities led to economic collapse.

This was a time when termination had become government policy, but there was no possibility of terminating the Navajo's federal recognition under the conditions then prevailing. The Krug report of 1948 outlined the government's vision of how to deal with the problem.[28] The report estimated that only a little more than half the people currently on the reservation could be supported there. Others would have to move elsewhere: to cities or to reservation land belonging to other tribes along the Colorado river on the Arizona–California border. The recommendations of the report were embodied in the Navajo–Hopi Long Range Rehabilitation Act (PL 81-474). Money was authorised for the construction of schools and health facilities, roads and trails, communication systems and service facilities, domestic water supplies and irrigation systems, industrial and business development, off-reservation relocation, and a revolving loan fund for small businesses. Of the money authorised by the legislation, virtually the full amount was allocated for construction and water projects, and virtually none for industrial and business development or the revolving loan fund. What was created was not an economy capable of being productive and self-supporting but one that was based upon social services (both for income and for jobs) and the extraction of natural resources (coal, oil, uranium and forest products). That has continued to be the pattern right into the present.

A number of manpower studies in the 1960s and 1970s showed that unemployment and underemployment were high, of the order of 50–60 per cent, and that of the people who were employed about two-thirds worked for the service sector or the government, excluding tribal employees who worked for such enterprises as the forest products industry.[29] It was in this context that the War on Poverty of the 1960s and Indian Self-determination and Educational Assistance Act (PL 93-638) and the Indian Health Care Improvement Act (PL 94-437) of the mid 1970s assumed particular significance, for, quite apart from the benefit to the health of the population, they reinforced the pattern of employment in government and service jobs that had come to characterise the reservation economy by 1960. Little has changed since then. The Navajo tribe estimated unemployment (not including underemployment) in 1991 to be 36 per cent. Of employed Navajos, 64 per cent worked in services and government.[30]

The health care system on the Navajo reservation

Like health care on other reservations in the 1920s and 1930s, that provided to Navajos by the Bureau of Indian Affairs was regarded by many observers as sadly deficient. Hospitals were described as 'shabby and derelict' and 'rattle traps', and many of the staff as 'no-account' and 'stupid'.[31] Many were unsympathetic to Navajos, to their health beliefs and practices in particular. One physician wrote of Navajo ceremonialists and healers:

> The real harm caused by these men comes from the perpetuation of superstitions and failure to recognize the limits of their usefulness as healers ... It is my conviction that they are to blame for much crippling and many deaths which could be averted by proper medical care. Time and again they call for physicians when the patients are about to die; the reason for calling a doctor at the last moment is to have an opportunity to shift the blame, or to gain the help of the agency or the local missionary for the burial.[32]

It was partially to counteract attitudes like these among field staff that Collier encouraged what many Bureau employees scoffingly called 'the anthropological approach.' On the Navajo Reservation this resulted in two classic ethnographic monographs, Clyde Kluckhohn and Dorothea Leighton's *The Navaho* and Leighton and Kluckhohn's *Children of the People*. It also resulted in a less well known volume by Alexander and Dorothea Leighton, *The Navaho Door*.[33] This was intended specifically as a guide book for Bureau personnel, particularly those concerned with providing health care. The authors attempted to encourage a more tolerant, even collegial, attitude among staff towards traditional Navajo healers. They also attempted to explain why Navajos were often reluctant to come to hospitals:

> It is well to bear in mind that the Indians' experience with hospitals extends over a period of less than one lifetime. Only recently have they brought in a patient before he was moribund; they commonly hold the opinion that a hospital is a place to go to die. A generation ago this was the view of most people in our culture and it still is the view of many people today.[34]

In fact, until the era of sulphonamides and antibiotics, which began in the late 1930s, the Navajos' view of hospitals as a place to go to die was not at all unreasonable. Moreover, there is some evidence that at least some Navajos drew distinctions between different sorts of doctors. Elinore Gregg, a public health nurse in the Bureau of Indian Affairs in the 1920s and 1930s, reported that on a trip to the Navajo reservation in the 1920s:

> I was interviewed by two old Navahos who had heard by the grapevine that I was coming, and they had ridden one hundred miles from Bluff, Utah, on horseback, to ask 'Washington' to send them a new doctor who 'could cut'. They had only an internist, Dr Gillespie. Their Navaho med-

> icine men could take care of other illnesses, but they had only a piece of glass to cut with, and that was not very successful even with an appendix abscess. They wanted a surgeon, not an internist! ... The Indians knew the difference.[35]

By the 1920s anaesthesia and sterile technique had been developed, and surgery had become the first hospital-based speciality. Non-surgical specialists had not nearly as much to offer patients at the time, and clearly some Navajos even in places as remote as Bluff were well aware of the distinctions. After World War Two, when antibiotics became widely available and as hospital and clinic facilities were improved and the number of staff increased, and as roads were paved and motor vehicles became more common, Navajo utilisation of both in-patient and out-patient services increased dramatically, as it did throughout the Indian Health Service.[36] Navajos have been quite willing to make use of the Euro-American health care system when it has been perceived to be accessible and effective.[37] This is not to say, however, that there have not been conflicts and misunderstandings between patients and providers of care, an issue to which we return in the final part of this chapter.

We have observed that the Indian Health Service has been one of the major employers on the reservation. With Indian preference in hiring, and with more Navajos receiving professional training, the jobs they now occupy are not simply lower-level ones such as aides, licensed practical nurses or maintenance and cafeteria staff. Navajos now occupy many positions at all levels of the bureaucracy, including the Navajo area directorship.

In addition to this indianisation of the federal bureaucracy, the availability of funds for the tribe to contract with the Indian Health Service to manage health programmes of its own has resulted in the growth of a Division of Health within the tribal government, which has the largest budget of any branch or division, $46.4 million in fiscal year 1994, 80 per cent of which comes from federal sources.[38] Much of the money is used for substance abuse prevention and treatment programmes, some of which are subcontracted to other organisations, some of which are run by the Division of Health itself. It is in the area of substance abuse that one sees most clearly the emergence of generically Indian or specifically Navajo treatment modalities within formal programmes. Before describing this process, however, we turn to a discussion of changing Navajo health beliefs and practices.

Navajo health beliefs and practices

Authors describing the ceremonial patterns of the Southwestern culture area have emphasised the contrasts between the shamanistic and individualistic religious practices of hunters and gatherers and the communally-oriented priestly religions of the sedentary Pueblos, despite the fact that both were based upon a common foundation of belief about the nature of supernatural power and the causes of disease.[39]

Throughout the continent disease was thought to be caused by *soul loss, spirit possession, intrusive object, breach of tabu* or *witchcraft*. Curing rituals, whether conducted by priests or shamans, sought to remove the cause of disease rather than the symptoms, which, if the cure was successful, would disappear of their own accord. Disease, caused by supernatural agents, was treated by religious practitioners who controlled supernatural power. Symptoms, by contrast, could be treated by naturalistic methods. Herbal remedies, setting broken bones, massage, heat treatment, and the cauterisation of wounds were administered by various knowledgeable individuals who did not necessarily control supernatural power, and did not preclude the need for a ritual cure.

Traditional Navajo religion is an amalgam of hunter–gatherer and Pueblo agriculturalist traditions directed toward the maintenance of harmonious relationships between men, nature and the supernatural. As illness is a major indicator of disharmony, Navajo ritual is predominantly health-oriented and thus is congruent with the emphasis of hunting societies upon personal religious participation and upon the health and well-being of the individual. There are many references to crops in the rituals, 'but Navajo ceremonialism does not show the intense preoccupation with maize and its life cycle which characterizes the true farming peoples'.[40] Whereas hunting societies tend to seek visionary experiences and have shamans whose powers are received direct from the realm of the supernatural, agricultural societies tend 'to create standardized ritual with an hereditary officiant whose power is not the result of a vision but of memorizing a formula, both in words and behavior.'[41]

The most prestigious figure in the Navajo hierarchy of religious practitioners is the singer (*hatałi*), whose knowledge of a particular ritual is gained over long years of apprenticeship with another practitioner. The singer cures but does not diagnose the illness. Below him is the diviner, or diagnostician. Diagnosis is done by 'listening', 'star gazing' or 'hand trembling'. By far the most common method of diagnosis today is hand trembling, which is practised by both men and women, although, in our experience, women outnumber men. The singer most closely approximates the Pueblo priest; the diagnostician is more like the shaman. Hand trembling is said to be an unsought gift signalled by the involuntary shaking of the right arm. The person so chosen is thought to be possessed by the spirit of the supernatural Gila Monster. A ceremony must then be performed to control the shaking so that it does not become a disease and, at the same time, to introduce the individual to the diagnostician's role.

We have already noted that Navajos are not reluctant to use modern medical services when they perceive them to be accessible and effective. This is congruent with the separation of symptom treatment from supernatural cure, and the use of a physician's services does not indicate a change in the patient's belief in the efficacy of the native system. Unfortunately, Anglo-Americans have tended to see changes in Navajo behaviour as direct indicators of corresponding changes of beliefs. For example, when Navajos were reluctant to use the hospital, calling it a 'house of death', health providers believed that it was owing to the belief in dangerous 'ghosts' (*chindi*) of the dead. They did not consider that Navajos also made decisions based upon the very real observation that a high proportion of hospital patients were not cured. Later, with the advent of antibiotics after World War Two, when Navajos began to use the hospital in ever increasing numbers, physicians attributed this to a change of belief rather than to improved cure rates.

Sources of conflict

It has been only in the past twenty-five years that Anglo attitudes toward Navajo religion have become somewhat less ethnocentric and more tolerant. Most physicians thought the Navajo inferior and steeped in ignorance and superstition. The death of a Navajo child taken from hospital for a ceremony was invariably regarded as proof of this, and the mother would be lectured severely on the need to rely exclusively on modern medicine. The death of a child in the paediatric ward, however, was seen only as an unfortunate event that did not reflect on the quality of medical care. Such exchanges left the physician frustrated and the mother angry and more distrustful of the hospital than before.

We have already seen that increased use of the hospital was taken to mean that Navajo belief in malevolent ghosts was waning when, in fact, it was the accurate perception that fewer patients were dying in hospital that had lessened Navajos' fears. In general, the tendency for Anglos to see any desired change in Navajo behaviour as evidence of a corresponding change in beliefs created more frustrations when seemingly 'acculturated' Navajos continued to act on traditional beliefs in other situations.

If physicians were confused by Navajo behaviour, it is equally true that Navajos had little understanding of the behaviour of the Anglos with whom they came into contact. We have seen that Navajo healing ceremonies are used to remove the cause of a disease and that the treatment of symptoms could be sought anywhere. As physicians dispensed medicines and treated symptoms, Navajos perceived them to be the equivalents of native herbalists and bone-setters and not of equal status with native ceremonialists. This perception was strengthened by the fact that Indian Health Service physicians were generally young men just out of medical school who had chosen to do their military service in the IHS. This was in sharp contrast to the ceremonialist, who was an older man and who had taken years to learn his profession. Navajo patients were willing to accept the symptomatic treatments offered by physicians but would then contract for a ceremonial to effect a cure. Physicians, defining themselves as healers qualified to diagnose, treat and cure the disorder, were angered by the Navajos' persisting tendency to rely on their own ceremonials.

The growing reliance on modern medicine for symptomatic treatment is attested to by a study of medical decision-making in a large Navajo kin group during the 1960s.[42] In 48 per cent of choices to seek treatment only modern medical care was utilised. Thirty-nine per cent of decisions involved utilising both native healers and physicians, while only 13 per cent involved the exclusive use of native practitioners. Faints, vague symptoms and culturally defined illnesses without symptoms were never treated by physicians alone. Conversely, no childbirths or traumas were ever treated exclusively by ceremonialists, and the hospital was utilised for childbirth and trauma significantly more often than for other conditions.

Especially frustrating was the tendency for Navajos to refuse elective surgery and any treatment regimen requiring a protracted period of time, many visits to hospital or transfer to a specialty hospital away from the reservation. The resulting conflicts with patients often involved a rhetoric that had little to do with the issue at hand. Navajos claimed that surgery was an invasion of the body and that 'true' healers, i.e. Navajo *hatali*, had no need to cut into the body but could effect a cure without invasive practices which were taken as evidence that physicians were inexpert and only 'experimenting' on them. Physicians prevailed upon to allow a patient to have native treatment in conjunction with the recommended procedure, however, most often found them happy to follow the doctor's recommendations.

Navajo nurses in the Tuba City hospital in the early 1960s complained that an elderly Navajo ceremonialist with colon cancer was refusing to have a colostomy; evidence, certainly, of his ignorance and stubborn refusal to abandon his superstitions. They asked the Health Education staff to persuade him to follow medical advice.[43] An appointment with the surgeon was arranged and the procedure was explained in detail: its risks, benefits, and the fact that after the surgery the patient would have to evacuate excrement through a tube. The patient asked for a few days to think it over. Upon his return, he thanked the staff for their efforts on his behalf. It was, he said, the first time anyone had taken the time to explain things to him. He continued, saying that he had decided not to have the operation and explained that in the Navajo way he would have a nickname given him by the community, and that he had not spent his life as a respected ceremonialist only to have his children and grandchildren known in the community as the descendants of the 'old man who shits in a bottle'. The surgeon, satisfied that the patient had made an educated choice, accepted his decision and the encounter was concluded with good feeling on both sides.

In another case, a ten-year-old haemophiliac refused to take his medication and his mother suggested to the Field Health nurse that the choice was his to make. The nurse could not understand how any mother could show such lack of concern for the health of her child and angrily attributed her attitude to the Navajos' callousness toward human life generally and their children in particular. Once again, the Health Education staff were prevailed upon to persuade the boy and his mother. The boy recognised the seriousness of his condition and knew his mother loved him and would do anything she could to help him. But, he said, frequent trips to the hospital drained family resources and he did not want his siblings' needs to be slighted just to keep him alive as a semi-invalid. In this instance, also, the patient's choice appeared mature and well thought out. The value Navajo placed upon kindred as well as individual autonomy differed considerably from the attitudes and values of the average Anglo and had to be explained carefully to the medical staff.

With careful and detailed explanation, and willingness on the part of a physician to deal with patients as rational and mature, conflicts can most often be resolved satisfactorily. Such conditions, however, are not easily attained. The attitudes of the Navajo nurses in the first example provide a case in point. Trained Navajo health professionals have accepted the physician as source of knowledge and have, until very recently, labelled the more traditional members of their own society as backward. As these are the people who might serve as mediators between physicians and patients, the conflict is increased when they also treat the patient as an inferior. Unfortunately, physicians who do not speak Navajo assume that Navajo employees are performing this role and assume further that patients have been adequately educated.

One of the most persistent popular non-Indian terms for Indian languages is 'the Indian dialect', which implies not only that Indians do not speak a fully developed language but also that all tribes speak some variant of the same language. Even among health professionals there seems to be a tendency to believe that, if there is no single word in Navajo that precisely translates an English term or concept, Navajo is somehow deficient. This misapprehension is clearly born of ignorance, but the negative connotation derives from the perception of things Indian as being somehow less than things White. It is doubtful whether similar inferences would be drawn about German or French. In the early 1960s the language barrier was sufficient to make communication between health personnel and Navajo patients dangerously inadequate. An interpreter training programme was developed which was to serve as a model for similar programmes to be established in all reservation hospitals.[44]

At the time of the programme's inception only 3 per cent of deaths occurring in the Tuba City hospital resulted in autopsies. Because hospital accreditation demanded a considerably higher rate, there was some incentive for the medical staff to support a programme which promised a solution to this as well as several other problems. By physicians' accounts, Navajos refused permission to conduct a post-mortem because they were superstitious about the dead and nothing one could tell them seemed to change their minds. Moreover, families of the deceased seemed unwilling to accept the physician's condolences. According to Navajo employees there was no way to say 'I am sorry' in Navajo and the literal translation of autopsy as 'to cut into the body to find the cause of death' only served to agitate Navajos further. Both the Navajo and the Anglo staff were content to leave it at that: Navajo just did not have the words to convey the physicians' meanings, and Navajos were ignorant and unwilling to accept modern ways because of their mistaken fears and beliefs.

Using an approach that sought to calibrate concepts rather than to provide literal, word-for-word translations, Navajos and Anglos were asked to define the concept of the autopsy. The physicians had taken for granted that everyone understood that modern scientific medicine was based upon constant learning and that an autopsy was a way to discover new facts and expand knowledge. The Navajo staff confessed they had not known this, thinking that the physicians wanted to determine the cause of death to make sure they had not made a mistake. The solution was found by explaining to patients and their families the difference between modern medicine, which was constantly learning and expanding, and the Navajo system, which was self-contained and complete. Once the context of the concept was clarified there was little difficulty getting Navajo families to understand and accept the reason for the request.

Translating 'I am sorry' rested on the understanding that the word used by Navajos also meant 'worried', and 'anxious', so that its meaning was determined by the context in which it was used. Navajo society is based on kinship, and, as a general rule, those who are not kinsmen are not expected to take a personal interest in each other's affairs. When physicians said, 'I am worried that your baby died and would like your permission to cut into the body to find the cause of death', Navajos could only take it to mean that the doctor was incompetent and was afraid he had made a terrible mistake. By instructing the Navajo interpreter to say, 'This White doctor knows how you must feel and he wants you to know that, because his life has been devoted to saving the lives of patients, he too feels a sense of loss and is sorry it has happened,' condolences were adequately conveyed. Within a year the autopsy rate had risen from 3 per cent to over 80 per cent.

The point is that interpreting from one language to another involves some understanding of the cultures of which each language is a part, and that the Navajo interpreters had never gone beyond telling the physicians there was no 'word for that' in Navajo until a training programme treated the Anglo and the Navajo as equal members of a team which had a common goal in the medical encounter. Not only did Navajo modes of communication have to be examined as important and complex elements in the process, but Anglo concepts also had to be analysed in the same manner.

At no level of the structuring of Navajo–Anglo interactions was there a context in which a Navajo could communicate with an Anglo and have his or her views taken seriously. The subordinate position of the Navajo was set not only by status as an Indian in American society but also by position in the medical hierarchy. Navajos who were pressed into service as interpreters were employed in such lowly positions as janitors, nurses' aides or driver–interpreters in the field health programmes. These positions rarely demanded more than a high-school education and the pay was commensurate with the skill demanded by the job. Navajos were not employed or paid to be skilled medical interpreters, yet the non-Indian staff felt no compunction about taking them from their assigned tasks without warning and asking them to perform as interpreters in what was often a delicate medical situation. The Navajos felt that their medical knowledge, their knowledge of the health programmes and their command of English were inadequate to the task and wondered what the doctors really expected of them.

Thus, at the personal level of interaction, the Anglo staff operated as if interpreting was a simple affair, to be accorded no respect or extra consideration. At the institutional level this attitude was set in bureaucratic concrete. Despite the fact that in the 1960s there were about eight times as many Navajo-speakers as there were a century before, when Navajos were put on their reservation, the official position was that Navajo was a dying language and there was not and would not be a well paid position of medical interpreter in the Indian Health Service. The interpreter training programme was conceived of as a form of in-service training for Navajo personnel that would not even lead to promotion in the positions they held. In any event, no funds were provided to establish interpreter training programmes throughout the reservation and, after a few years, the routines developed in Tuba City were no longer in use.

Genuine conflicts and their escalation

Upon occasion, conflicts between patients and physicians would escalate until tribal politicians or US Congressmen became involved. In one instance an old man required to wear a catheter was discharged from hospital because the ward was full. The patient complained bitterly, maintaining that he would not receive proper care at home. The local trader advised the family to contact the chairman of the Tribal Health Committee and complain of malpractice. Traders and other Anglos who resented the free medical care provided for Indians often fostered an antagonistic view of the IHS, claiming that the physicians were incompetent and were experimenting on Indians.

The issue could have been amicably resolved if (a) the physician had thought to have the social worker or the field health staff evaluate the home conditions before discharging the patient, or (b) the chairman of the Tribal Health Committee had demanded that physicians should learn to utilise a team approach to such problems. Unfortunately, by claiming malpractice, the Navajo politician sought to enhance his reputation as defender of Navajo rights against the federal government. The medical staff could show, however, that malpractice was not involved, and a stalemate was reached with bad feeling lingering on both sides.

Problems like this have often resulted from the unresponsiveness of IHS physicians, not simply as a result of some personal or professional deficiency. They are a consequence of the structure of the system itself. Care is free, physicians are salaried, and there are few other health care providers competing to serve Indians. Without oversight or independent advocates for patients such a system may well become insensitive to the needs of patients.

One of the only alternative sources of medical care has been the few mission hospitals located on or near the reservation. The primary goal of these hospitals has typically been to gain converts. In consequence they were especially responsive to their clients and sought to give them as pleasant an experience as possible.

The distinction between client-dependent and colleague-dependent practices is useful here,[45] for it suggests the strengths and weakness of each system. For example, in one case the health education staff of the Tuba City hospital were sent to check on an elderly diabetic who had not come to hospital to refill her medication for some time. Arriving at the patient's home, they were informed that the patient had received medication from the mission hospital, to which she had been given a ride. They were then shown a several months' supply of multivitamins she had been given. The family maintained that the mission hospital gave better service than the IHS because waiting times and physician encounters were brief. To take another example, patients at the IHS have been known to threaten to go to a mission hospital to get the shot they were demanding if the IHS physician refused to give it because it was not medically indicated. The mission hospitals would generally accede to the demand.

Client-dependent practices such as the mission hospitals are at risk of giving unnecessary and sometimes harmful treatment to satisfy their patients' demands and keep them coming back. Colleague-dependent practices, on the other hand, may deliver technically better medicine but may be unresponsive to the emotional or other needs of their patients precisely because they are insulated from them.

Recent changes in the health care system

The past thirty years have seen significant changes in IHS programmes. Starting in the late 1960s, a younger and more idealistic cadre of well trained doctors who chose IHS instead of serving in Vietnam were more ready to sympathise with Navajos. Although their understanding of Navajo culture was not significantly improved, they were more friendly and sympathetic. Then, as the universal military draft of physicians was discontinued, the IHS encouraged young medical students to practise on the reservation during the summers. Many of them subsequently entered the IHS and some stayed on the reservation for a number of years.[46] Navajo patients were now able to establish more stable relationships with physicians, a situation that fostered more trust and co-operation.

As infectious diseases were brought under control the IHS turned its attention to a variety of chronic problems. Mental health services were established in the mid 1960s, followed by substance abuse treatment programmes. As surgery and antibiotics were accepted earlier, so too Navajos increasingly utilised these new services and, in so doing, began to learn new ways of thinking about their health. In the alcohol treatment programmes women especially began to learn that there was something they could do about physical and sexual abuse, and men learned that other men feel the same fears, frustrations and despair as they do. In short, Navajos began to perceive that the new knowledge was beneficial and to utilise the new services in ever increasing numbers. Sometimes, of course, knowledge valued by some was contested by others. Women, for example, sought more information about birth control while many men objected.

Although declining rates of fertility and increased use of contraceptives among the Navajo appear to parallel similar trends at the national level, other changes in behaviour suggest that there is increasing sensitivity and responsiveness to the educational messages of the IHS.[47] Before 1950 breast feeding was virtually universal among the Navajo, and children were fed on demand for at least a year. By 1977, however, only 10 per cent of mothers were breast feeding at the time of discharge from hospital. This decline parallels the national decline in breast feeding from 65 per cent in 1946 to 25 per cent in 1971, much of it due to increased levels of education and hospital births as well as exposure to national culture generally.[48] In all likelihood, however, the decline was made more precipitous by the formula manufacturers' practice of distributing free formula and bottles to Navajo mothers in IHS hospitals.

National trends reversed during the 1970s until, by 1980, 62 per cent of mothers were breast feeding upon discharge from hospital.[49] By 1989, however, the national rate had declined to 52 per cent. By contrast, Navajo rates increased from 10 per cent in 1977 to 70 per cent in 1980 and continued to rise until, in 1994, they had reached approximately 80 per cent. We attribute this significant reversal to the fact that the IHS discontinued the distribution of free formula and began a concerted effort to encourage breast feeding in all hospitals after 1977.

Changing Navajo life

The shift from a pastoral to a wage work economy that began with the stock reduction programmes in the 1930s has had significant effects on social organisation as well as on religious life. The Kaibeto plateau (Land Management District 1) was, in 1936, the area most reliant on stock raising on the reservation. At the time over 50 per cent of subsistence was derived from stock raising and only 23 per cent from wage income. By the 1970s livestock accounted for only 7 per cent of income, wage work for 50 per cent and welfare for 42 per cent.[50] In areas where jobs were more accessible the proportion of income derived from wage work was often over 90 per cent. The subsequent breakdown of co operating kin groups led to a lessened ability to pay for costly ceremonies. At the same time, the demands of wage work made it difficult for young men to apprentice themselves to ceremonialists. In large part, the decline in the number of ceremonialists and the growth of the Native American Church (peyote religion) as well as of Christianity can be traced to the transformation of the economy.

In a study of Navajo ceremonialists on the Kaibito Plateau, Eric Henderson notes that young men, unable to train as ceremonialists, began to adopt alternative routes to status.[51] Peyotism spread rapidly through the western reservation during the 1950s and 1960s. Younger men, engaged in wage work, can gain ceremonial prestige and additional income by studying the less demanding 'peyote way' rather than becoming traditional ceremonialists, and all of the men identified by Henderson had steady wage work during the 1950s and 1960s. It is clear that a knowledge of peyote ceremonialism bestows a degree of prestige, that learning is less demanding than learning a Navajo song and the peyote ceremony is less time-consuming. In short, it is more fitted to the constraints on weekly wage labourers.

Becoming a Christian lay preacher is also a route to prestige for some younger Navajo males. Between 30 per cent and 50 per cent of the District 1 population may be adherents of Christianity, although only about 10 per cent are relatively regular churchgoers.[52] Nor do such conversions necessarily indicate radical changes in values or beliefs. Among fundamentalist Protestants, Jesus has become the 'poor man's shield against witchcraft', and young Navajo lay preachers tend to bring all their relatives with them into their congregations. A young preacher told us that the peyotists in his community once attempted to witch his congregation. In the middle of Sunday service the congregation began to faint and it was only by concerted prayer that they were able to turn the witchcraft back upon the peyotists. That conversion does not always signal a radical change of belief is also attested to by the fact that 60 per cent of 147 heads of households surveyed on the western part of the reservation claimed adherence to traditional Navajo religion.[53] Of these, however, only 24 per cent claimed not to combine their traditionalism with some form of Christianity or with peyotism.

As religious heterogeneity has increased so the number of traditional ceremonialists has decreased.[54] In 1905 there were twenty ceremonialists on the Kaibito Plateau and there was a ratio of one ceremonialist to thirty patients. By the 1950s the number had increased to forty-eight but, with the rapidly increasing population, there were fifty patients to each ceremonialist. By 1980 there were only twenty-four ceremonialists serving a population of 4,244; a ratio of 1:176. For a number of years, however, this shortage of ceremonialists was not noticeable, owing to the expanding road network and the growing number of automobiles. Not only has the number of ceremonialists declined but so has the number of different ceremonies. Although there were twenty-four ceremonialists alive on the Kaibito plateau in 1980, only eighteen were still practising. Six of these men only did the Blessingway, which is not a curing ceremony. Another six knew only the Evilway, the special treatment against witchcraft and ghost contamination. Only two men knew two or more ceremonies in addition to the Blessingway; both were in high demand in their own and in neighbouring communities. Residents of the area have lamented the decline in the number of ceremonialists and the abbreviated repertoire of ceremonial skills.

Despite these declines, it would be premature to predict the demise of Navajo religion. Many Navajos, aware of the trend, are attempting to counter it. There is now a 'Navajo Nation Medicinemen's Association' and school training new ceremonialists.[55] Navajos' penchant for combining different forms of religion, the tendency for people as they age to return to traditionalism and the rise of 'nationalist' sentiment all serve to keep some form of religion and healing alive. Wagner has documented instances of Blessingway rituals incorporated into peyote ceremonies.[56] And we have found some hand trembler diagnosticians who have included some Blessingway and Evilway prayers in their rituals so that they can diagnose as well as cure in a single, short, inexpensive ceremony. This argues for the development of a folk religion in the midst of competing various Christian denominations, with many Navajos satisfied with a syncretistic approach to their religious lives.

III. The 'indianisation' of Indian health care[57]

We have described changes in the way services are provided, with the tribal government contracting with the Indian Health Service to manage substance abuse treatment and several other programmes. We have also shown that there have been major changes in the traditional Navajo religious/healing system. In this section we should like to suggest some of the ways in which the changes are related.

Recall that in the 1960s government policy began to emphasise the importance of community control. The purpose was not simply empowerment but the creation of jobs ('new careers in human services'). Not only was the purpose to reduce unemployment, but it was said that only people from the community understood the people and their problems well enough to provide appropriate services. Indeed, this belief legitimated the preferential hiring of local people in a variety of human service occupations. In substance abuse treatment this resonated with the position of Alcoholics Anonymous, that sober alcoholics were the people best suited to help those who were still drinking. Moreover, because trained professionals in such treatment programmes were hard to find (nation-wide as well as on Indian reservations), this ideology was particularly attractive.

Through the 1970s these ideas evolved into 'self-determination', which involved Indian tribal entities contracting to run a variety of programmes. Combined with the Indian Health Care Improvement Act, this meant more money, jobs, education and responsibility for Indians in health care. One of the areas that got special attention was substance abuse prevention and treatment. The Senate Committee on Interior and Insular Affairs explained its intent with regard to the expansion of these programmes as follows:

> The essential aspect of these projects would be the integration of Indian cultural patterns into the rehabilitative and learning processes. This would be accomplished, in part, by hiring Indian staff, working through individual tribal entities, and emphasizing the Indian's image of himself.[58]

Because the high rate of substance abuse in Indian communities was attributed to the loss of traditional culture, treatment, to be effective, required the restoration of that culture. Thus programmes began to incorporate various elements of both Navajo and pan-Indian treatments. More than that, however, along with the school system these treatment programmes began to be seen as a means by which traditional Navajo culture could be preserved. But because so many ceremonies have become extinct and only short versions of many others are still performed, what is being preserved is only a fragment of what had been a complex religious/healing system. In addition the very process of introducing elements of traditional healing into formal treatment programmes changes the traditional system, for, like other treatment modalities, they must be fitted into the regular schedule of programmes, and their use must be reported to the Indian Health Service and the Navajo tribe on the same forms that are used to report individual and group therapy sessions and other therapeutic encounters. No longer are they part of a complete system integrated into other aspects of people's lives.

One of the reasons most commonly invoked for preserving traditional Navajo healing rituals is that, unlike Western medicine, which separates mind from body, Navajo beliefs are holistic. Indeed, many of them bear an uncanny resemblance to New Age ideas as well as to alternative traditions within orthodox medicine. This is not simply because New Age ideas and psychosomatic medicine draw upon Indian cultural beliefs but because many Navajos, like many non-Indian Americans, have absorbed such ideas as part of the ambient cultural atmosphere. More specifically, some contemporary Indians working in health and social service bureaucracies have accepted as an accurate rendering of their traditional culture the ideas of non-Indian New Age savants and psychosomaticists. For example, a Navajo woman described the substance abuse treatment programme in which she worked as using 'cultural therapy'. 'We use the biopsychosocial model,' she continued. This model of health and disease has long been promulgated by George Engel,[59] a professor emeritus of psychiatry and medicine at the University of Rochester. It does not draw its inspiration from any Native American religious tradition, but in the thinking of our informant it has been assimilated to an understanding of Navajo religion. More than that, it has become a way of describing and explaining the healing characteristics of 'cultural therapy'.

To take another example, a Navajo man who is responsible for administering an alcohol treatment programme, in distinguishing traditional Navajo beliefs from the mind–body duality characteristic of Western medicine, described the traditional Navajo view of each human being as a circle divided into quarters, representing the physical body, the emotions, the mind and the spirit, all surrounded by another circle representing the family and society. This is precisely one of the assumptions on which New Age thought is based and, we would argue, represents a diffusion into Navajo culture of formulations of personality organisation that were not there previously.

That ideas about the value of traditional healing have been introduced into the formal health care system is, then, the result of several factors. First, the system itself has changed: an increasing proportion of staff at all levels is Indian, and in contrast to many of the Indian professionals of a generation ago – a few of whom we described in the previous section – many of them wish to recover and use traditions that have been lost to them.

Second, not only does the assertion of the importance of traditional knowledge reinforce ethnic pride, but it helps legitimate claims to control the institutionalised treatment system itself. For to the degree that healing techniques can be said to depend upon indigenous local knowledge rather than professional and presumably universal knowledge, local people rather than cosmopolitan professionals can claim the unique expertise necessary to provide it. It is no accident that such claims are made particularly in the areas of mental health and substance abuse, not surgery and internal medicine, for the claims to universally valid knowledge have been asserted more successfully in the latter than in the former domains.

Finally, we may regard this integration of Navajo and pan-Indian healing rituals into treatment programmes as an innovation. There is some reason to think that organisations which adopt innovations are more likely to be complex and loosely organised than those that do not.[60] Such organisations tend to have a diverse group of employees, and there may be relative autonomy among various groups of them to institute innovations that do not have a significant impact on other units. The various agencies on the Navajo reservation form such a loosely integrated system, and many of the agencies themselves are characterised by considerable autonomy among their divisions. It is therefore of little concern to some units if others wish to innovate by making traditional modes of treatment available to their clients. If alcohol treatment programmes provide sweat lodges for their clients the surgical services will not care.

Thus changes in the government's health care system and changes in the Navajos' traditional religious healing system have resulted in attempts to use the formal bureaucracy as a means of preserving Navajo culture. The paradox is, of course, that the very act of bureaucratic institutionalisation will itself accelerate change.

IV. Conclusions

Historically federal Indian health policy has been made without substantial consultation with Indian tribes, and that still is often the case even though individual Indians increasingly hold positions of responsibility within the Indian Health Service. It is federal policy which shapes the context in which Indians as individuals and Indian tribes as corporate bodies confront Anglo medical institutions and ideologies. The confrontation has often been adversarial: sometimes based on honest misunderstandings between well intentioned people; sometimes the result of prejudice; sometimes fomented by politicians seeking to create an issue rather than solve a problem. Generally it has not been the actual content of knowledge that has been contested. Historically Navajos have regarded Anglo medical concepts as separate and different from their own, and when Anglo treatments provided relief they were widely used without threatening core Navajo beliefs.

This pattern has changed as Indian policy and the reservation economy have changed. The traditional religious/healing system is fast becoming a folk system, one among many syncretistic religions. And a large number of Navajos work at all levels of the health care system for both the tribe and the federal government. All these changes have made Western medical institutions and their accompanying intellectual and ideological supports increasingly important. In response some Navajos argue that Western biomedicine is reductionist, and that traditional Navajo religion is holistic and spiritual, just as many non-Indians do. Indeed, we have said that these claims draw on similar sources and are part of a larger cultural critique of Western science and medicine. But this is a new critique. A generation or more ago many Navajos regarded Anglo medicine as a separate domain, one that was useful for some purposes but not for others, and their critiques had to do with the way care was provided – for instance, with the compassion, competence, adequacy or accessibility of the doctors, nurses and dentists who served them – not with the content of the knowledge. For most people that is still the case.

Notes

1 S. J. Kunitz, *Disease and Social Diversity: the Impact of Europeans on the Health of non-Europeans*. New York: Oxford University Press, 1994; see especially chapters 2 and 7.

2 Division of Resource Management (Finance), Indian Health Service, US Public Health Service, Department of Health and Human Services, Rockville, Maryland. The figures do not include allocations for the construction of facilities, only for the provision of services.

3 Figures on federal outlays are not shown. They appear in the following sources. US Bureau of the Census, *Historical Statistics of the United States, Colonial Times to 1970, Bicentennial Edition*, Part 2. Washington, D.C.: US Government Printing Office, 1970, tables, Series Y457–465. US Bureau of the Census, *Statistical Abstract of the United States: 1992*. Washington, D.C.: US Government Printing Office, 1992, table No. 494, p. 317.

4 F. S. Cohen, *Handbook of Federal Indian Law*. Albuquerque, N.M.: University of New Mexico Press (1942) 1971: 243–4.

5 US Congress, Office of Technology Assessment, *Indian Health Care*, OTA-H-290. Washington, D.C.: US Government Printing Office, 1986: 53.

6 National Tuberculosis Association, *Tuberculosis among the North American Indians: Report of a Committee of the National Tuberculosis Association appointed on October 28, 1921*. Printed for the Committee on Indian Affairs, 67th Congress, 4th Session. Washington, D.C.: US Government Printing Office, 1923: 93.

7 Office of Technology Assessment, *Indian Health Care, ibid.*: 43.

8 Institute for Government Research, *The Problem of Indian Administration*. Baltimore, Md: Johns Hopkins University Press, 1928.

9 See L. C. Kelly, *The Assault on Assimilation: John Collier and the Origins of Indian Policy Reform*. Albuquerque, N.M.: University of New Mexico Press, 1983. See also K. Philp, *John Collier's Crusade for Indian Reform, 1920–54*, Tucson, Ariz.: University of Arizona Press, 1977.

10 Institute for Government Research, *The Problem of Indian Administration*, p. 51.

11 Philp, *John Collier's Crusade*: 96.

12 *Ibid.*: 97.

13 Kelly, *The Assault on Assimilation*; Philp, *John Collier's Crusade*; S. J. Kunitz, 'The social philosophy of John Collier', *Ethnohistory* 18 (1972): 213–29.

14 J. W. Mountin and J. G. Townsend, *Observations on Indian Health Problems and Facilities*, Public Health Bulletin No. 223, Washington, D.C.: US Government Printing Office, 1936: 6.

15 *Ibid.*: 14–15, 22–3, 27.
16 Philp, *John Collier's Crusade*: 204–6.
17 For a statement of the assimilationists' view of the importance of improved health and education programmes see F. Foard, 'Health services for the North American Indians', *Medical Woman's Journal* 57 (1950): 9–16. Foard was Director of Medical Services of the Bureau of Indian Affairs at the time.
18 S. J. Kunitz, *Disease Change and the Role of Medicine: the Navajo Experience*. Berkeley and Los Angeles, Cal.: University of California Press, 1983: 151–2.
19 US Department of Health, Education and Welfare, Public Health Service, Office of Surgeon General, Division of Public Health Methods, *Health Services for American Indians*, Public Health Service Publication No. 531, Washington, D.C.: US Government Printing Office, 1957: 117–18.
20 P. H. Stuart, 'Financing self-determination: federal Indian expenditures, 1975–88', *American Indian Culture and Research Journal* 14 (1990): 1–18 at p. 2.
21 Kunitz, *Disease Change*: 47.
22 Stuart, 'Financing self-determination': 9.
23 *Ibid.*: 8. Italics in original.
24 J. Jorgensen, 'Federal policies, American Indian polities and the 'New Federalism', *American Indian Culture and Research Journal* 10 (1986): 1–13.
25 At the time of writing (autumn 1994) the Clinton administration has attempted to reduce IHS staff numbers and funding. Indian tribes and the Indian Health Service have resisted the policy. In the short term the result has been demoralisation. The long-term results are still unknown. See also S. J. Kunitz, 'The history and politics of US health care for American Indians and Alaskan natives', *American Journal of Public Health* 86 (1996): 1464–73.
26 G. and R. G. Bailey, *A History of the Navajos: the Reservation Years*. Santa Fe: School of American Research Press, 1986.
27 D. Aberle, *The Peyote Religion among the Navaho*, second edition, Chicago: University of Chicago Press, 1982.
28 J. A. Krug, *The Navajo: a Long-range Program for Navajo Rehabilitation*, Washington, D.C.: Bureau of Indian Affairs, Department of the Interior, 1948. This period is discussed in greater detail in Kunitz, *Disease Change*: 39–44.
29 Forest products are the one example of an extractive enterprise run by the tribe: all the others were controlled by large corporations, with low royalties and few jobs coming to the tribe. This period is covered in Kunitz, *Disease Change*: 44–51.
30 Navajo Nation Division of Economic Development, *Overall Economic Development Plan 92–93*, Window Rock: The Navajo Nation, 1991.
31 E. D. Gregg, *The Indians and the Nurse*, Norman, Okla.: University of Oklahoma Press, 1965: 104. See also Kunitz, *Disease Change*: 145–76.
32 S. J. Tillman, 'Health among the Navajos', *Southwestern Medicine* 20 (1936): 355, 388, 432. See also L. Schnur, 'Navajos train ward aides to counteract "medicine man"', *Modern Hospital* 59 (1942): 80.
33 C. Kluckhohn and D. Leighton, *The Navaho*, Cambridge, Mass.: Harvard University Press, 1946; D. Leighton and C. Kluckhohn, *Children of the People*, Cambridge, Mass.: Harvard University Press, 1948; A. H. and D. C. Leighton, *The Navaho Door: an Introduction to Navaho Life*, Cambridge, Mass.: Harvard University Press, 1944.
34 Leighton and Leighton, *The Navaho Door*: 56.
35 Gregg, *The Indians and the Nurse*: 105.
36 Indian Health Service. *Trends in Indian Health – 1993*, US Department of Health and Human Services, Public Health Service, Indian Health Service, Office of Planning, Evaluation and Legislation, Division of Program Statistics, Rockville, Md, 1993.
37 Kunitz, *Disease Change*: 161–2.
38 Navajo Nation Division of Economic Development, *Overall Economic Development Plan*: 13.
39 R. Underhill, *Ceremonial Patterns in the Greater Southwest*, American Ethnological Society Monograph 13, New York: Augustin, 1948; L. Lamphere, 'Southwestern

ceremonialism', in A. Ortiz (ed.), *Handbook of North American Indians* 11, *Southwest*, Washington, D.C.: Smithsonian Institution, 1983: 743–63.

40 Underhill, *Ceremonial Patterns*: x. For a more detailed discussion of the development of Navajo religion see J. E. Levy, R. Neutra and D. Parker, *Hand Trembling, Frenzy, Witchcraft, and Moth Madness: a Study of Navajo Seizure Disorders*, Tucson, Ariz.: University of Arizona Press, 1987, chapter 2.

41 Underhill, *Ceremonial Patterns*: viii.

42 J. E. Levy, 'Traditional Navajo health beliefs', in Kunitz *Disease Change*: 143.

43 Between 1959 and 1962 Levy was the resident anthropologist in a health education project run by the School of Public Health of the University of California, Berkeley.

44 J. E. Levy, 'Interpreter Training Program', Window Rock, Ariz.: USPHS, Division of Indian Health, Window Rock Field Office. Window Rock, Ariz., 1964.

45 E. Freidson, *Profession of Medicine*, New York: Dodd Mead, 1970.

46 The attractiveness of these arrangements differs among Indian Health Service regions. The Southwest seems better able to retain physicians than some other regions.

47 S. J. Kunitz, 'Navajo and Hopi fertility', *Human Biology* 46 (1974): 435–51, *id.*, 'Factors influencing recent Navajo and Hopi population change', *Human Organization* 33 (1974): 7–16.

48 E. G. Yencho, 'Social factors associated with the mother's decision to breastfeed her firstborn infant', University of Arizona, School of Nursing, M.A. thesis, 1977; A. M. Wright, A. M. Bauer, C. Clark, F. Morgan and K. Bagishe, 'Cultural interpretations and intracultural variability in Navajo beliefs about breastfeeding', *American Ethnologist* 20 (1993): 781–96.

49 A. S. Ryan, *et al.*, 'Recent declines in breastfeeding in the U.S., 1984–89', *Pediatrics* 88 (1991): 719–27.

50 E. B. Henderson and J. E. Levy, 'Survey of Navajo community studies, 1936–74', *Lake Powell Research Project Bulletin* 6 (1975): 130–1.

51 E. B. Henderson, 'Kaibeto Plateau ceremonialists, 1860–1980', in D. M. Brugge and C. J. Frisbie (eds), *Navajo Religion and Culture: Selected Views. Papers in honour of Leland C. Wyman.* Santa Fe: Museum of New Mexico Press, 1982: 164–75.

52 *Ibid.*: 173.

53 J. J. Wood, 'Western Navajo religious affiliations', in Brugge and Frisbie, *Navajo Religion and Culture*: 176–86.

54 Henderson, 'Kaibeto Plateau ceremonialists': 167.

55 This is the Navajo Healing Arts Training Program at Rough Rock Demonstration School, which has been supported by the National Institutes of Mental Health since 1970. D. F. Aberle, 'The future of Navajo religion', in Brugge and Frisbie, *Navajo Religion and Culture*: 219–31.

56 R. M. Wagner, 'Pattern and process in ritual syncretism: the case of peyotism among the Navajo', *Journal of Anthropological Research* 31: 162–81.

57 The material in this section is based upon S. J. Kunitz and J. E. Levy, *Drinking Careers: a twenty-five year follow-up of three Navajo populations*, New Haven, Conn.: Yale University Press, 1994, chapter 9.

58 Committee on Interior and Insular Affairs, *Report of the Committee on Interior and Insular Affairs, United States Senate, together with Additional Views to accompany S. 2938 (Indian Health Care Improvement Act)*, Washington, D.C.: US Government Printing Office, 1974: 87.

59 G. L. Engel, 'The need for a new medical model: a challenge for biomedicine', *Science* 196 (1977): 129–36.

60 A. L. Greer, 'Advances in the diffusion of innovation in health care organizations', *Milbank Memorial Fund Quarterly* 55 (1977): 505–32 at 517.

CHAPTER FIVE

What/who should be controlled? Opposition to yellow fever campaigns in Brazil, 1900–39

Ilana Löwy

The eradication of yellow fever was one of the central goals of public health activity in Brazil in the first half of the twentieth century. The means adopted, may, however, seem excessive. Yellow fever had a high mortality rate during epidemic outbreaks; it was nevertheless far from being the most important public health problem. Mortality from diseases such as tuberculosis, gastroenteritis, typhoid fever, diphtheria or measles was much higher, while the efforts to control them were incomparably smaller than those invested in anti-yellow fever campaigns. The disparity may be more easily understood if we accept Michael Worboys's assertion that tropical medicine did not concentrate on all the diseases present in the tropics, or even those which killed the greatest number of persons, but only on those which periodically brought about a great rise in mortality.[1] High mortality from endemic diseases, particularly among the young and the poor, was often quasi-invisible. By contrast, deviations from the 'normal' pattern of morbidity and mortality acquired high visibility and became the target of energetic sanitary intervention. In addition, the sudden rise in mortality from yellow fever was observed above all among newcomers to an endemic area, that is, among Europeans or North Americans. The spectacular course of yellow fever (black vomit, delirium) and high mortality among the sick during epidemics also contributed to the transformation of this disease into a symbol of the 'curse of the tropics' and an important target of sanitary efforts.

The symbolic image of yellow fever was particularly important in Brazil, where yellow fever became identified with backwardness, while victory over the disease was transformed into an icon of progress. In the early twentieth century, Brazil was an independent state with strong nationalist trends. Its urban elites, concentrated in a few major cities in the south, strove to emulate the Western model of scientific and technological development. On the other hand, early twentieth-century Brazil was an underdeveloped country, with a vast interior in which conditions of life (e.g. the brutal exploitation of the local population by rubber and coffee plantation owners) were little different from those in colonial countries. The publication of Euclides da Cunha's novel *Os sertoes* in 1902[2] is often seen as the event which 'revealed' the existence of the interior of Brazil to urban elites. The novel, a fictionalised report of the repression by the Brazilian army in 1896–97 of a rebellion led by a religious mystic, Anthonio Conselhero, depicted the inhabitants of the interior (*sertanejos*, that is, inhabitants of the *sertao*, the semi-desert zones of the Brazilian north-east) as primitive, backward, fanaticised and racially degenerate, but also as brave, persevering and faithful. Da Cunha's novel opened a debate on Brazilian national identity. Intellectuals who identified with the 'brasilianismo' movement wrote about the misery of the north and stressed that Brazil is also *os sertoes* and Jeca Tatu (the prototypical Brazilian backwoodsman). Gradually the official discourse incorporated the notion of 'two Brazils', urban and rural, and of the huge gap which separated them. Many educated Brazilians viewed medicine and hygiene as one of the central means of closing that gap. The diffusion of a health message aimed at decreasing human suffering but also at the transmission of the norms and values of the organisers of the sanitary campaigns, such as the transformation of Jeca Tatu into an efficient agricultural worker.[3] The anti-yellow fever campaigns – those conducted by Brazilian public health officials and those conducted by the experts of the Rockefeller Foundation (RF) – need to be understood, I propose, within the general framework of tensions between coastal Brazil and the interior, between the cities and the countryside, between the federal government of Brazil and local authorities, between the small educated elite and the masses of poor Brazilians, between a wish to adopt a Western (European, then North American) model and an aspiration to develop Brazilian national identity.

In the absence of efficient therapies for yellow fever the only meaningful sanitary action was prevention. The Reed Commission – sent in 1900 by the US army to investigate yellow fever epidemics in Cuba – confirmed the observation (first made by the Cuban, Carlos Finlay) that yellow fever is transmitted by the mosquito *Aedes aegypti* (then called *Stegomyia fasciens*). The conclusions of the Reed Commission were rapidly confirmed by other researchers, and the control of yellow fever was identified with the control of its vector.[4] In the early twentieth century the anti-yellow fever campaigns combined fumigation, which killed adult mosquitoes, anti-larval work to prevent mosquito breeding, and the isolation of sick persons from insects. Opposition to this type of anti-yellow fever campaign consisted mainly of resistance to the compulsory reconstruction of the urban environment as part of the new anti-larval campaigns. By contrast, for RF experts control of yellow fever became identified with the control of *aegypti* larvae. *Aedes aegypti* breeds exclusively near human habitations, and the anti-larval measures imposed by the RF experts, in particular between 1930 and 1939, involved tight control over the inhabitants of endemic areas, both the living and – from 1930 on, with the introduction of obligatory sampling of cadaveric tissue (viscerotomy) – also the dead.

This chapter opens with a short description of opposition to Oswaldo Cruz's campaign in Rio de Janeiro (1903–07), then describes the reactions to the first RF-directed anti-yellow fever campaign (1923–30), and follows in detail the opposition to the second RF campaign (1930–39). Resistance to these anti-yellow fever campaigns, I argue, was mainly opposition to what was perceived by the inhabitants as an unjustified, arbitrary and often brutal intrusion into their private lives by an authoritarian power.

Early control: Oswaldo Cruz's anti-yellow fever campaign, 1903–07

The anti-yellow fever campaign organised by Oswaldo Cruz was both a demonstration of the efficacy of certain scientific concepts and a political action.[5] Oswaldo Cruz (1872–1917) was trained as a bacteriologist at the Pasteur Institute, Paris (1896–98), and became an enthusiastic advocate of new approaches to the control of infectious diseases. In 1902 the progressive governor of the state of Sao Paolo, Francisco Rodriguez Alves, was elected President of Brazil. When he settled in the capital, Rio de Janeiro, Alves was appalled by the poor sanitary status of the city. He identified the struggle against epidemic diseases with the struggle against the backwardness and underdevelopment of Brazil, and was particularly concerned about the persistence of yellow fever and its consequence, the reluctance of foreign ships to call at Rio de Janeiro harbour.

Shortly after his election Alves appointed Oswaldo Cruz head of the National Department of Public Health (DNSP). Cruz immediately started an energetic campaign against three infectious diseases: smallpox, yellow fever and plague.[6] There was little opposition to anti-plague measures, i.e. the cleaning of the city streets and elimination of rats. By contrast, both the compulsory vaccination to eliminate smallpox and the anti-yellow fever measures were resisted by the inhabitants of Rio de Janeiro. Protests against compulsory vaccination against smallpox reached their peak in November 1904 with an organised rejection of the vaccination, anti-vaccine street riots and a revolt in the military academy of Prahia Vermelha. The main argument of opponents of the obligatory vaccination and hygiene measures was that 'the compulsory aspect was an attack against human dignity. Persuasion and conviction, yes. Coercion, never. It was arbitrary and despotic. A sanitary dictatorship.'[7] President Alves was obliged to revoke the compulsory vaccination law.[8]

The opposition to anti-yellow fever measures was less organised. It was expressed at two levels: popular opposition to the forcible implementation of sanitary measures, doubled by opposition from medical professionals to what they viewed as an excessive faith in the mosquito hypothesis.[9] The Rio de Janeiro press strongly criticised 'the dictatorship of the new administration', characterised by a mixture of 'direct political violence and violence mediated through sanitary measures'. The newspapers complained about the brutal implementation of the sanitary measures, which did not take into account the population's feelings. Rio de Janeiro inhabitants, some journalists claimed, were victims of a 'tentacular arbitrary power which limits their freedom in the streets, in their houses, in the exercise of their professions, in their right to private property'.[10] The press articles reflected popular anger. The government of President Alves and the prefect of Rio de Janeiro, Pereira Passos, decided to use Cruz's sanitary campaign to modernise the federal capital. The main victims of the modernisation efforts were the inhabitants of the poor quarters of the centre of the city. Their houses were sometimes demolished, their possessions thrown out, street trading was banned, and their usual way of life was totally disrupted. Opposition to this sanitary campaign, later presented by some Brazilian authors as the expression of the ignorance of the poor, had in fact a precise social and economic context.[11]

In addition, the presentation of opposition to Cruz's sanitary measures as a reflection of the 'backwardness' of the masses did not account for some experts' opposition to Cruz's campaign. This opposition was led by the previous director of DNSP, Nuno d'Andrade. He summed up his ideas in a series of articles published in 1903 in one of the main Rio de Janeiro newspapers, *Jornal do Commercio*. D'Andrade thought that the 'mosquito theory' of transmission of yellow fever was a useful hypothesis, but he was sceptical about its universal validity. He protested against the 'tyranny of new doctrines' and their uncritical acceptance by physicians and politicians. The new 'scientific' view of yellow fever was, he proposed, highly simplified. It did not take into consideration the important seasonal and local variability of morbid forms of the disease. D'Andrade supported the efforts to eliminate mosquitoes, but he proposed that the traditional anti-yellow fever measures – disinfecting the clothes and bedding of the sick, and isolating them not only from mosquitoes but from other people – should be maintained at the same time.[12]

One might argue that d'Andrade was merely an old-fashioned physician unable to accept new theories. The pathological entity 'yellow fever' (as defined through the isolation of its causal agent, a specific virus) is indeed, as all the experts agree today, transmitted to man exclusively by mosquitoes. On the other hand, in the early twentieth century scientists did not knew how to isolate, cultivate or visualise viruses, and the diagnosis of yellow fever was based solely on clinical observation. Consequently, in endemic areas, yellow fever was often confused with other pathologies which induced jaundice.[13] D'Andrade's warning not to abandon all 'traditional' anti-infection measures when dealing with a suspected case of 'yellow fever', and not to rely on extermination of the mosquitoes alone, may be seen in retrospect as reasonable advice, at least in an endemic area. In 1903 however, Rio de Janeiro was an epidemic, not an endemic, area. The constant influx of non-immunised immigrants, combined with the high density of the *aegypti* mosquitoes in the city, created optimal conditions for repeated outbreaks of yellow fever. The outbreaks mainly affected foreigners, who frequently developed the typical symptoms of that disease. Energetic anti-mosquito measures – such as those undertaken by Cruz – were indeed the most efficient way to stop a yellow fever epidemic in a city.

From 1907 on Oswaldo Cruz's campaign was seen as a clear-cut triumph. In 1903 there were 584 declared cases of yellow fever in Rio de Janeiro; in 1906, forty-two; in 1907, thirty-nine; in 1908, four; and in 1909 none.[14] From 1907 on the press hailed Cruz as a national hero. His anti-yellow fever campaign was transformed into an emblem of the achievements of Brazilian science. Consequently, one of the main characteristics of this campaign, the systematic extermination of adult mosquitoes by squads of *mata mosquitos* (mosquito killers) who fumigated houses, became the hallmark of the correct way to control yellow fever. This method combined the advantages of breaking the chain of infection during epidemics, (temporarily) ridding the population of (*aegypti* and other) mosquitoes, and enhancing the visibility both of the public health officials who conducted fumigation campaigns and of the politicians who supported them. While at first some inhabitants of Rio de Janeiro opposed the fumigations, later the periodic interventions of uniformed *mata mosquitos* became identified with energetic and efficient public health policy.[15] Attempts by RF experts to eliminate fumigation and concentrate exclusively on antilarval steps were at first viewed by Brazilian public health officials and politicians as a dangerous departure from the established (and, they believed, well tried) way to fight yellow fever.

Loose control: the Rockefeller Foundation's first anti-mosquito campaign, 1923–28

The RF started its anti-yellow fever work in Brazil in 1923. The general policy of the International Health Board (IHB; from 1928, the International Health Division, or IHD) of the RF was to fight diseases (such as yellow fever) which could, they believed, be eradicated rapidly, and therefore demonstrate the efficacy of their sanitary approaches.[16] The RF experts were present in Brazil from 1918 on, but at first they concentrated their efforts on the eradication of hookworm, a sanitary activity which, they believed, would greatly improve the health and the work capacity of coffee plantation workers.[17] In 1923 the increase in the incidence of yellow fever in Brazilian coastal cities attracted the attention of IHB directors to the disease.[18] The foundation signed an agreement that year with the Brazilian government according to which the IHB, together with DNSP, would take over the elimination of mosquitoes in the north of Brazil, in the framework of the RF–DNSP co-directed Co-operative Yellow Fever Service (YFS). The anti-mosquito campaign would be funded by the RF.[19]

RF anti-yellow fever activities in the years 1923–28 were based on two assumptions. The first was that the elimination of mosquito larvae was the only efficient anti-yellow fever measure. The fumigations were spectacular, and eliminated bothersome insects. They were expensive, however, and – except in the case of an acute epidemic outbreak – inefficient. Only systematic elimination of the breeding sites of the *aegypti* mosquito could reduce the density of these mosquitoes to a level which would interrupt the transmission chain of yellow fever. The second assumption, named the 'key focus' theory, was that large cities were the only permanent reservoir of the yellow fever virus.[20] The virus, the RF specialists believed, was specific to humans, and a minimum density of population was necessary for its continuous transmission. If eliminated from the larger cities, yellow fever would 'burn itself out' in less populated areas, in which anti-larval work was not feasible anyway, because of the increasing conditions of poverty, filth, ignorance and general wretchedness of the inhabitants'.[21] Neither assumption was shared by Brazilian specialists. They were sceptical about the efficacy of the anti-larval measures introduced by the RF. They also thought that yellow fever was endemic in rural areas. US experts did not observe yellow fever in the countryside, Brazilian doctors suggested, because they were looking only for 'typical' forms of the disease, usually observed in the cities where recent immigrants lived. By contrast, the inhabitants of endemic areas suffered from 'atypical', milder forms of yellow fever, often misdiagnosed by RF specialists.[22] Between 1923 and 1928 the RF implemented anti-larval posts in all the major cities of the north of Brazil. The Ministry of the Interior issued instructions to the YFS, but the instructions gave only a vague outline of the service's activities. The (short) instruction sheet stated, for example, that 'the inspectors will call on all houses of their respective zones, taking the requisite steps so that all larvae foci are immediately destroyed', but did not make explicit what the 'requisite steps' were. It did not explain either what the duties, obligations and limits upon the intervention of YFS officials were.[23] The YFS was formally co-directed by the RF and DNSP, but in fact the RF experts did not include local DNSP employees in their decision-making. A few DNSP officials resented the undermining of their authority by the RF staff. Thus Sebastio Barroso, responsible for the DNSP office in Salvador (Bahia), resigned in 1923, because, he explained, he had discovered that the supposed partnership with RF experts was in fact an invitation to put all responsibility in their hands, and to adopt without question their methods of eliminating larvae.[24]

Barroso's opposition to the anti-larval methods of the RF reflected a widespread feeling. These methods relied, in the years 1923–28, mainly on the control of containers for drinking water. Brazilian cities at that time did not usually possess a general underground system of water distribution, and even in neighbourhoods in which such a system existed the water supply was often interrupted. The inhabitants relied on storing water for domestic use in smaller *jarras* (jars) or bigger *caixas d'agua* (cisterns). The RF specialists believed that the most efficient method to prevent the breeding of *aegypti* mosquitoes in water receptacles was to put in them small fish which eat mosquito larvae. The introduction of fish was, however, often perceived by the inhabitants as an intolerable interference with their water supply – a particularly explosive subject in a hot climate, and in regions which suffered from periodic dry spells. White, who directed the RF's anti-yellow fever work, complained in 1924 about 'the villainous propaganda against fish which cuts our efficiency by probably 33% and increases our costs at least 20%'.[25] The inhabitants complained of faecal matter and dead fish in their drinking water. Water from receptacles into which fish were introduced, they claimed, was stinking and, moreover, was contaminated and dangerous to health because the fish were collected from streams heavily polluted by sewage. The 'oiling' of water receptacles, that is, spreading a thin layer of oil on the surface of a receptacle in which *aegypti* larvae had been found, met with even greater opposition because it made the water unfit for domestic use. The inhabitants also complained about the invasion of their privacy. Some YFS *guardas* (inspectors), inhabitants of Bahia claimed, asked to be admitted to private rooms as early as 7.00 a.m.[26]

> Certain localities, such as Victoria (Esprito Santo), were described as a hard station to work. Complaints against the service were numerous and the people were usually opposed to anti-larval routine. ... The people in Victoria like the type of service that they have now. I am told that the guarda enters, says '*Bom dia Senora, a jarra esta limpa hoje? Si Senor, esta limpa. Bom, muito obrigado, ate logo, Senora*' ('Good day, Madam, is the water recipient clean today? Yes, Sir, it is clean. Very good, thank you, see you next time, Madam').[27]

The RF experts also complained about the need to 'humour' local populations and the representatives of the Rural Prophylaxy Service by agreeing to 'traditional' (and to them inefficient) anti-yellow fever measures such as fumigation and the isolation of the sick.[28] Their difficulties notwithstanding, the RF staff believed in 1927 that anti-larval work in the larger cities was progressing well, thanks mainly to the improvement of the water supply and the replacement of old drinking water receptacles by new ones fitted with covers.[29] The initial opposition to YFS measures, the RF experts stated in 1928, had disappeared thanks to a suitable blend of firmness and diplomacy.[30]

From loose to tight control: yellow fever epidemics in Rio de Janeiro and the Rockefeller Foundation's second anti-mosquito campaign, 1928–32

The number of declared cases of yellow fever in the coastal cities decreased markedly in 1925 and 1926, and during the first three quarters of 1927 no single case of yellow fever was reported. The RF experts believed that they were very close to the goal of totally eradicating yellow fever from Brazil. In 1927 the RF closed sixty-one mosquito eradication stations, leaving only four.[31] The appearance of yellow fever in Rio de Janeiro, in spring 1928, however, put an end to hopes that the disease had disappeared. The epidemic spread rapidly in the city. The DNSP director, Clementino Fraga, attempting to imitate Oswaldo Cruz, induced large-scale fumigations conducted by thousands of *mata mosquitos*.[32] At the end of the summer of 1928 Fraga announced that the epidemic had been halted.[33] The announcement was premature, however, and in 1929 the epidemic started anew. Several neighbouring countries had forbidden Brazilian ships access to their ports, again transforming the epidemic of yellow fever into a symbol of 'contagious backwardness'.[34] The epidemic was finally stopped in 1929, but the demonstration of the inefficacy of the DNSP in preventing it, combined with the observation that cities in the north of Brazil (where the RF worked) had resisted yellow fever relatively well, strengthened the bargaining power of RF experts.[35]

In January 1929 the RF and the Brazilian government signed a new agreement, according to which the RF became responsible for yellow fever control north of the state of Sao Paulo, and the DNSP south of the state. The government agreed to pay half the RF's expenses. A modified agreement, signed in December 1929, gave the RF responsibility for yellow fever throughout Brazilian territory, except for Rio de Janeiro State. In summer 1930 Fred Soper became head of the IHD office in Brazil, and set out to radically reorganise the yellow fever service, which was, Soper decided after three months of travel in the north, cumbersome and inefficient.[36] In October 1930, following a 'revolution' (or, rather, a *coup d'état*), Getulio Vargas became the President of Brazil.[37] Vargas's regime, authoritarian and populist, advocated modernisation and close co-operation with the United States.[38] Consequently it strongly supported the RF's anti-yellow fever work; in Soper's words, 'Dr Getulio Vargas was both father and mother of the present yellow fever service.'[39]

A new agreement between the RF and the government, signed in early 1931, stipulated that the government would pay 80 per cent of the expenses of the YFS, but at the same time would allow the RF experts full administrative autonomy (e.g. in hiring and firing employees and fixing their salaries and working conditions) and immunity from control. In the years 1931–39 the RF experts thus directed a government agency sustained by Brazilian laws and funded almost exclusively by taxpayers' money but were not accountable to any Brazilian institution. This duality of the RF-directed YFS – US philanthropic organisation and Brazilian government agency – was reflected in an exchange between Soper and Wilbur Sawyer (then the director of the IHD). Sawyer argued (in 1935) that the responsibility for (future) anti-yellow fever vaccination campaigns should be transferred to Brazilian authorities, who, as the recipient of the benefits, should also carry responsibility for the risks. Soper's answer was that Sawyer 'overlooks completely the fact that *we* are the Brazilian authorities'.[40]

The reorganisation of the yellow fever service under Soper reflected changes in the beliefs of the RF specialists. The 1928–29 epidemic had discredited the 'key focus' theory. The RF experts became convinced that yellow fever was, after all, endemic in rural areas. Some also suspected that the hypothesis (advanced by some Brazilian doctors) was correct that other mosquitoes, and not only *Aedes aegypti*, and other mammals, not only humans, were involved in its transmission. Consequently, Soper and his colleagues decided to extend the network of anti-larval posts to the interior of the country. Precise epidemiological knowledge about the prevalence of yellow fever was needed in order to decide where to locate such posts. It was obtained through systematic autopsies of all those deceased from a sudden 'fever' and the development of a network of 'viscerotomy posts', which sampled cadaver tissue with a special instrument – the viscerotome – and sent it for diagnosis to a central laboratory. Systematic examination of cadaver livers confirmed that yellow fever was present in many localities previously held to be free from the disease.[41] In 1932 the RF experts described a non-*aegypti*-transmitted yellow fever in rural areas ('jungle yellow fever').[42] The (suspected, then proved) existence of a reservoir of the virus responsible for 'jungle yellow fever' outbreaks in wild animals shifted the goal of RF experts from eradication to control. It did not, however, lessen their dedication to the goal of control of the mosquito *Aedes aegypti*. The *aegypti* mosquito, Soper and his colleagues explained, was solely responsible for epidemic forms of yellow fever. In the absence of a vaccine the strict control of *aegypti* breeding was the only way to prevent the spread of yellow fever virus from isolated cases of 'jungle yellow fever' to densely populated areas.[43]

The anti-mosquito work of the 'new' YFS, Soper believed, should have a firm legal basis. RF experts worked closely with Brazilian officials to elaborate such a basis. A draft of YFS regulations, prepared by the RF staff, stated in its first paragraph that YFS employees must have the right 'to inspect premises all the time, to destroy mosquito foci, to remove roof gutters, to autopsy all suspected cases, to fine householders who fail to obey the service orders, who obstruct premise inspections or who do not maintain premises free from mosquito breeding'. The memorandum stated that 'the aim of course is to put the onus of mosquito prevention on the householder and not on the service'.[44] The official regulations of the YFS (decree No. 21434 of 23 May 1932) follow closely the RF experts' original proposal.[45] The first paragraph states the principle of the YFS's omnipresence:

> Personel of the Yellow Fever Service shall visit weekly ... all premises inhabited or not, private and collective dwellings, including yards, patios, tile-roofs or other; factories; shops; commercial and industrial establishments; colleges; retreats; convents; churches; monasteries; cemeteries; hospitals; sanatoriums; maternity hospitals; markets; hotels; restaurants; boarding houses; stables; barns; barracks; prisons; forts; islands; dry-docks; stores of every kind, including explosives or inflammable materials; military and civil aviation fields; all means of

> transport whether by land, sea, river or air; lots, parks and public places; gardens and all other places.[46]

The regulations of the YFS further specified that all the water containers:

> must conform to the models approved by the Service ... these must be either mosquito-proof or constantly supplied with larvivorous fish of the species approved by the Service. ... Where there is a constant supply of water, domestic wall tanks shall not be permitted.

Roof gutters were allowed only where absolutely indispensable. Statues and embellishments on buildings, and flower vases, jardinieres, urns and other ornamental articles in cemeteries must not be such as to collect water. YFS staff had the right to destroy all receptacles in which mosquito foci were found or, alternatively, to apply larvicide to such receptacles. Persons who failed to conform to YFS regulations, those who abandoned 'tin-cans, pans, dishes, glassware, bottles, hardware, coconut shells, pottery and other articles capable of collecting water ... and anyone who opposes, hinders or objects in any way to the sanitary work defined in these regulations' could be fined, and recidivists condemned to three to thirty days of imprisonment. 'When persuasive or coercive measures fail, recourse shall be made to the police authorities ... In case of disrespect or insolence, proceeding in the criminal court should be commended.'[47] The repressive apparatus was necessary because the YFS officials were often confronted with hostile local populations who opposed both anti-larval measures and viscerotomy.

Viscerotomy and the opposition to the control of the dead

Brazilian investigators from the Oswaldo Cruz Institute observed specific histological changes in the livers of persons who had died of yellow fever.[48] These observations, which at first did not interest the RF experts, later became the basis of the diagnosis of 'silent' cases of yellow fever. Systematic autopsies of persons deceased from suspected 'fever' less than eleven days following the onset of disease were first introduced in 1930 by the director of the DNSP in Rio de Janiero State, Deicio Pareiras.[49] In order to carry out such autopsies in remote rural areas, one of the RF officials, Rickard (according to another version, Deicio Pareiras) developed an instrument for rapid sampling of liver tissue which could be used even by lay persons.[50] The 'liver punch', later renamed 'viscerotome', was composed of an external tubing and a sliding steel blade. It allowed, Rickard explained, sampling of liver tissue in less than a minute, even from a partly clothed cadaver.[51] The YFS rapidly developed a network of viscerotomy posts. There were twenty-six such posts in 1930, 199 in 1931 and more than a thousand in 1937. The Viscerotomy Service representative received a fixed sum for each sample of liver tissue sent to the central laboratory, and an additional bonus if the sample was found to be positive for yellow fever.[52] RF staff frequently complained about fraudulent practices by the representatives of the Viscerotomy Service. Several specimens of the same liver would be sent under different names, fragments of liver from animals were presented as human, rumours of yellow fever were spread to increase payments for liver samples, samples were taken from cadavers which had not died of sudden 'fever', and cadavers that should have been punctured escaped viscerotomy because the family bribed the person in charge of the viscerotome post. The RF officials therefore elaborated a complex system of surveillance of the employees of the Viscerotomy Service.[53]

Controlling the viscerotome operators was difficult enough, controlling the population even more so. The drilling of a hole in the abdomen of a recently deceased person was often perceived as an indecent violation of a dead body. It was nevertheless imposed by law. The decree of 23 May 1932 prohibited burial without the visa of the representative of the Viscerotomy Service, made death certificates and official burial permission a requirement and stipulated that if family or friends of the deceased were opposed to viscerotomy they would be fined and the tissue sample taken compulsorily under police protection.[54] In order to limit negative reactions, Rickard recommended that:

> the viscerotome should not be shown to persons having no connection with the Viscerotomy Service. In most cases such people do not understand the true significance of the service and react unfavorably at the sight of the instruments. The rumors that such people spread may cause unnecessary opposition from the families concerned.

The Viscerotomy Service representative, Rickard recommended, should always bear in mind that viscerotomy was an obligatory legal service maintained for the benefit of the public, and should overcome opposition by his courteous but firm manner.[55]

The 'firm and resolute' attitude of the Viscerotomy Service representatives was not always sufficient to prevent opposition. This opposition took different forms, some of them peaceful – such as the bribing of representatives or the development of clandestine cemeteries – and some more violent.[56] Stories about opposition to viscerotomy are abundant in the letters, diaries and memoirs of RF officials.[57] 'The wall of fanaticism they were up against to get livers,' Wilson Smillie explained, 'was tremendous. Everybody advised against it. As a surgeon one could do what one wanted, but the dead body was sacred, at least under the immediate impact of death.' The RF experts tried to fight this opposition, invariably labelled 'superstition', by a 'counter-superstition'. They addressed a local 'saint', Padre Cicero (1844–1934), venerated in the north of Brazil as a miracle worker.[58] Padro Cicero, who had a long record of favouring anti-government revolts but also of supporting right-wing politicians, befriended the RF officials in the 1920s and later used his influence to convince his followers that a liver punch did not hamper their chances of resurrection.[59]

The 'counter-superstition' tactics were not always effective, and the police protection for Viscerotomy Service representatives was not always sufficient. Bruce Wilson summarised in his diary the fights, difficulties and fatalities during the introduction and the maintenance of the Viscerotomy Service (five Service workers were killed by angry families). He also noted that in some localities political factions took advantage of opposition to viscerotomy to start a fight with government supporters.[60] The diary reached the Director of the IHD, Sawyer, in 1938. Sawyer was distressed, and ordered Soper to reduce the number of viscerotome posts immediately:

> the continued violence which seems almost inseparable from the widespread system of viscerotomy is a matter of concern and has reached a point at which it seems there should be a modification of our program. The total experience ... brings into serious question the advisability of a method which invites such violent resistance and offends the sensibility of the public.[61]

Soper strongly disagreed. For him the opposition to viscerotomy was a marginal phenomenon, much less important than he and his colleagues had initially feared. Five persons killed, he explained, 'is indeed a remarkably low score, considering the conditions under which the work has been done. When we consider that over 100,000 punctures have been made, many of them in regions of extreme religious fanaticism, the result is surprising.' On the plus side, Soper stressed, the network of viscerotomy posts was of invaluable help in bringing updated epidemiological information about the spread of yellow fever: 'positive livers are hot evidence, and get results from the local authorities'.[62] The viscerotomy posts in endemic areas were maintained.

Anti-larval measures and the opposition to the control of the living

The co-operative yellow fever service, remodelled by Soper, was a strictly hierarchical organisation. The 'old' YFS already had a pyramidal structure. At the base were the inspectors (*guardas*), then district and regional inspectors. The inspectors wore uniform, insignia marked their rank, and flags indicated their presence in a house. The uniforms did not, however, constitute legal permission to enforce anti-*aegypti* regulations. The 'new' YFS, armed with adequate legal powers, markedly improved the external control of inhabitants, and the internal control of its employees. Only such strict control could, Soper believed, lead to the efficient control of yellow fever. Later observers noted the resonance between Vargas' authoritarian regime and Soper's authoritarian way of conducting the anti-*aegypti* campaign.[63] Soper – nicknamed 'the dictator' by some of his colleagues – readily admitted that:

> a certain amount of almost religious fanaticism is essential for the work ... The longer a region passes without yellow fever, the more necessary this fanatical spirit becomes, since governmental and public memories are short, and to continue insisting on the application of rigorous control measures in an area apparently free from yellow fever is difficult.[64]

The basic unit of control of inhabitants was a zone – a group of houses visited once a week by a zone inspector. Five or six zones were grouped in a district and controlled by a district inspector. Districts were under the supervision of a general inspector whose work was controlled in turn by the regional director, nearly always a North American.[65] The zone inspectors were entitled to examine every room in the house (the right to visit bedrooms and bathrooms was explicitly included in the inspectors' instructions), and to empty or to coat with oil (occasionally, to destroy) offending water receptacles.[66] The district inspectors systematically surveyed the work of each zone inspector, examining houses either before his visits (to compare observations) or after them (to verify that all the larvae foci had been detected). The general inspector paid surprise visits to controlled areas, sometimes accompanied by the regional director. In addition, special groups – 'hidden foci squads' and 'adult mosquito capture squads' – verified the overall efficiency of anti-*aegypti* measures in a given area. The repeated inspections of houses and yards were viewed by many inhabitants as an intolerable intrusion into the privacy of their lives.[67]

Opposition to YFS anti-larval campaigns and to RF-directed epidemiological surveys – like the opposition to viscerotomy – was systematically 'folklorised', that is, explained by the belief that RF staff were 'always fighting superstition among the ignorant natives'.[68] Stories about the RF's anti-yellow fever campaign were enriched with anecdotes (often repeated) about the primitive religious feelings of local populations: fear of spirits and devils, superstitions linked with blood (hence opposition to the drawing of blood), the conviction that population surveys were an activity of the Antichrist.[69] A typical story was told by Smillie, who recalled that during a health survey in Pernambuco the *guardas* met with opposition and doors were slammed in their faces. Smillie rode down with a colleague to see what the problem was. In the woods they met a man with a gun who told them to keep away from his house or he would kill them. Asked why, he pointed to their shoes and dared them to take them off. He could not imagine a normal foot like his in a pointed shoe and suspected cloven-hoofed emissaries of the devil. Smillie took off his shoes.[70]

The backwardness of the local population was given as the main reason for opposition to YFS work. Suspected epidemics of yellow fever in Novo Exu (Pernambuco) were not investigated, Soper explained, because 'the people in this area are very suspicious and very superstitious. Repeatedly specimens have not been taken and probably could be secured only at grave personal risk.'[71] Occasionally, however, middle-class Brazilians, who could not be so easily 'folklorised' and described as 'primitive', also complained about the attitude of the YFS staff. The US consul in Victoria reported in 1932 that commercial associations in that city complained about YFS employees who 'are throwing kerosene in perfectly clear water, breaking tiles and gutters. The main complaint is the lack of respect for the property of others.' Inhabitants viewed the sealing of water cisterns as particularly offensive; the cisterns were on the roof, so it meant breaking into houses and commercial premises. The consul noted that 'it is significant of the attitude of the public here toward the work of the Mission that no slightest tribute is paid for its gratuitous and efficient work in the prevention of the propagation of the yellow fever mosquito'. One may note, however, that while the opposition of poor people to anti-larval measures was quickly dismissed as 'superstition', the US consul in Victoria recommended RF officials to conduct a press campaign to put across their point of view.[72]

Conclusion

The opposition to anti-yellow fever measures reflects the intrinsic ambiguity of 'sanitary campaigns' which aimed at bringing 'civilisation' to the interior. The campaigns combined the wish to improve the health of the population and to eradicate epidemic diseases with the drive to attain economic goals, such as the free circulation of people and merchandise in Brazilian ports, an improvement in the capacity of plantation labourers for work, or elimination of the image of 'backwardness' which deterred foreign investors. These ambiguities, present in the sanitary campaigns conducted by Brazilian experts, were amplified by the activities of the RF's 'missionaries of health', who worked in the grey zone between the sincere wish to improve the lot of indigenous populations, the belief that the most efficient way of doing so was to export the North American model of society (to make 'them' like 'us') and the desire to forward the economic interests of US companies.[73] Racism occasionally increased the ambiguity of the RF's sanitary campaigns. Some RF leaders held straightforwardly racist opinions. Wickliffe Rose, the first director of the IHB, explained after his visit to Brazil in 1920 that the backwardness of the northern part of the country should be attributed to the fact that its population 'is composed of shiftless blacks, parasitic whites of Portuguese origin and a large percentage of their hybrid progeny with traces here and there of Indian characteristics'.[74] One should hasten to add, however, that Brazilian intellectuals often held equally racist views. Adolpho Lutz and Astrogildo Machado from the Oswaldo Cruz Institute stated after their scientific expedition to the north in 1912 that the northern regions were backward because 'the black race is a major factor, and in some places the white element is totally absent. This naturally influences the character of the population, which generally lives by very primitive means.'[75]

The racial question influenced perceptions of yellow fever. Celebrating Oswaldo Cruz's achievements, the politician Rui Barbosa stressed that yellow fever exterminated the white race and spared the blacks: 'the yellow plague, negrophile and xenophobic, attacked the existence of the nation in its marrow'.[76] The influence of racial views was not, however, universal, unidirectional or simple. Some RF experts (e.g. Connor) believed that the 'racial factor' played an important role in the epidemiology of yellow fever and that blacks were immune to the disease.[77] By contrast, other specialists did not believe in racial differences in susceptibility to yellow fever. To Fred Soper the decisive epidemiological factor was endemicity and not race.[78] Soper's unrelenting – in his own words, 'fanatical' – drive to eradicate the *aegypti* mosquito from the South American continent was motivated by the belief that yellow fever was extremely harmful to native populations, and might be a great danger to all the inhabitants, not only to foreigners, new immigrants or city dwellers. Moderate coercion and some bruising of people's sensibilities were, Soper believed, not too high a price for the elimination of a major epidemic disease. He considered his anti-*aegypti* campaign in Brazil a great success, and a worthy example for imitation in other countries as well.[79]

Not all his colleagues agreed, and some estimated that the immense effort put into anti-yellow fever campaigns had hampered the development of public health measures. Yellow fever had (nearly) disappeared, but inhabitants of poor areas continued to suffer from a myriad of other acute and chronic pathologies. Andrew J. Warner, who was on the RF staff in Brazil in the 1930s, explained later that:

> Yellow fever suffocated general public health work in Brazil not only by diverting interest and funds and by lining up the IHD on the Federal side in the contests with Sao Paolo, but more subtly, by causing us to abandon our traditional anonymity and allowing limelights to play steadily for years on our own contribution of administrative talent. We exercised autocratic authority in a great national campaign toward which the Brazilians made major contributions in funds and personnel.

His colleague Coggenshall agreed. The main trouble with the anti-yellow fever campaign, he explained, was that it had become an end in itself, and did not lead to any further developments in public health.[80] But perhaps the problem was larger than the debate over whether the campaign was the most efficient way to use RF funds and expertise to promote public health. Summing up thirty years of public health work in developing countries in 1951, the former director of the IHD, Wilbur Sawyer, explained that:

> Early in the half-century it was surmised that improvement in health would promptly be followed by increased production, and a better economic position would result in fuller social development. Probably the health work would have had this effect, except for the periodic setbacks by war and by interference with international trade, travel and communications. *The problem is much broader than health, which cannot flourish in an adverse socioeconomic environment.*[81]

It is not impossible that, all their 'backwardness' notwithstanding, the inhabitants of regions in which yellow fever was endemic may have been able to grasp more rapidly than the former IHD director the link between their 'adverse socioeconomic environment' and their poor health. The perception might have affected their opposition to the RF's anti-yellow fever campaign. Yellow fever was perceived by them as but one among numerous 'fevers' and other diseases from which they suffered. The efficient control of the disease, an impressive achievement from the epidemiologist's point of view,[82] was not necessarily viewed in the same way by the inhabitants of infected areas. In their eyes the search for (infrequent) cases of yellow fever did not justify the offensive practice of viscerotomy, while the anti-larval campaigns (unlike the old-fashioned fumigations) imposed severe constraints without even offering relief from bothersome insects. One may reasonably assume that for many inhabitants the 'freedom from yellow fever' which resulted from the success of Soper's campaign was perceived mainly as freedom from control of their houses by inspectors of the YFS, and from the fear that their dead would be 'punched' by officials of the Viscerotomy Service.

Michael Worboys has proposed that what counts in the term 'tropical medicine' is not the 'tropical' location but the colonial status of the countries in which 'tropical medicine' developed.[83] The specific variant of 'tropical medicine' developed in Brazil reflected the combined influence of underdevelopment – of economic and social structures not very different from those of colonised countries – and of political independence, which brought nationalist feelings to the fore. The latter element affected policies towards populations. Western medicine developed the ideal of public health 'with populations', that is, education of the lay public, who would then become the active auxiliaries of public health officials. By contrast, Worboys explains, in colonial countries medical experts either wished to control epidemic diseases 'without populations', that is, through methods which did not involve the active participation of the natives, or, alternatively, through 'social engineering'.[84] The anti-yellow fever campaigns in Brazil – in particular the campaign directed by Soper in 1930–39 – were based on a specific variant of 'social engineering' which indissolubly linked public health measures with unusually tight control over the population.[85] The inhabitants of controlled areas contested the very principle on which the anti-yellow fever campaigns were based: the assumption that political authorities had the right to discipline their subordinates and to supervise, 'for their own good', all the intimate details of their life – food and drink, ornamentation and waste disposal, even the way they mourned their dead. The antagonism to these campaigns expressed, *in fine* – to follow Foucault – opposition to the 'transmission of the effects of power even to the most remote elements', such as the poorest inhabitants of the interior of Brazil.[86]

Notes

I am indebted to the archivists of the Rockefeller Archive Center and of the Casa Oswaldo Cruz, Fiocruz, and to researchers from the Casa Oswaldo Cruz for their help. This study was partly subsidised by a Rockefeller Archives research grant, and by the INSERM/FIOCRUZ agreement.

1 Michael Worboys, 'Colonial medicine and tropical imperialism: a comparative perspective', paper delivered to the Conference on Dutch Tropical Medicine, Amster-

dam, September 1989.

2 Euclides da Cunha, *Os sertoes* (Rio de Janeiro, 1902). French translation Jorge Coli and Antone Seel (Paris: A. M. Metallié, 1993).

3 Paolo Gadelha, Jaime Benchimol *et al.*, *Science Heading for the Backwoods* (Rio de Janeiro: Casa Oswaldo Cruz, 1992).

4 On the origins of the 'mosquito hypothesis' see Nancy Stepan, 'The interplay between socio-economical factors and medical science: yellow fever research, Cuba and the United States', *Social Studies of Science* 8 (1978): 397–423; François Delaporte, *History of the Yellow Fever* (Cambridge, Mass.: MIT Press, 1992); and on its confirmation in Brazil, Ilana Löwy, 'Yellow fever in Rio de Janeiro and the Pasteur Institute mission, 1901–05: the transfer of science to the periphery', *History of Medicine* 34 (1990): 144–63.

5 Nancy Stepan investigated the interaction between public health and politics during Oswaldo Cruz's sanitary campaign: N. Stepan, *The Beginning of Brazilian Science: Oswaldo Cruz, Medical Research and Policy* (New York: Science History Publications, 1976): 69–104. See also Oswaldo G. Cruz, *Opera Omnia* (Rio de Janeiro: Impressora Brasileira, 1971): vi–x; E. Sales Guerra, *Oswaldo Cruz* (Rio de Janeiro, Vecchi, 1940).

6 Stepan, *The Beginnings of Brazilian Science*: 85–91.

7 Carlos da Silva Aranjo, *The Immortalized Cow: Smallpox Vaccine and Wright Vaccines in Brazil* (Rio de Janeiro: Grafica Olimpica, 1972): 29.

8 Placido Barbosa and Casio Barbosa de Resende (eds), *Os servicios de saude publica no Brasil, especialemente na ciudad de Rio de Janeiro de 1808 a 1907* (Rio de Janeiro: Imprensa Nacional, 1909); Octavio G. de Oliveira, *Oswaldo Cruz e suas actividades na direçao da saude publica brasileira* (Rio de Janeiro: Seriçao Grafico do Instituto Brasileiro de Geografia e Estatistica, 1955).

9 Yellow fever was a serious health problem in Rio de Janeiro at the end of the nineteenth century, in particular for new immigrants (more than a thousand dead in epidemic years). Carlos Seidel, 'Dados estatisticos applicaveis au estudo etiologico da febre amarella', *O Brazil Medico* 16 (21 1900): 181–4.

10 *A Noticias*, 10 July 1903; 'Kaledoscopia', *A Tribuna*, 9 July 1903; *O Pais*, 11 July 1903; *Jornal do Commercio*, 22 July 1903. Press cuttings, Archives Oswaldo Cruz, Casa Oswaldo Cruz, Fiocruz, Rio de Janeiro.

11 Simon Schwartzmann, *A formaçao da comunidade cientifica no Brazil* (Sao Paolo: Editora Nacional, 1979): 130–1.

12 They were later collected in a booklet. Nuno d'Andrade, *Febre amarella e o mosquito* (Rio de Janeiro: Jornal do Commercio, 1903).

13 For example, experts agree today that the Rockefeller Institute yellow fever expert, Hideyo Noguchi, confused leptospiral jaundice with 'true' (that is, viral) yellow fever in the 1920s. Hideyo Noguchi, Henry R. Muller, Octavio Torres *et al.*, *Experimental Studies of Yellow Fever in Northern Brazil* (New York: Rockefeller Institute for Medical Research, Monograph No. 20, 1924); Paul Franklin Clark, 'Hideyo Noguchi, 1876–1928', *Bulletin of the History of Medicine* 33 (1959): 3–20.

14 Oswaldo Cruz, 'The sanitation of Rio', *The Times*, 28 December 1909.

15 Stepan, *The Beginning of Brazilian Science.*

16 Rockefeller Foundation, *Annual Report, 1925* (New York: Rockefeller Foundation, 1925).

17 Roy E. Nash, 'Selling public health in Brazil', *Brazilian American* (official organ of the US delegation to the Brazilian Centennial Commission), 4 April 1922, Rockefeller Archive Center (hereafter RAC), Record Group (R.G.) 5, series 2, box 23, folder 137.

18 Steven Williams studied the relations between RF officials and Brazilian authorities in the years 1925–30. S. Williams, 'Nationalism and public health: the convergence of Rockefeller Foundation technique and Brazilian authority during the time of yellow fever, 1925–30', in Marcos Cueto (ed.), *Missionaries of Science: the Rockefeller Foundation and Latin America* (Bloomington, Ind.: Indiana University Press, 1994): 23–49.

19 The agreement was confirmed by the Brazilian government. Decree No. 16300, 31 December 1923.

20 This theory was first formulated by Henry Carter. Carter to Russell, 11 August 1923. RAC, R.G. 5, series 1, box 73, folder 1073; Carter to White, 23 February 1923, RAC, R.G. 5, series 1, box 73, folder 1035. See also Joseph H. White, 'Memorandum descriptive of method of work against yellow fever', RAC, R.G. 5, series 305, box 23, folder 138.

21 Lucian C. Smith, 'Report on a trip to the Joazeiro area', 14 March 1927, RAC, R.G. 1.1, series 305, Box 19, folder 155.

22 Odair Franco, *Historia de febre amarelle no Brasil*, Rio de Janeiro: Ministerio da Saude, 1969; Joao Cribelli Guimares, 'Febre Amerella Silvestre', unpublished habilitation thesis, Institute de Microbiologia, Universidade Federal do Rio de Janeiro, 1974.

23 'Instructions approved by the Minister of Interior Affairs and laid down by the National Department of Public Health, concerning the execution of the Services of Yellow Fever', Rio de Janeiro, 11 September 1923; RAC, R.G. 5, series 305, box 24, folder 142.

24 Memorandum by Homer Brett, on 'Anti-yellow fever work in Bahia by the Rockefeller Foundation', 11 December 1923, RAC, R.G. 5, series 305, box 24, folder 142.

25 White to Russell (the director of IHD), 29 January 1924, RAC, R.G. 5, series 305, box 23, folder 1212.

26 *Ibid.*

27 A. V. Burke to M. Connor, 23 March 1927, RAC, R.G. 1.1, series 305, box 19, folder 155.

28 Connor to Soper, 7 March 1929, RAC, R.G. 1.1, series 305, box 20, folder 160.

29 Connor to Soper, 1 June 1927, RAC, R.G. 1.1, series 305, box 19, folder 155.

30 Soper to Russell, 8 February 1928; Russell to Soper, 1 March 1928, RAC, R.G. 1.1, series 305, box 20, folder 158.

31 IHB report on its activities in Brazil, last half-year, 1927, RAC. Williams discusses IHB efforts to promote extensive urban waterwork projects in northern Brazil (to be carried out by the US firm Ulen & Co.). Williams, 'Nationalism and public health': 35.

32 Clementino Fraga, *A febre amarella no Bresil: notas e documentos de uma Grande Campanha Sanitaria* (Rio de Janeiro: Officia Graphica da Inspection de Demographia Sanitaria, 1930); Clementino Fraga Filho (ed.), *Clementino Fraga, intinerario de uma vide, 1880–1971* (Rio de Janeiro, 1973); Fraga's correspondence 1928–29, Fraga file, Archives of Casa Oswaldo Cruz, Rio de Janeiro.

33 Ludwig Rajchman (Director of the Hygiene Office of the League of Nations), to Fraga, 21 December 1928, Fraga file, Archives of Casa Oswaldo Cruz, Rio de Janeiro.

34 Dr Abt, from the International Hygiene Office, to Fraga, 3 March 1929; letter from the Uruguayan Minister of Foreign Affairs to the Brazilian Foreign Affairs Minister, 24 July 1929, Fraga file, Archives of Casa Oswaldo Cruz, Rio de Janeiro.

35 Letter from Connor, director of RF in Brazil, to Russell, 6 November 1929, RFA, R.G. 1.1, series 305, box 20, folder 121.

36 Hackett's interview with Soper, 17–18 February 1951, RAC, R.G., 3.1, series 908, box 1, folder 8. Lewis W. Hackett, one of the founders of the IHB, planned to write a history of IHB/IHD and in the early 1950s interviewed numerous participants on their IHD activities. Hackett died before completing his project.

37 Thomas E. Skidmore, *Politics in Brazil, 1930–64* (London, Oxford and New York: Oxford University Press, 1967): 4–47.

38 The RF experts were not always advocates of democracy abroad. Thus Wickliffe Rose (the founder of the IHB) explained in 1920 that 'Brazil is a democracy only in name ... Under the present condition it is best so; with more than 80 per cent of the people illiterate there can be no intelligent public opinion.' W. Rose, memorandum of 25 October 1920, p. 11, RAC, R.G. 5(2), series 305, box 25, folder 153.

39 Soper, Diary, 25 September 1934, p. 231, RAC, R.G. 1.1, series 305, box 28, folder 209.

40 Soper to Sawyer, 27 March 1935, RAC, R.G. 1.1, series 305, box 21, folder 176. (Italics mine.)

41 The 'mouse protection test', which revealed the presence of anti-yellow fever antibodies in the blood (and thus of past prevalence of yellow fever) was an additional tool of epidemiological surveys. See W. A. Sawyer and Wray Lloyd, 'The use of mice in tests of immunity against yellow fever'. *Journal of Experimental Medicine* 54 (1931): 533–55.

42 F. Soper, H. Penna, E. Cardoso *et al.*, 'Yellow fever without *Aedes aegypti:* study of a rural epidemic in the Valle do Chanaan, Esprito Santo, Brazil, 1932', *American Journal of Hygiene* 18 (1933): 555–87.

43 Anti-yellow fever vaccine, developed by IHD scientists in their New York laboratory, was first tested in Brazil in 1938.

44 Bruce Wilson, memorandum ('A project of legal instruction for the YFS') sent to Russell, director of the IHD, on 21 July 1931, RAC, R.G. 1.1, series 305, box 21, folder 167.

45 The sixty detailed articles in this text may be contrasted with the sixteen imprecise paragraphs of the instructions for the 'old' YFS approved by the Brazilian Ministry of the Interior in September 1923.

46 Decree 21434, 23 May 1932, approving the regulations of the services for the prevention of yellow fever in Brazil', RAC, R.G. 1.1, series 305, box 21, folder 167.

47 *Ibid.*

48 H. Roche Lima, 'Da importancia pratica das lessoes do higado na fabre amarelle', *Rev. Med. Hambourg* 2 (1921): 336–9; C. Marginos Torres, 'On the importance in post-mortem diagnosis of yellow fever of microscopic lesions described by Rocha Lima and Hoffman', *Memorias Instituto Oswald Cruz* 19 (1926): 13–18.

49 Rickard to Hackett, 23 October 1951; Hackett's interview with Soper, 17–18 February 1951; RAC, R.G. 3, series 908, box 1, folder 7.

50 Hackett's interview with Rickard and Kumm, RAC, R.G. 3, series 908, folder 8. F. L. Soper, E. R. Rickard and P. J. Crawford, 'The routine post-mortem removal of liver tissue from rapidly fatal yellow fever cases for the discovery of silent yellow fever foci', *American Journal of Hygiene* 19 (3 1934): 549–66; Decio Pareiras, 'The creation of the viscerotomy service for the diagnostic of yellow fever and the first viscerotome', in L. Ribeiro (ed.), *Brazilian Medical Contributions* (Rio de Janeiro: Olympio, 1939): 106–7.

51 E. R. Rickard, 'The organization of the Viscerotomy Service of the Brazilian Co-operative Yellow Fever Service', *American Journal of Tropical Medicine* 17 (1937): 163–90.

52 Rickard, 'The organization of the Viscerotomy Service'; Rockefeller Foundation, *Annual Report, 1937* (New York: Rockefeller Foundation, 1937).

53 Soper's diary, entry of 22 April 1932, RAC, R.G. 1.1, series 305, box 28; Rickard, 'The organization of the Viscerotomy Service'; Hackett's interview with Dr Wilson G. Smillie, 10 November 1950, RFA, R.G. 3, series 908, folder 19.1. RF officials saw fraudulent practices as resulting exclusively from employees' greed, and did not consider the possibility that they might also reflect popular opposition to viscerotomy.

54 Soper to Russell, 15 July 1932, RAC, R.G. 1.1, series 305, box 21, folder 170; 'Decree 21434, 23 May 1932, approving the regulations of the service for the prevention of yellow fever in Brazil'.

55 Rickard, 'The organization of the Viscerotomy Service': 181–2.

56 Hackett's notes on viscerotomy (based on information supplied by Rickard), RFA, R.G. 3, series 908, box 3, folder 19.1.

57 Hackett's interview with Dr Wilson G. Smillie, 10 November 1950, RFA, R.G. 3, series 908, box 3, folder 19.1.

58 Hackett's interview with Bruce Wilson, RFA, R.G. 3, series 908, box 3, folder 19.1; P. Gadelha, Jaime Benchimol *et al.*, *Science Heading for the Backwoods*; Lourenço Filho, 'Padre Cicero Baptista' (manuscript, dated 1926), RFA, R.G. 3, series 908, box 3, folder 19.1.

59 A visit to Padre Cicero in Joazario became a ritual stop for the RF staff. The Americans noted with amusement that the living symbol of the primitive faith of the north became, under their influence, an admirer of John D. Rockefeller and an avid reader of *National Geographic Magazine*. Smillie to Russell, 31 May 1927, RAC, R.G. 1.1, series 305, box 21, folder 155.

60 In the 1930s the RF emissaries in peripheral posts were required to keep a regular diary, and to send a copy to their immediate superior.

61 Sawyer to Soper, 6 May 1937, RAC, R.G. 1.1, series 305, box 23, folder 182. See also Hackett's interview with Dr Wilson G. Smillie, 10 November 1950, RFA, R.G. 3, series 908, box 3, folder 19.1; Hackett's interview with M. E. Tennant, *ibid.*

62 Soper to Sawyer, 12 May 1937; Soper to Sawyer, 30 June 1937. RAC, R.G. 1.1, series 305, box 23, folder 182. Sawyer disagreed, and claimed that 'the number of persons murdered is doubtless insignificant when compared to thousands of persons who feel they are being imposed upon'. Sawyer to Soper, 6 June 1937, *ibid.*

63 Greer Williams, *The Plague Killers: Untold Stories of Three Campaigns against Disease* (New York: Scribner, 1969): 265–6.

64 Soper to Russell, 14 May 1932, RAC, R.G. 1.1, series 30, box 21, folder 170.

65 F. L. Soper, B. D. Wilson, S. Lima and W. S. Atuens, *The Organization of Nation-wide Anti-*Aedes aegypti *Measures in Brazil* (New York: Rockefeller Foundation, 1943).

66 The RF experts gradually abandoned their faith in fish as a general solution to the larvae problem.

67 Soper *et al., The Organization of Nation-wide Anti-*Aedes aegypti *Measures in Brazil.*

68 Hackett's notes from his interview with W. A. Sawyer, RAC, R.G. 3, series 908, box 3, folder 19.1, page 49.

69 Hackett's interview with Kumm; Hackett's interview with Rickard; RAC, R.G. 3, series 908, box 1, folder 9.

70 Hackett's interview with Smillie.

71 Soper to Sawyer, 23 June 1933, RAC, R.G. 1.1, series 305, box 21, folder 170.

72 Report from the US embassy in Brazil to the State Department, 23 November 1932, RAC, R.G. 1.1, series 305, box 21, folder 170. In the 1930s the financial burden of anti-yellow fever work was carried almost entirely by the Brazilian government. Klotz to Russell, 3 April 1933, *ibid.*

73 Williams, 'Nationalism and public health': 26–7.

74 W. Rose, memorandum of 25 October 1920, on p. 7, RAC, R.G. 5(2), box 25, folder 153.

75 A. Lutz and A. Machado, 'Journey along the Sao Francisco river', *Memoirs of the Oswaldo Cruz Institute*, 1919, p. 185, quoted in P. Gadelha, J. Benchimol *et al., Science Heading for the Backwoods.*

76 Quoted by Sidney Chalhoub, 'The politics of disease control: yellow fever and race in nineteenth-century Rio de Janeiro, Brazil', *Journal of Latin American Studies* 25 (3 1993): 441–63, at p. 462.

77 Russell to Flexner, 10 August 1928, RAC, R.G. 1.1, series 305, box 20, folder 159.

78 Hackett's interview with Soper, 6 June 1951, RAC, R.G. 3, series 908, box 4, folder 20.

79 Fred L. Soper, 'The newer epidemiology of yellow fever', *American Journal of Public health* 27 (1 1937): 1–14.

80 Hackett's interview with A. J. Warner, 1950, RAC, R.G. 3; series 908, box 3, folder 19.1; Hackett's interview with Coggenshall, 18 September 1950, *ibid.*

81 Wilbur A. Sawyer, 'Medicine as social instrument: tropical medicine', *New England Journal of Medicine* 244 (6 1951): 217–24, at p. 224. Italics minc.

82 Soper, 'The newer epidemiology of yellow fever.

83 Worboys, 'Colonial medicine and tropical imperialism'. See also Harish Naraindas, 'Poisons, putrescence and the weather: a geneaology of the advent of tropical medicine', paper presented at the ORSTOM/UNESCO conference 'Twentieth Century Science beyond the Metropolis', Paris, 19–23 September 1994.

84 Worboys, 'Colonial medicine and tropical imperialism'.

85 'Social engineering' was an important goal of the RF, in particular after its reorganisation in 1927. Raymond B. Fosdick, *The Rockefeller Foundation* (New York; Harper, 1952); Robert Kohler, *Partners in Science: Foundations and Natural Sciences* (Chicago and London: Chicago University Press, 1991).

86 'Permettant de conduire des effets de pourvoir jusqu'au éléments les plus ténus et les plus lointains'. Michel Foucault, *Surveiller et punir* (Paris: Gallimard, 1975): 252.

CHAPTER SIX

The hook of hookworm: Public health and the politics of eradication in Mexico

Anne-Emanuelle Birn and Armando Solórzano

In an engaging book entitled *The Empire's Old Clothes* the Chilean author Ariel Dorfman has analysed the way in which twentieth-century children's literature reflects the era's varying forms of imperialism.[1] This argument can be extended to the sphere of medical imperialism. The most salient example is Jean de Brunhoff's series of stories about Babar the elephant, which began with the capture of Babar and his friend Celeste in Africa. Transported against their will, the elephants were forced to become show animals in a grand European circus. Upon their escape, they were befriended by the 'Old Lady' who gave them an accelerated course in 'civilised' behaviour.[2] She taught the elephants to stand upright, to wear clothes, and to eat with forks and knives. When Babar and Celeste returned to Africa, they brought along Western medicine. According to de Brunhoff, the elephant community readily accepted a new hospital with its particular rules and practices. In order to demonstrate the value of European medicine, Babar was the first to be admitted after having broken his trunk, and he readily accepted the authority of the Old Lady, now in the guise of a nurse.

While the Rockefeller Foundation's endeavours to 'develop' Mexico required a greater effort than the Old Lady's moulding of Babar, in both cases relatively small-scale endeavours had a tremendous impact on respective terrains. Beginning in the late nineteenth century, the medical optimism and armamentaria spawned by bacteriological discoveries led, for the first time, to potentially realisable dreams of disease eradication. In 1909 John D. Rockefeller, attracted by the technical challenge, social utility and romance of eradication, launched the Sanitary Commission for the Eradication of Hookworm Disease in the United States. Hookworm, the so-called 'germ of laziness', was believed to be a key factor in the south's lower productivity; its eradication would pave the way for the industrialisation of this large section of the country. The brainchild of a maverick medical zoologist, a powerful philanthropy officer and a prominent educator (respectively Charles Wardell Stiles, Frederick Gates and Wickliffe Rose), the Sanitary Commission marked the beginning of a long and romantic affair between philanthropy and scientific public health.[3] From 1910 to 1914 teams of physicians and technicians travelled to countless rural communities in eleven states in a bid to educate more than a million poor southerners about hookworm, to administer hundreds of thousands of treatments, and to convince inhabitants to wear shoes and to build and use latrines to avoid the spread of hookworm. This extended effort, costing about US$800,000 (US$11.3 million in 1991 dollars), relied on the co-operation of local governments and boards of health, as well as on the participation of agricultural clubs and churches.[4] Though only moderately successful (resistance stemmed in part from suspicion that the shoes being peddled were made in Rockefeller-owned factories), the Sanitary Commission awakened the Rockefeller Foundation to a variety of public health needs, including professional training, the permanent organisation of health departments, and popular health education. In addition, it served as a model for international efforts in public health for over four decades.

The Sanitary Commission was incorporated into the new Rockefeller Foundation (RF) in 1913 and reincarnated as the International Health Commission (rechristened the International Health Board, or IHB, in 1916 and the International Health Division, or IHD, in 1927).[5] Eager to extend its public health plan around the world, the new Commission soon initiated hookworm control programmes in the Caribbean, Latin America and the Orient. These projects illustrated the Progressive Era's confidence in science's ability to systematically solve humankind's secular problems. The ready response to the Rockefeller invitation by the governments of over ninety countries of varying political hues was not always shared by the popular classes, and the public health campaigns generated a varying combination of resistance, suspicion, hostility, acquiescence and popularity. This chapter examines how and why the RF exported its hookworm eradication programme to Mexico in the early 1920s and explores the social and political reaction to the campaign.

Long-term turbulent relations between Mexico and the United States, the instability generated by more than a decade of warfare during the Mexican Revolution, and the threats to US economic interests provided ample basis for both the diplomatic and the development components of the RF's involvement. Following an expensive yellow fever campaign managed entirely by the RF,[6] the foundation assured Mexican health officials that a hookworm programme would be a more co-operative endeavour.[7] Financially this was true, for the RF's annual budget in Mexico plunged by over 90 per cent, from $100,000 per year in 1921–24[8] to under $10,000 per year subsequently.[9] Footing less than a sixth of the hookworm campaign bill, the RF retained virtually all decision-making powers.

The hook of hookworm

The IHB was more interested in promoting the establishment of public health institutions and spreading the 'knowledge of scientific medicine' – which linked each disease to a specific microbe – than in reducing the burdens of illness and death, and each IHB disease activity served a specific purpose in reaching that goal. Hookworm served as a 'preliminary survey' of health and disease conditions, a 'demonstration of cure and prevention' and an introduction to the role and value of a community health organisation.[10] Diseases chosen needed a rapidly demonstrable, economical cure. Costly projects, like diarrhoea control through the construction of water and sewage systems, did not serve as effective propaganda. Yellow fever, regarded an imminent threat to world commerce, served as an expensive exception to the rule of reasonably priced programmes.[11]

The IHB initiated its leverage over Mexico in the planning stages of a hookworm programme. In early 1923 Wickliffe Rose, the IHB's influential first director, solicited Mexico Health Department chief Alfonso Pruneda for his country's participation in a co-operative hookworm campaign. Rather than proposing a joint plan, however, the IHB insisted that Mexico should request assistance, promising that the invitation would 'receive sympathetic consideration'.[12] The IHB called this process a mere formality, but it immediately turned the Mexican government into a subservient player. In place of IHB gratitude to Mexico, Pruneda had to obsequiously thank the RF.[13] Mexican President Alvaro Obregón, pleased with the outcome of the yellow fever campaign, overlooked this affront. He quickly approved the hookworm programme, hoping that it would help quell continuing unrest and strengthen his political position.[14]

In the next phase of negotiation RF officials demonstrated their mastery of administrative tactics. The 'invitation' by the Mexicans involved the acceptance of a lengthy list of RF requirements. The Mexican government was to maintain a central office, provide clinic sites around the country, pay the salaries of Mexican officials, furnish a chauffeur-driven car for the IHB representative, and lift customs fees for both programme and personal materials. Most important, virtually all decision-making (including budgeting, personnel and project planning) was relinquished to the RF representative, even once the Mexican government was funding the entire hookworm budget.[15] Each year of the five-year hookworm project the RF reduced its contribution to the $24,000 budget by 20 per cent, the first year paying 80 per cent and the fifth year, when the project was incorporated into the Health Department, paying nothing.[16] Notwithstanding its extensive control, the publicity-shy RF insisted that the host government should receive all credit for programme accomplishments[17] as compensation for considerable concessions. The Foundation's anonymity also allowed it to avoid controversy, such as accusations that it was interfering with local affairs or threatening national sovereignty.

Why did nationalistic Mexico acquiesce to these conditions? For the Mexican elite and Western-trained physicians,[18] RF programmes offered professional and technological advance, international interaction and a means of improving the health and strength of the working population.[19] The chance to modernise overshadowed concern about foreign interference. Revolutionary politicians, anxious to fulfil their promises to the Mexican people, believed that science and public health were neutral forces that would bring progress when coupled with social and political measures such as land redistribution and worker protection.[20] The strict conditions imposed by the RF appeared an inevitable part of a desired public health model that would eventually be implemented, with or without foreign participation.

Once the hookworm campaign was approved in November 1923, the first task was to survey hookworm prevalence and general conditions around Mexico in order to select a locale. Secretary of Health Pruneda's proposal that a survey should be conducted by an IHB physician with two Mexican assistants[21] was rejected by the RF home office, even though IHB officers in Mexico strongly endorsed the idea.[22] RF home office administrator Frederick Russell pictured the 'place' of Mexican doctors in the 'office doing routine campaign work … so they can take it over when we leave', insisting that IHB officer Henry Carr must carry out the hookworm survey alone, for 'he will do it properly'.[23]

Carr was born in Milledgeville, Georgia, in 1895 and graduated from Harvard Medical School in 1920. Three years later he joined the International Health Board, and he spent over thirty years working for the RF in Mexico, Greece, the Dominican Republic, Bolivia, Cuba, Peru and New York.[24] Dispatched to conduct the survey, Carr was warned that, as he travelled through isolated communities, he might be asked to examine people with a variety of ailments unrelated to hookworm; his refusal to provide care could jeopardise the survey, but the provision of too much free care would impede his progress.

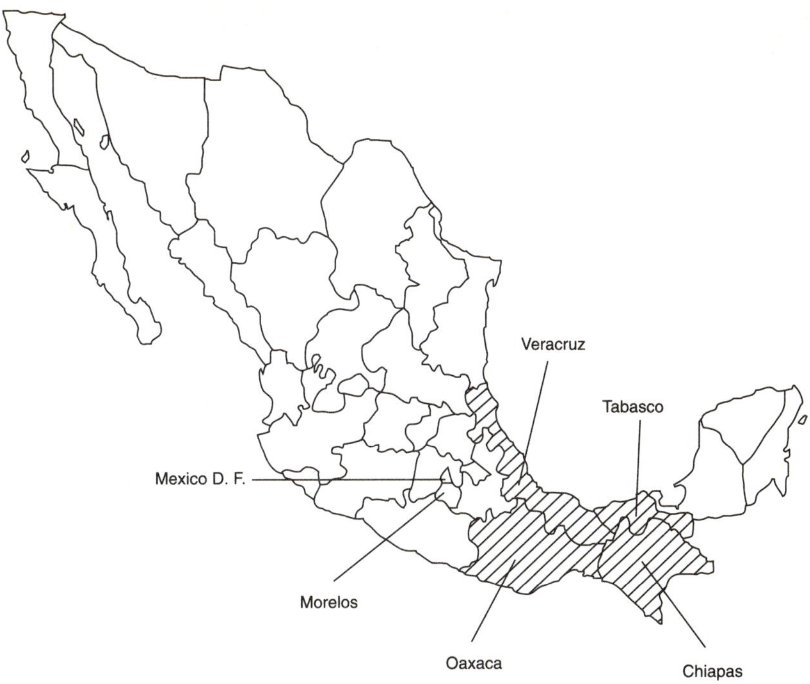

Figure 6.1 Sites of the Rockefeller Foundation hookworm campaign in Mexico, 1 January 1925–30 June 1928 (shaded area).
Source José Amézquita *et al.*, *Historia de la Salubridad y de la Asistencia en México* (Mexico, D.F.: Secretaría de Salubridad y Asistencia, 1960) II, p. 280

In early 1924 Carr set out to examine the geographical distribution of hookworm, the demographic make-up of the infected population, general living and working conditions, the severity of the disease, the source of the infection, the species of hookworm implicated and the overall 'effect of the disease on the individuals involved'.[25]

In Mexico City, the Revolution appeared to have ended with Alvaro Obregón's coup and subsequent election to the Presidency in 1920, but for the rest of the nation a decade of war-time strife left a legacy of rural discontent, violence and peasant uprisings. The main foci of regional conflict were in the states of Michoacán, Zacatecas, Guanajuato and Veracruz.[26] In addition to these agrarian revolts, the militant Cristeros, who opposed the 1917 Constitution's separation of Church and state, instigated open revolts from 1926 through the late 1920s, particularly in the states of Guanajuato, Jalisco, Colima and Michoacán.[27] In 1924 General Plutarco Elias Calles replaced Obregón as President, but challenger Adolfo de la Huerta accused Calles of fraud and collusion with his predecessor. With the support of rebel forces, de la Huerta left the capital and organised insurrection in Veracruz.[28] Peasant militarisation, political turmoil, and Catholic rebellion, together with the United States's repeated threats that it would invade Mexico unless the Constitution's repudiation of foreign oil holdings was overturned, meant that the problems leading to the Revolution – monopolisation of land, low wages, poor education and political instability – remained unresolved. From 1923 to 1928 Mexico lived 'on the brink of catastrophe and in the midst of a profound inner stress that threatened to snap at any time'.[29]

Only casually alerted to which areas might be perilous, Carr apprehensively outlined the criteria he would follow, promising to survey troubled states as soon as they were free of conflict between rebel and federal forces.[30]

After several months surveying hookworm prevalence in coastal communities, Carr was most struck by the relatively *low* level of hookworm infestation, compared with the south of the United States or the West Indies.[31] This observation was overlooked by the home office, which was committed to a hookworm programme regardless of the ailment's epidemiological importance. The RF was convinced that state and local authorities need only be exposed to the hookworm campaign in order to 'create ... a desire for a local health service capable of dealing with the more pressing public health problems'.[32]

In fact the IHB had pinpointed the desired campaign locale before the survey was even begun. Veracruz, the focus of the yellow fever campaign, remained strategic for both the Mexican government and the IHB as a hub of oil production, international commerce, and agriculture. Health activities could increase popular morale, diminish the threat to exports and keep productivity high. Second, a powerful group of anti-Obregón rebels was based in Veracruz. The federal government wished to intensify its activities to gain the support of the general population and counter the rebels.[33] In Veracruz the RF could carry out a federally supported health programme while maintaining relations with the revolutionary forces. Like a magnate who donates money to rival political campaigns, the RF painstakingly courted both the Huertista rebels and the Obregón government.

Though Carr sought to stay in Mexico following the survey, the IHB quickly replaced him with the more seasoned officer, Andrew Warren, who had spent several years with the IHB setting up health demonstration projects in rural Kansas and Oregon. With hookworm staff selected and trained, and supplies arriving, Warren was expecting to go to Veracruz, but owing to 'military disturbances', the programme was instead launched in Tlaxcala in April 1924. The RF maintained that sites were selected for the scientific and practical reasons of high disease prevalence and co-operative local authorities, yet Carr's survey showed virtually no hookworm in Tlaxcala.[34] However, Tlaxcala was accessible to Veracruz, located part way from Mexico City, adjacent to the main artery.[35] Thus the hookworm demonstration programme began in a region known to be hookworm free.

As soon as conditions permitted, the campaign moved its mobile brigades into rural Veracruz. The IHB pursued two approaches, one preventive, the other curative. First, health education strategies were used to try to induce rural Mexicans to wear shoes and build and use latrines. Poverty precluded both options, but peasants gradually began to use the latrines that were built for them. Second, uniformed IHB officers administered an oral dose of chenopodium and a purgative either in a clinic or in the home. The medicine 'magically' cured the hookworm, not unlike the herbs of local healers, but otherwise the treatment was completely alien to rural Mexicans. Most villagers did not perceive themselves as sick, because the symptoms of anaemia were an accustomed part of life. Moreover, the IHB health officers sought patients, not vice versa.

According to medical understanding since the 1920s,[36] hookworm, or uncinariasis, stems from the presence of hookworms (*Necator americanus* in the Americas) in the human digestive tract, with more severe symptoms appearing in persons suffering from malnutrition. Anaemia, stunted growth, fatigue and weakness particularly target children. Other symptoms include yellowed skin, and swollen legs and bellies. The hookworm enters the body where the skin is tender, often between the toes, then migrates through blood vessels to the lungs, where it is coughed out and swallowed into the alimentary tract. There it is nourished by blood sucked through the wall of the upper small intestine; it reproduces and is periodically expelled with faeces. Anyone walking barefoot in places strewn with hookworm-ridden human faeces can come into contact with the disease.

The campaign to promote the use of latrines posed a great challenge to the hookworm brigades. Warren lamented, 'On account of the poverty and the lack of intelligence ... no type [of latrine] suits the needs of the people here.'[37] Only the common earth pit was feasible, but Warren deemed even the wooden platform beyond the means of peons. For a peasant to spend a large sum to construct 'a place to defecate when he and his ancestors have for hundreds of years used the open spaces without apparent cost, is almost too much for us to expect him to comprehend'.

Over the long term, Warren argued, the cost of the *excusado* would be far smaller than the costs of disease and death, but this was not a 'tangible thing'.[38] Warren finally decided on a pit latrine as the 'simplest, the cheapest, the most practical'. With an inclined platform for squatting rather than sitting, because even North Carolina farmers 'could not defecate when sitting ... upon the seat of a water closet', Warren began to perfect the technique. Comparing the peasants to rabbits who were not attracted to brightly-coloured hutches, Warren claimed to understand why peons refused to use sleek new pit latrines which were 'much better than the houses in which they lived'. IHB personnel quickly perfected the construction of rudimentary pit latrines, enclosed by wobbly walls.

Warren argued against offering material support to peons in building latrines because 'they are a tricky, trifling lot and they will do nothing they can make some one else do'.[39] Peons could be instructed, but if supplied with wood, Warren argued, they would sell it rather than build latrines for their families. The Veracruz governor and state health officer, Agustín Hernández Mejía, issued a decree requiring *excusados*. This was a necessary step, Warren argued, because 'The people here are so accustomed to doing things only when they are compelled to.'

Reports from Mexican officials reflected more understanding of the cultural norms surrounding shoe-wearing and defecating. Future Minister of Health Bernardo Gastelum's report on Alvarado, Veracruz, explained that although girls defecated only in one place, they began wearing shoes at the age of ten, which reduced their rates of infection. Young boys always defecated in a new place, but as they grew older they began to concentrate their scatological deposits in one place. Because they did not customarily wear shoes, infection rates increased among older boys.[40]

As John Ettling has noted for the southern United States, before the RF 'could set about the business of destroying' hookworm it had to expend energy and money to 'create the disease in the minds of the people'.[41] Most people with anaemia considered hookworm not an illness but an unavoidable (and largely unrecognised) fate, like hunger. Yet IHB officers expected their illustrated, house-to-house seminars on the life cycle of hookworm to replace popular conceptions of sickness. Villagers stared at the posters, intrigued by the practices of the newcomers and often pleased at the new government activities, but there is no evidence that any subscribed to the germ theory.[42]

Health education efforts employed persuasion strategies that were less alien to rural Mexicans. A pamphlet entitled *La historia de un niño* played on the stereotypes of Mexican men's pride in being bigger and stronger than women. On the front cover of the pamphlet was

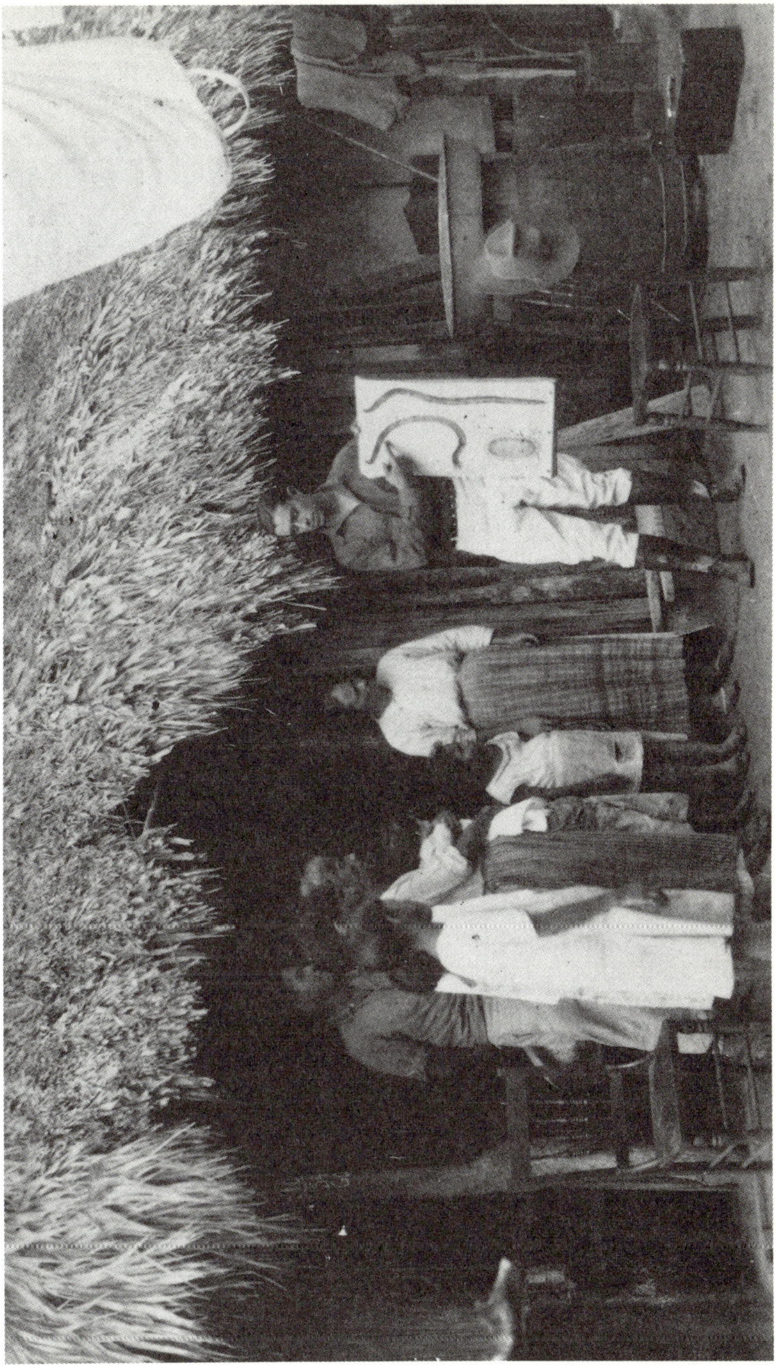

Plate 6.1 Demonstrating the life cycle of the hookworm. *Courtesy* The Rockefeller Archive Center

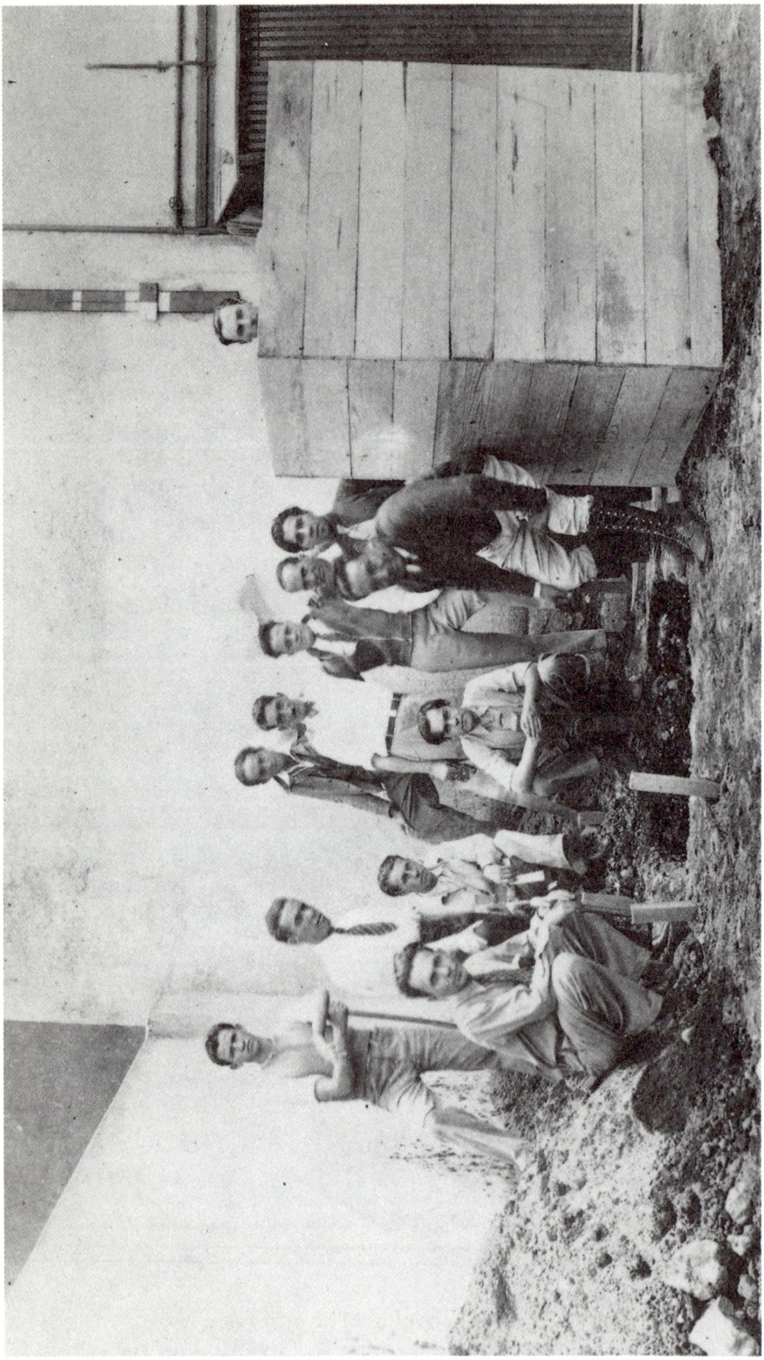

Plate 6.2 Pit latrine construction. *Courtesy* The Rockefeller Archive Center

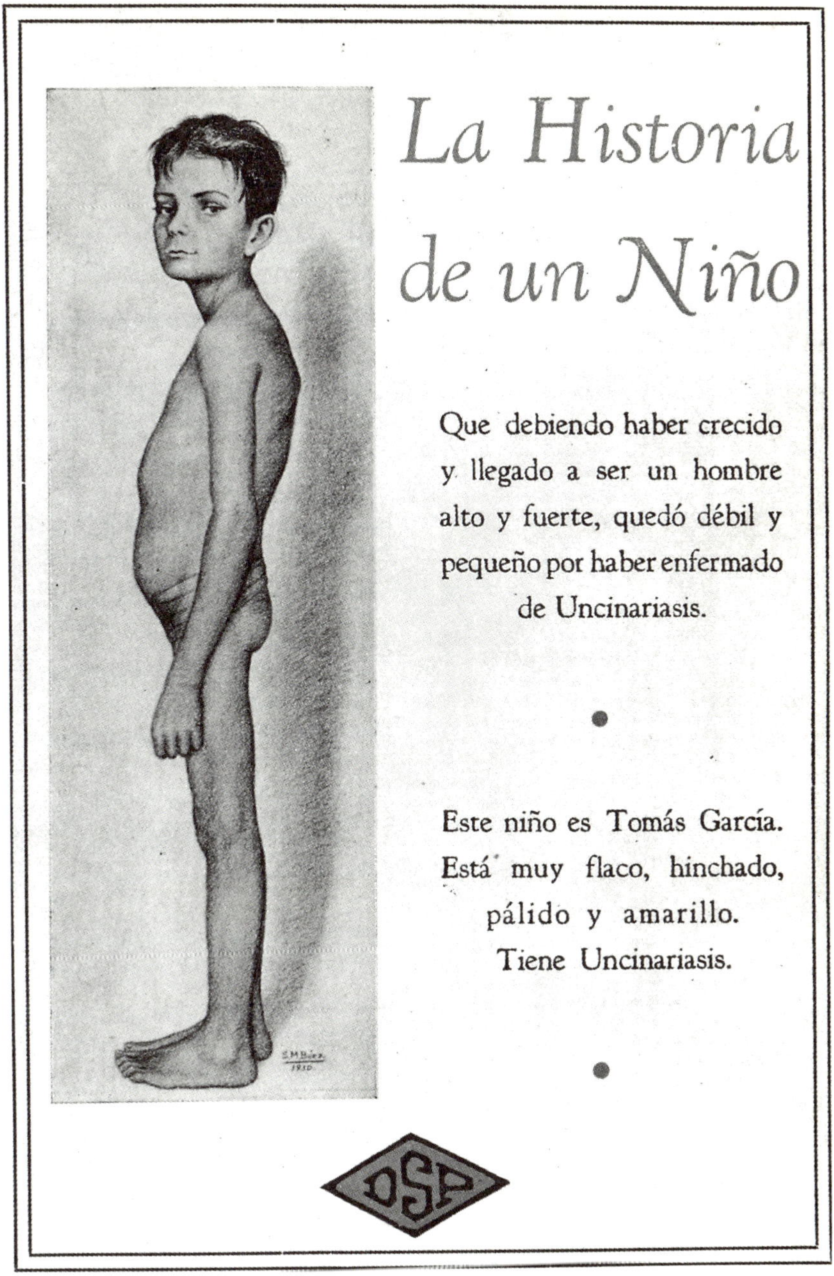

Plate 6.3 Front cover of 'The story of a boy'.
Courtesy The Rockefeller Archive Center

Como recobró sus fuerzas después de curado, trabajó bastante y con diligencia, ahorrando dinero. Poco a poco edificó una casa amplia y alegre. Años después los niños crecieron, pero Tomás, como consecuencia de la enfermedad sufrida, no pudo crecer y quedó pequeño de cuerpo, debiendo haber sido un hombre alto y fuerte, de no haber enfermado de uncinariasis.

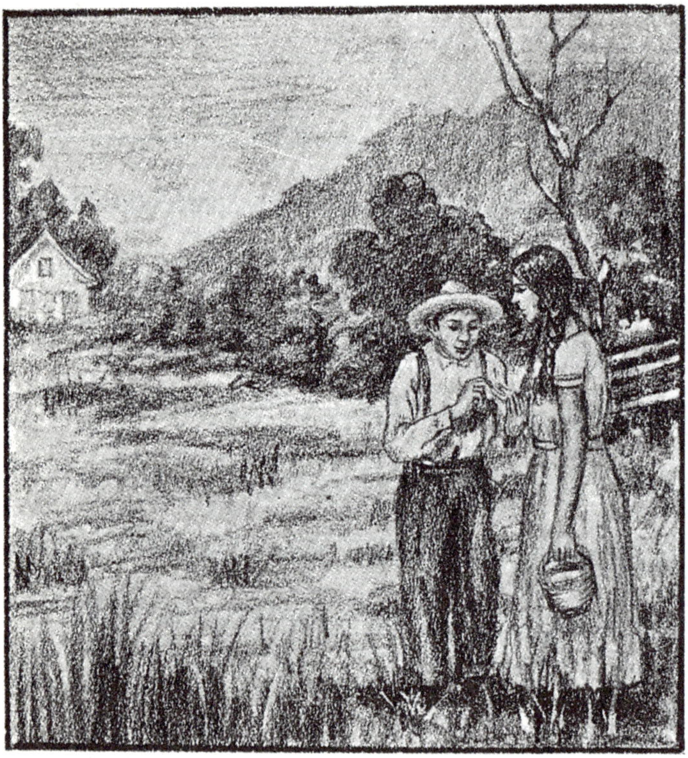

Tomás y Elena ya crecidos. Está sacando una espina del dedo de Elena.

Su hermana Elena, que estaba muy pequeña cuando enfermó y que fué curada a tiempo, sí creció y llegó a ser una joven sana y hermosa.

Plate 6.4 Inside cover of 'The story of a boy'.
Courtesy The Rockefeller Archive Center

Tomás García, a 'skinny, swollen, pale, and yellow' boy. Tomás 'should have grown up to be a tall and strong man but was left weak and small because he had hookworm'. On the next page Tomás was shown cured, but he never grew to the expected manly size. His younger sister Elena, cured of hookworm at an earlier stage, had grown to be a beautiful and healthy young woman, taller and stronger than her elder brother.[43]

The dangers of treatment

At the beginning of 1925 the Rockefeller Foundation's central office was shifted to Veracruz so that Warren could save money on travel and keep a closer eye on the hookworm team now headed by Dr Juan Solórzano Morfin, the respected former chief quarantine officer for Veracruz (who had been extremely supportive of the yellow fever effort). By this time, the campaign had discontinued the use of the dispensary method that required the population to come to the doctor, because people could not be supervised during the hours after they swallowed the medicine and because many failed to return to the clinic for subsequent treatments.

The replacement intensive method required the hookworm brigades to travel from house to house. The anti-helminthic, but not the purgative, was administered under the eye of a trained inspector directly in the home of the individuals being treated. Assistants returned during the course of the day to monitor the condition of those treated. Preliminary fecal examinations were only administered to individuals who refused treatment. Positive results gave 'an added weight to [the inspector's] already heavy argument, and the individual usually takes the medicine'.[44]

In the Veracruz town of Córdoba, the infection rate was approximately 60 per cent, but Warren advocated the use of mass treatment to gain results more quickly, a strategy routinely employed only in areas of high infection (over 75 per cent), where a lower cost per capita could be achieved in this manner. Mass treatment forewent the preliminary diagnosis, treating the entire population regardless of the actual fecal presence of hookworm. However, the occasionally unpleasant, or even fatal, aftereffects of treatment meant that up to one fourth or more of the population would be faced with an unnecessary risk. If the drugs were entirely harmless, Warren noted, this mass 'shotgun method' would be less objectionable.[45]

Notwithstanding this position, Warren employed mass treatment at doses 'not advocated by the [International Health] Board'.[46] He justified the concentrated dose of chenopodium (2 cc at one time, instead of 1 cc per hour during three successive hours) by its efficiency. Because the entire dose was taken in front of unit personnel, he argued, its correct administration was assured. Warren was so convinced of the efficacy of his method that he failed to see its potential dangers. A man believed to be heavily infected with hookworm almost suffocated under Warren's care, but he viewed the absence of the 'distressing consequences' of intoxication as a signal of success.

Warren did recognise that the 'rate and degree of infection in the area probably was not of sufficient gravity to absolutely justify' the mass treatment procedure, but he believed that by eliminating 'time-consuming preliminary examinations', the campaign could quickly provide a large number of treatments, thus gaining popular recognition.[47] Warren acknowledged that 'making an impression with the campaign' was of 'paramount' importance, far greater than the actual value of the treatments.

While IHB director Frederick Russell praised his men for the hurdles they overcame in latrine construction,[48] he paid little attention to the not infrequent instances of poisoning by anti-helminthics. Young children were often the victims of these overdoses, generally dying within hours of chenopodium administration. RF teams did their best to muzzle publicity about the cases lest the hookworm campaign be jeopardised.[49] Officers were required to report any deaths linked with IHB programmes. While candid, the reports were defensive. A nine-year-old girl 'should not have been killed' but she was suffering from malnutrition. Warren denied responsibility for her nutritional state instead of admitting that the hookworm team ought to have recognised her condition and barred treatment.[50] Carr, who returned to Mexico in 1926 to replace Warren, later found that a castor oil purge made the chenopodium less toxic, especially for children. Because the chenopodium also became less efficient, a second dose needed to be given.[51] Rather than facing the social, economic and health problems of malnutrition, the RF came up with technical solutions, ever varying the dose size, drug mix and interval between treatments.

In another case, Warren reported that a seven-year-old boy from San Andrés Tuxtla died from intestinal obstruction, not from the anti-helminthics, using the argument that his entire family was infected with hookworm as (unverified and irrelevant) evidence. In this case, Warren also accused the *ayudantes* (assistants) of improper administration of the drugs. Normally, Warren asserted, the hookworm staff was both well paid and well trained, attracting high quality men. However, the unavoidable hiring of lower paid *ayudantes* had led to the deaths. These *ayudantes* could 'not be trusted … When a $100.00 peso indian [*sic*] tells me he has done something I do not believe him until I have seen the results.'[52] Dr Solórzan Morfín had a different interpretation, complaining that the 'medically ignorant' Warren had attempted to increase the volume of treatments given and overcome his problems in overseeing three brigades and the central office by hiring *ayudantes* and assigning them a minimum quota of weekly treatments.[53]

In trying to keep costs down, Warren explained, 'We have had a very unusual experience that involves the question of the advisability of allowing non-technical men of limited secondary education to administer highly toxic drugs.'[54] After receiving chenopodium and carbon tetrachloride, ninety-three people became ill, thirty severely. Warren identified the probable cause as pulque, a home-made drink made from fermented maguey plant, consumed in large quantities, he maintained, by the majority of the population. Because of the difficulty in changing the popular pulque-drinking custom, Warren's best safeguard was to discontinue the use of carbon tetrachloride, which caused adverse effects when mixed with alcohol. Problems with hookworm treatment were systematically blamed on the habits of Mexican peasants rather than on the campaign's administration.

Resistance and acceptance

In June 1927 the Veracruz newspaper *El Istmo* published an article saying that the IHB campaign had been poorly managed, causing several people to die at the hands of charlatans. Striking at Carr via RF administrator Russell, the article accused Carr of not supervising the clinics and of entrusting Juan López, 'the one who is not a doctor', with patient care. The newspaper promised to investigate further and to 'fight for humanity'.[55] Russell was not fazed by the accusations, attributing the views to a single individual who opposed the campaign's methods. Carr identified the author as an alcoholic physician turned down for a job with the campaign. While ignoring the source of the 'untrue charges', Carr controlled further damage by entertaining the editor and his family, who promptly published 'two nice, sensible articles commending our work'.[56] Warren, too, was plagued by criticism of the dire consequences of hookworm treatment and defensively decried stories 'originated by charlatans and the few we have encountered who were not in sympathy with the work'.[57]

In terms of formal correspondence, the RF's detractors were outnumbered by its fans. Literate citizens and businessmen wrote to the RF in New York to express admiration and to ask 'God that all the benefits that this noble Institution has spread throughout the entire world may be converted into blessings on behalf of the great North American people'.[58]

However, even among elites the hookworm campaign engendered

opposition. In larger towns the IHD units faced the unexpected opposition of another group of practitioners – allopathic physicians. In Minatitlán and Puerto México local physicians charged the unit with 'trying to diminish the amount of disease in the area, jeopardizing their livelihood'.[59] The frustrated IHD officers tried to argue that the clinics would boost rather than diminish the doctors' clientele, for 'as the people become more "health conscious" they will be more ready to consult the physician'.[60] Local doctors were also irritated by the modern equipment used by the sanitary units. They feared that their patients would begin to demand similar sophisticated apparatus. Carr, of course, viewed this as a positive development, but many physicians believed that the new technology would put them out of business, leaving rural populations without even basic medical services.[61]

An evaluation of the campaign

In 1926 the IHB placed Mexican doctors at the head of each of the hookworm brigades, which by then had expanded into the states of Oaxaca and Chiapas. These physicians, who later held important positions in the Health Department, became committed advocates of hookworm control. As evidenced in Table 1, their involvement led to a significant increase in the number of latrines constructed and treatments administered. Warren believed that the expanded role of Mexican physicians increased public confidence in the campaign.[62]

IHB officers recognised treatment as the 'best sort of propaganda for good health'. Each cure of hookworm was 'a very obvious and dramatic occurrence', which became 'an advertisement for better hygiene'.[63] Yet the hookworm brigades served to convince local and state government officials and health officers of the effectiveness of public health measures more than the people. Because the brigades were in each community for a few weeks only, they served more as a novelty to villagers than as proof of the value of health services. The limits to acceptance of health authorities by peasants was demonstrated in a town in Morelos over a decade after the hookworm campaign ended; when a local health officer tried to close down the annual fair to prevent a meningitis epidemic, five soldiers were mobbed and killed and the health officer 'barely escaped hanging'.[64]

The RF viewed the popularity of its efforts more positively. Halfway through the campaign the RF became pleased with the 'good co-operation from district peons'.[65] RF officer Andrew Warren boasted, 'the confidence of the people is such that we can kill a member of the family with chenopodium and the other members will demand that they continue to receive their treatment'.[66] At this level the RF's diplomatic achievements appeared to outweigh the benefits in health.

At the same time, the RF home office was highly satisfied that 'public health work will help to clarify ... a new relationship between the peon and the state and federal governments, and help the peon to understand and appreciate the duties and responsibilities of government to the people and convince him that the government has a real interest in his welfare, health and happiness'.[67] By enabling peasant identification with the new organisations developing in Mexico at the time, the RF at once assisted in legitimising the state and increasing its responsibility for the health of the population.

Hookworm, however, was only a beginning. Carr realised that although his hookworm talks and clinics were well-attended, most villagers suffered from a range of health problems.[68] He proposed the transformation of the hookworm campaign into permanent rural health departments. Simultaneous Mexican interest led to the rapid opening of co-operative sanitary units, but the early activity of the Minatitlán-Puerto México units heavily emphasised hookworm diagnosis and treatment, the testing of anti-helminthic drugs, latrine construction and popular health education lectures, despite Carr's promises to attack the most important diseases. The continued emphasis on hookworm long after the establishment of the co-operative health units rested on the need to show concrete achievements. Hookworm's easy identification and treatment made its control far simpler than any other disease eradication endeavour. At seven each morning, dozens of empty-stomached people would line up for hookworm treatment, receiving 'the same attention as in the private office of the best physician', but for free.[69] Through the 1930s Mexican reports repeatedly stressed the importance of hookworm in Mexico's excess morbidity and mortality rates. The first was an exaggeration and the second close to a lie, but years of hookworm propaganda had convinced many Mexican health officials that hookworm control was the nation's most valuable public health crusade.

IHB officer Warren, and even Carr, became as convinced as these officials in the primacy of hookworm control. Though Warren was aware that hookworm prevalence could not compare with other more fatal diseases, and though he had been repeatedly solicited for co-operation in tuberculosis control (which the home office routinely rejected because 'it takes too many years to show results'[70]), he came to regard hookworm as a root cause of poverty in Mexico. Likewise, Carr, who had witnessed the epidemiological insignificance of hookworm first-hand when he conducted the hookworm survey, became committed to hookworm control after taking over from Warren. Despite evidence to the contrary, Carr deemed hookworm 'more important than malaria'.[71]

Table 6.1 *Hookworm campaign activities, 1924–28*

Year	*Persons treated*	*No. of treatments*	*No. of latrines built*	*Cost ($)*	*1991 equivalent*
1924[a]	21,529	28,763	337	43,836	350,040
1925[b]	44,917	79,228	631	35,694	276,880
1926[c]	53,527	97,660	6,328		
1927[d]	61,877	126,799	5,179		
1928[e]	32,557	78,420	2,768	45,000	357,590

Note Blank spaces indicate missing data.
Sources

[a] Warren, 'The First Annual Report of the Activities of the Hookworm Campaign for Mexico during the Year 1924'. RG 5. Series 3. Box 143. RFA. The *per capita* cost of the hookworm campaign was $1.03 ($8.22 in 1991 terms), which included the population both of persons who received treatment and of those not infested with hookworm (and not receiving treatment).

[b] Warren to Russell, 31 December 1925. Rockefeller Foundation Archives. RG 5. Series 3. Box 144. By the second year of the programme the *per capita* cost dropped by more than half, to 43 cents.

[c] Carr, 'Annual report of the Lucha contra la Uncinariasis', Section for Tropical Diseases of the Departamento de Salubridad Pública, for the year 1926. Rockefeller Foundation Archives. RG 5. Series 3. Box 144.

[d] Carr, 'Annual report of the Lucha contra la Uncinariasis', Section for Tropical Diseases of the Departamento de Salubridad Pública, for the year 1927. Rockefeller Foundation Archives. RG 5. Series 3. Box 144.

[e] Carr, Annual Report of the Lucha contra la Uncinariasis, Section for Tropical Diseases of the Departamento de Salubridad Pública, for the year 1928. Rockefeller Foundation Archives. RG 5. Series 3. Box 144.

Discussion

In the late 1940s, as the IHD was deciding on its future in the post-war era, dozens of officers wrote to offer suggestions on the organisation's continuing responsibilities. Henry Carr advocated the IHD's return to 'fundamentals', especially hookworm control, for:

> there is just as much hookworm disease in countries where the climate is favorable for it, as there was in 1913 when the Foundation was established. I know because I have seen it all, and there is no public health work that benefits so many people and in such a real and vital way.[72]

Finally, in 1951, after much soul-searching, the IHD was collapsed into a scaled-down Division of Medicine and Public Health (which was headed by the Mexico hookworm campaign director Andrew

Warren from 1951 to 1954), with international health work limited to scientific consultation to, for example, UNICEF projects.

Though a preliminary survey found hookworm to be an epidemiologically minor problem in Mexico, the RF expended considerable energy on adapting its campaign to local conditions. Numerous obstacles, including the resistance of local doctors and populations, the death of villagers undergoing treatment, and the health officers' limited ability to understand the scatological practices of rural Mexicans, delayed widespread support for the hookworm campaign.

Throughout the campaign there were different levels of resistance, from peasant refusal to build and employ latrines to the Mexican government's attempts to shape the organisation of activities to physician opposition to outside intervention for corporatist reasons. Resistance must be defined broadly in order to incorporate both hierarchical and substantive distinctions. Following the hookworm campaign, the RF used increasingly sophisticated means of fending off opposition. Once the novelty of the hookworm campaign had worn off, hostile groups of traditional healers organised in hilltop towns in Morelos through the early 1930s, with enough popular support to prevent the RF from establishing local health units for several years.[73] Displeased at the new providers who had begun to displace them, the *curanderos* and their communities held to a unified concept of spiritual and physical well-being as opposed to the bifurcated beliefs of the outsiders, who failed to attend to the spiritual needs of the ill.[74] Public health measures exported not only the curing, repairing and pain mitigation roles of Western science but also its ideological and philosophical orientation: the Cartesian duality between mind and body, a mechanistic view of the body, and the allopathic duality between prevention and cure – notions incompatible with the philosophies of numerous Mexican cultures.

While *curanderos* were brushed aside as superstitious witches, empirical midwives were brought into the units for modern sanitary training, for they provided a service that the units could not fulfil. Through the 1930s dozens of barefoot midwives were equipped with black bags, taught how to use forceps and persuaded that supine mothers delivered the healthiest babies.[75]

Many of the most lasting changes in the conceptualisation and practice of public health following the hookworm campaign were effected through the grants the RF offered to individual health professionals for study in the United States. Over three decades these prestigious fellowships went to forty-two physicians, six nurses and twenty sanitary engineers.[76] During the same period dozens of Mexican health officials, including each incoming Minister of Health, received travel grants to visit North American public health offices and research centres.[77] These administrators would assure that the IHD models would stay firmly in place and that a new generation of public health officers would be trained similarly. Fellows were selected for their intelligence, capacity to work and, especially, the likelihood that they would dedicate their career to government service.[78] Such guarantees seemed unattainable, yet in 1940 IHD representative George Payne could proudly report that, of thirty-nine Mexican fellows, thirty-six were serving in the government. Most occupied influential positions, including secretary-general, director of epidemiology and head of the Institute of Hygiene.[79] The home office was elated: 'If infiltration of the governmental health structure of Mexico with trained personnel continues ... the outlook is with real optimism'.[80] Thus, in the years following the hookworm campaign, the RF relied more on subtle hegemonic techniques to avoid opposition than on direct confrontation.

Once hookworm control was accepted by rural Mexicans, however, no other public health activity could surpass its popularity and efficacy. Mexican leaders and health officials recognised the political benefits of hookworm control, gaining credibility for bringing popular social programmes to the people. Long after the RF had begun to develop local health units to handle a wider and more pressing range of health needs, the hookworm campaign's educational, therapeutic and latrine-building activities remained key elements of public health efforts in rural Mexico.

Ultimately, and perhaps ironically, the elimination of hookworm disease was not the goal of the hookworm campaign. Instead it offered an effective means of igniting interest in public health among the Mexican political establishment, physicians and rural inhabitants through a dramatic demonstration of hookworm control. The hookworm campaign also set the terms of the relationship between Mexico and the RF. The foundation maintained administrative control even though its representatives were officially in subordinate positions within the Department of Public Health; it set budget incentives that assured Mexico's long-term commitment to the disease control endeavours launched by the RF; it promoted a public health orientation that favoured the control of diseases amenable to individualised medical interventions; it encouraged the replacement of traditional health practices and practitioners with their 'scientific medicine' counterparts; and it began to stimulate the professional training and full-time commitment of health personnel. These transformations began during the hookworm campaign, but were only strengthened during subsequent RF programmes, through the development of a modern, US-style network of local public health departments and the moulding of a cadre of promising young doctors to lead the transition.

In the end, opposition to the hookworm campaign was muted by the enthusiasm of intermediary Mexican officials, just as Babar smoothed the way for acceptance of an elephant hospital. In accordance with the RF's intentions, and despite considerable resistance, hookworm's demonstrable, dramatic cure and the technical feasibility of eradication, regardless of hookworm's secondary medical importance, made Mexico's acceptance of modern public health possible by laying the groundwork for the founding of local sanitary units and the training of a vast network of health personnel in RF-supported institutions in both the United States and Mexico. Hookworm served as an 'entering wedge', but the wedge became lodged in Mexican soil.

Notes

1 Ariel Dorfman, *The Empire's Old Clothes: What the Lone Ranger, Babar and Other Innocent Heroes Do to Our Minds*. New York: Pantheon Books, 1983.

2 Jean de Brunhoff, *Le Voyage de Babar*. Paris: Hachette, 1952.

3 For a thorough account of the Rockefeller Sanitary Commission see John Ettling, *The Germ of Laziness Rockefeller Philanthropy and Public Health in the New South*, Cambridge, Mass.: Harvard University Press, 1981. An engaging study is Stephen J. Kunitz's 'Hookworm and pellagra: exemplary diseases in the new south', *Journal of Health and Social Behavior* 29 (1988): 139–48. Also see Mary Boccaccio, 'Ground itch and dew poison: the Rockefeller Sanitary Commission, 1909–14', *Journal of the History of Medicine and Allied Sciences*, 27 (1972): 30–53; James H. Cassedy, 'The "Germ of laziness" in the south, 1900–15: Charles Wardell Stiles and the progressive paradox', *Bulletin of the History of Medicine* 45 (1971): 159–69; and William Link, 'Privies, progressivism, and public schools: health reform and education in the rural south, 1909–20', *Journal of Southern History* 54 (1988): 623–42. For the most extensive portrait to date of the Rockefeller Foundation see Raymond Fosdick, *The story of the Rockefeller Foundation*, 2nd edn, New Brunswick, NI, Transaction Publishers, 1989. Also see Robert Shaplen, *Toward the Well-being of Mankind: Fifty Years of the Rockefeller Foundation*, New York: Doubleday, 1964.

4 John Ettling's fascinating study of the Sanitary Commission reveals the development of important working relationships and campaign strategies that served as a model for later endeavours in international health.

5 The history of the IHD has been incompletely told by Lewis Hackett, 'Once upon a time', *American Journal of Tropical Medicine and Hygiene*, 9 (2 1960): 105–15; Greer Williams, *The Plague Killers*. New York: Scribner, 1969; and Fosdick, *Rockefeller Foundation*. There are numerous memoirs by physicians who worked with the International Health Board. For instance, M. E. M. Walker, *Pioneers of Public Health: the Story of some Benefactors of the Human Race*, Edinburgh: Oliver & Boyd, 1930; Wilder Penfield, *The Difficult Art of Giving: the Epic of Alan Gregg*, Boston: Little, Brown and Company, 1967; Benjamin E. Washburn, *As I Recall*, New York: Rockefeller Foundation, 1960; Hugh H. Smith, *Life's a Pleasant Institution: the Peregrinations of a Rockefeller Doctor*. Tucson, Ariz., 1978; Victor Heiser, *An American Doctor's Odyssey: Adventures in Forty-five Countries*. New York: Norton, 1936; Fred Soper, *Ventures in World Health: the Memoirs of Fred Lowe Soper*, ed. John Duffy, Washington, D.C.: Pan-American Health Organization, 1977.

6 Armando Solórzano, 'The Rockefeller Foundation in Mexico: nationalism, public health, and yellow fever, 1911–24, Ph.D. dissertation, University of

Wisconsin–Madison, 1990.

7 This chapter is based in large part upon A. E. Birn, 'Local health and foreign wealth: the Rockefeller Foundation's Public Health Programs in Mexico, 1924–51', Sc.D. dissertation, Johns Hopkins University, 1993.

8 Report by John A. Ferrell on visit to Mexico, 14 March–13 April 1941. Statement corrected 28 September 1942. Rockefeller Foundation Archives. RG 2 – Stacks. Box 561. Folder 3814.

9 The RF budget for Mexico in 1927 was $6,855.39; in 1928, $2,239.15.

10 International Health Board, Summary of Politics in Force, Public Health Work, 25 May 1927. Rockefeller Foundation Archives. RG 3.1. Series 908. Box 11. Folder 123.

11 Through the 1920s a 'yellow' journalist could earn a sizable bonus by exposing a yellow fever outbreak in a Mexican or Brazilian port. Yellow fever also served as an entering 'wedge' into a country, but the urgency of its elimination dictated different operating conditions. In Mexico, for example, the RF shouldered almost the entire cost (over $100,000 per year) and did not mask its commanding role in the campaign.

12 Wickliffe Rose to Alfonso Pruneda, 4 December 1922. Rockefeller Foundation Archives. RG 5. Series 1.2. Box 137. Folder 1820.

13 Alfonso Pruneda to Wickliffe Rose, 19 February 1923; and Alfonso Pruneda to Frederick Russell, 20 March 1923. Rockefeller Foundation Archives. RG 5. Series 1.2. Box 162. Folder 2110.

14 Solórzano, 'Rockefeller Foundation in Mexico'.

15 'Proyecto para el plan en participación que deberá seguirse por un período de cinco años entre el Gobierno de México y la International Health Board para dominar la Uncinariasis', 12 November 1923. Archivo Histórico de la Secretaría de Salud y Asistencia. RG Public Health. Presidential Section. Box 8. Folder 17.

16 *Ibid.*

17 Vincent to Sheffield, 21 May 1925. Rockefeller Foundation Archives. RG 1.1. Series 323. Box 13. Folder 93.

18 Those at the top of the medical profession stood to gain in prestige through the expansion of the legitimacy of American-style allopathic medicine. Interview with Felipe García Sanchez, former RF fellow, Health Department official, Mexico City, 5 June 1991. See also Robert Lambert, 'Medical education in Mexico survey'. 14–30 November 1936. Rockefeller Foundation Archives. RG 1.1. Series 323. Box 13. Folder 95.

19 Private Mexican citizens and businessmen wrote to the RF in New York to express admiration and to ask 'God that all the benefits that this noble Institution has spread throughout the entire world may be converted into blessings on behalf of the great North American people', Tomas Perrín to George Vincent, 6 April 1926. Rockefeller Foundation Archives. RG 5. Series 1.2. Box 257. Folder 3272. Also see E. R. Brown, 'Public health in imperialism: early Rockefeller programs at home and abroad', *American Journal of Public Health* 66 (9 1976): 897–903.

20 See, for example, *Plan Sexenal, 1934–40, Partido Revolucionario Nacional*, Querétaro, 1933.

21 Pruneda to Vaughn, 14 March 1924. Rockefeller Foundation Archives. RG 5. Series 1.2. Box 193. Folder 2475.

22 Vaughn to Russell, 15 March 1924. Rockefeller Foundation Archives. RG 5. Series 1.2. Box 193. Folder 2474.

23 Russell to Vaughn, 25 March 1924. Rockefeller Foundation Archives. RG 5. Series 1.2. Box 193. Folder 2475.

24 Unsigned memo, circa 1955, Rockefeller Foundation Archives, RG 3.2. Series 908. Box 6. File 55.

25 The most laboured point in the survey was that the microscopic examination of faecal specimens for the presence of ova was a faulty measure because not all persons with positive stools had the disease, a discovery previously made by Darling, Smillie and Cort. See Warren and Carr, 'The incidence of hookworm disease in Mexico', technical report to the IHB, 1925. Rockefeller Foundation Archives. RG 5. Series 2. Sub-series 323. Box 33. Folder 199.

26 See Alan Knight, *The Mexican Revolution*, 2 vols, Cambridge University Press, 1986; Heather Fowler Salamini, *Agrarian Radicalism in Veracruz 1920–1938*, Lincoln: University of Nebraska Press, 1978; and Paul Friedrick, 'Agrarian revolt in Naranja', in W. Dirk Raat and William Beezley, eds, *Twentieth Century Mexico*, Lincoln: University of Nebraska Press, 1986, pp. 159–67.

27 David C. Bailey, *Viva Cristo Rey! The Cristero Rebellion and the Church-State Conflict in Mexico*, Austin: University of Texas Press, 1974; Jean A. Meyer, *The Cristero Rebellion: The Mexican People Between Church and State, 1926–1929*, Cambridge University Press, 1976.

28 Lyle C. Brown, 'The Calles-Cárdenas connection', in W. Dirk Raat and William Beezley, eds, *Twentieth Century Mexico*, Lincoln: University of Nebraska Press, 1986, pp. 146–58.

29 Frank Tannenbaum, *The Struggle for Peace and Bread*, New York: Alfred A. Knopf, 1950, p. 65. Also see Heather Fowler Salamini, 'Adalberto Tejada and the Veracruz Peasant Movement', in James W. Wilkie, Michael C. Meyer and Edna Monzón de Wilkie, *Contemporary Mexico: Papers of the IV International Congress of Mexican History*, Los Angeles: University of California Press, UCLA Latin American Center, 1976.

30 Carr to Vaughn, 19 April 1924. Rockefeller Foundation Archives. RG 5. Series 1.2. Box 193. File 2470.

31 Carr to Russell, 18 September 1924. Rockefeller Foundation Archives. RG 5. Series 1.2. Box 193. Folder 2470.

32 Ferrell to Carr, 8 October 1929. Rockefeller Foundation Archives. RG 1.1. Series 323. Box 17. Folder 140.

33 See Solórzano, 'The Rockefeller Foundation in Mexico'.

34 H. P. Carr, 'Observations upon hookworm disease in Mexico', *American Journal of Hygiene* (6 (July supplement) 1926): 42–61.

35 *Ibid.*

36 A current popular medical school text is Michael Katz, Dickson Despommier and Robert Gwadz, *Parasitic Diseases*, New York: Springer, 1982. Helminthological and entomological references from the first decades of the century include Robert Hegner and William Taliaferro, *Human Protozoology*, New York: Macmillan, 1924; Millard Langfeld, *Introduction to Infectious and Parasitic Diseases, including their Cause and Manner of Transmission*, Philadelphia, Pa.: Blakiston, 1907; and Ernest Carroll Faust, *Human Helminthology: a Manual for Clinicians, Sanitarians, and Medical Zoologists*. Philadelphia, Pa.: Lea & Febiger, 1929.

37 All citations in this paragraph are from Warren to Russell, 9 July 1925. Rockefeller Foundation Archives. RG 5. Series 1.2. Box 226. Folder 2875.

38 *Ibid.*

39 *Ibid.*

40 Bernardo Gastelum, 'Report of the Lucha contra la Uncinariasis', May 1925. Rockefeller Foundation Archives. RG 5. Series 3. Box 144.

41 J. Ettling, *The Germ of Laziness*: 23.

42 Interview with Alberto P. León, former RF fellow, Health Department official and current Institute of Health Tropical Diseases professor, Mexico City, 10 April 1991.

43 *La historia de un niño*, Departamento de Salubridad Pública, Servicio de Propaganda y Educación Higiénica, Lucha Contra la Uncinariasis, Mexico, 1930. Archivo Histórico del Estado de Morelos. Section II/021/241. Box 39. Folder 83.

44 Warren, 'Report of the Lucha Contra la Uncinariasis for the Quarter ending 31 March 1925'. Rockefeller Foundation Archives. RG 5. Series 3. Box 144.

45 Warren to Read, 26 July 1924. Rockefeller Foundation Archives. RG 1.1. Series 323. Box 17. File 139.

46 All citations in this paragraph are from: Warren to IHB, 28 August 1924. Rockefeller Foundation Archives. RG 1.1. Series 323. Box 17. Folder 139.

47 All citations in this paragraph are from: Warren, 'Narrative report of the work of the Lucha Contra la Uncinariasis for the Córdoba Area, 1925'. Rockefeller Foundation Archives. RG 5. Series 3. Box 144.

48 Russell to Warren, 19 March 1925. Rockefeller Foundation Archives. RG 5. Series 1.2. Box 226. Folder 2875.

49 The efforts to avoid publicity regarding treatment-related deaths were largely successful. In 1927 Juan Solórzano Morfín, who himself had administered a lethal dose of chenopodium when he was campaign director, complained about these reproachable mistakes, but he excused the RF because of the campaign's success in awakening both physicians and the public to the problem of intestinal parasites. See Juan Solórzano Morfín, 'Tratamiento de la uncinariasis', *Gaceta Médica de México*, 58 (6 1927): 331.

50 *Ibid.*: 363.

51 Carr to Russell, 3 September 1926. Rockefeller Foundation Archives. RG 5. Series 1.2. Box 257. File 3275.

52 Andrew Warren, 'Report of case of poisoning by antihelminthic', 29 March 1926. Rockefeller Foundation Archives. RG 5. Series 2. Subseries 323. Box 33. File 196.

53 Juan Solórzan Morfin, p. 336.

54 Warren to Read, 26 July 1924. Rockefeller Foundation Archives. RG 1.1. Series 323. Box 17. File 139.

55 *El Istmo* 4 June 1927. Rockefeller Foundation Archives. RG 5. Series 1.2. Box 296. File 3753.

56 Carr to Russell, 5 July 1927. Rockefeller Foundation Archives. RG 5. Series 1.2. Box 296. File 3753.

57 Warren, 'Narrative report of the hookworm work in Mexico for the year 1925'. Rockefeller Foundation Archives. RG 5. Series 3. Box 144.

58 See, for example, Thomas Perrín to George Vincent, 6 April 1926. Rockefeller Foundation Archives. RG 5. Series 1.2. Box 257. File 3272.

59 Carr to Russell, 19 August 1928. Rockefeller Foundation Archives. RG 1.1. Series 323. Box 19. Folder 156.

60 *Ibid.*

61 *Ibid.*

62 Warren to Russell, 27 May 1924. Rockefeller Foundation Archives. RG 5. Series 1.2. Box 258. File 3281.

63 Carr, 'Annual report of the Lucha Contra la Uncinariasis, Section for Tropical Diseases of the Departamento de Salubridad Pública, for the year 1926'. RG 5. Series 3. Box 144. RFA.

64 Bailey to Ferrell, 9 May 1940. Rockefeller Foundation Archives. RG 1.1. Series 323. Box 20. File 165.

65 Russell to Carr, 24 March 1927. Rockefeller Foundation Archives. RG 5. Series 1.2. Box 296. File 3753.

66 Warren to Russell, 15 July 1926. Rockefeller Foundation Archives. RG 5. Series 1.2. Box 258. File 3282.

67 Russell to Warren, 31 December 1925. Rockefeller Foundation Archives. RG 5. Series 1.2. Box 226. File 2876.

68 Carr, 'Lucha Contra la Uncinariasis of the Departamento de Salubridad Pública, for the 3rd Quarter of 1926'. Rockefeller Foundation Archives. RG 5. Series 3. Box 144.

69 'Report of the Hookworm Campaign, the Minatitlán-Puerto México Cooperative Sanitary Unit, and the Puerto México Antilarval Service for the Second Quarter, 1931'. Communicable Diseases Section, Departamento de Salud Pública, México, D.F. Archivo Histórico del Estado de Morelos. Section II/021/242. Box 39. Folder 84.

70 Russell to Warren, 26 March 1926. Rockefeller Foundation Archives. RG 5. Series 1.2. Box 258. File 3281.

71 Carr to Russell, 11 December 1928. Rockefeller Foundation Archives. RG 1.1. Series 323. Box 21. File 169. The RF did become involved in malaria activities in Mexico, but mostly form a research perspective. Malariologist Walter Earle and others investigated mosquito trapping methods, the links between rice cultivation and malaria, and the use of DDT as a household and human de-lousing insecticide. The first community-wide trials of DDT for typhus control were carried out in Mexico in the early 1940s, when the sashes worn by traditionally-dressed peasants were sprayed

with DDT. See Birn, 'Local health', for more details.

72 Henry Carr to G. K. Strode, 1 June, 1950. Rockefeller Foundation Archives. RG 3.1. Series 908. Box 14. Folder 148. In 1951, after much soul-searching, the IHD was collapsed into a scaled-down Division of Medicine and Public Health (which was headed by Mexico hookworm campaign director Andrew Warren from 1951 to 1954), with international health work limited to scientific consultation to, for example, UNICEF projects.

73 Hermillo Espinoza Canales, retired chauffeur for Cuernavaca Sanitary Unit, interview with Birn, Cuernavaca, Morelos, 15 April 1991.

74 Francisco Guerra, 'Pre-Columbian medicine: its influence on medicine today', in John Z. Bowers and Elizabeth F. Purcell, eds, *Aspects of the History of Medicine in Latin America*, New York: Josiah Macy, Jr. Foundation, 1979. Mexican officials and physicians were mostly the descendants of Spaniards, holding European religious and scientific views. Catholic *mestizos*, who assumed a larger role in public life following the Revolution, comprised the majority of the Mexican population. Numerous indigenous communities had been 'converted' to Catholicism, and Christian symbols were often incorporated into the traditional religion.

75 'La Guera' Colonel, retired nurse for Jojutla, Morelos sanitary unit, Cuernavaca, Morelos, interview with Birn, 15 February 1991. Also see Informe del Servicio de Higiene Rural por el primer trimestre, Sección de Enfermedades Comunicables, Departamento de Salubribad Pública, 1931. Archivo Histórico del Estado de Morelos. Section II/021/241. Box 39. Folder 83.

76 Table IIa, 'Public health fellowships and nursing fellowships for the years 1917–1950', in *The Rockefeller Directory of Fellowship Awards, 1917–1950*. New York: Rockefeller Foundation, 1950. Rockefeller Foundation Archives. RG 12. Series 100. Box 32. Folder 239.

77 Fellowship Recorder Cards. Rockefeller Foundation Archives. RG 10. IHB TG Mexico.

78 Ferrell to Carr, 31 January 1930. Rockefeller Foundation Archives. RG 2. Series 323. Box 41. Folder 341.

79 Payne to Ferrell, 25 October 1940. Rockefeller Foundation Archives. RG 1.1. Series 323. Box 20. Folder 165.

80 Ferrell to Payne, 28 October 1940. Rockefeller Foundation Archives. RG 1.1. Series 323. Box 20. Folder 165.

CHAPTER SEVEN

Unequal contenders, uneven ground: medical encounters in British India, 1820–1920

Deepak Kumar

> The countrymen of Manu, Confucius, Zoroaster and Mahomet cannot be said to be mere imitators. Philosophy, literature and the sciences and arts are not unknown to them. The difference between them and the nations of modern Europe is a difference of degree and number ... When we descend, however, from the concrete to the particular, the difference by no means appears to be so great as it would at first sight.

Thus wrote S. C. G. Chuckerbutty (1826–74), who, in 1855, was the first Indian medical graduate to join the Indian Medical Service (IMS).[1] This statement was a subtle and soft defence of what he had inherited *vis-à-vis* what he had acquired in the course of his training in modern medicine. The defence was a difficult project and perhaps doomed, given the colonial nature of the encounter he was witnessing. Differences were made to 'appear' great (though in some cases they were real enough). Colonial hegemony rested upon baring the differences, real or assumed, and stamping one's supremacy.[2] Medical discourse was an important tool to achieve this and at the same time 'a critical site of interaction and conflict'.[3] It was a double-edged weapon: it could distance and universalise simultaneously; one side emphasised the intrinsic difference between the two cultures while the other worked for a scientific hegemony.

Never before had India faced a challenge like this. Hindus and Muslims practised two different systems but they collaborated – at least in the field of medicine – and rarely fought over it.[4] *Madanul-shifa-Sikandarshahi* (an early sixteenth-century Indian medical text written in Persian) is an example of this composite culture, evolving over centuries of coexistence. Numerous medical texts and commentaries were written in Sanskrit, Arabic and Persian between the ninth and eighteenth centuries.[5] Indian medical traditions were fairly strong and epistemologically not dissimilar to those of the Europeans when they arrived. In Goa the Portuguese had appreciated the local physicians (vaidyas) and even licensed them.[6] The European doctors who accompanied every naval despatch from Europe emerged as powerful interlocutors (for both political and cultural purposes). They not only looked after the sick on board ship and on land, but were also the first to report on the flora, fauna, resources and cultural practices of the new territory. They were surgeon-naturalists and adventure-scientists, roles in which they felt superior in their encounters with medical practices of other peoples, although, intermittently, they did show respect for the latter.[7] Increasingly, however, the colonial doctors developed into a cultural force. They began to redefine what they saw in the colonies in terms of their own training and perceptions. Their work encompassed not only the understanding and possible conquest of new diseases but also the extension of Western cultural values to the non-Western world.[8] Gradual assimilation or synthesis was not on their agenda.

India came to be described as a vast pathological reservoir, overlaid perennially by a thick layer of maladies. The new code words were 'sudden', 'severe', 'decline', 'decadence', 'deterioration', 'degeneration' and, worst of all, 'putrefaction'.[9] Against this backdrop, there were signs of some ambivalence and some appreciation of the indigenous ethos at least until the mid-nineteenth century. In this category comes the work of J. Johnson (1813), B. Heyne (1814), H. Wilson (1825), W. Ainslie (1826), W. Twining (1832), G. Playfair (1833), J. R. Martin (1837, 1856), J. F. Royle (1837), T. W. Wise (1845) and many others.[10] However, it was the culture of ancient India that began to receive glowing tributes. Royle talked of 'a full and continued stream of light, which shows that the ancient Hindoos, with great acuteness and philosophical discernment, turned their attention successfully to almost every department of human knowledge'.[11] Medieval India, by contrast, came in for stinging criticism. Decadence and Muslim rule emerged as synonyms. Not many Indians would have agreed with these perceptions. But the educated Indians of the early and mid nineteenth century did show signs of restlessness and an acute sense of identity crisis. The language and practice of medicine were to play an important role in this.

Co-opting the new signs

From the Indian point of view the mid nineteenth century was a period of looking for fresh opportunities and acquiring new knowledge. Syncretism, not revivalism, was the agenda. Even among the British officials there were some who wanted the government to attempt a fusion of 'both exotic principles and local practices, European theory and

Indian experience', and thereby 'revive, invigorate, enlighten and liberalize the native medical profession in the mofussil'.[12] Similar views were echoed by the emerging Indian intelligentsia in ample measure. To illustrate, we cite three relatively less known (though important) Indians from the three presidency areas: Raja Serfoji (1798–1832, Tanjore), B. G. Jambhekar (1802–46, Bombay) and S. C. G. Chuckerbutty (1826–74, Calcutta).

Raja Serfoji, the last Maratha ruler of Tanjore, having surrendered real power to the British Resident, spent his time in the pursuit of knowledge. Father Schwartz, a German missionary, was his friend, philosopher and guide. Fascinated by the different medical systems, he had opened an institution for research in medical science and called it the Dhanvantri Mahal (abode of Lord Dhanvantri, the God of Medicine). He assembled leading physicians there from the Ayurvedic, Yunani, Siddha and Western systems. As a result of their interactions and investigations, the best among the tried and effective remedies were collected in a series of works named *Sarabendra Vaidya Muraigal*.[13] These were composed by the court poet in Tamil verse to facilitate easy memorising and popularisation. With the help of Father Schwartz and the British Resident, Serfoji procured hundreds of European medical books and even surgical instruments. He already had a large collection of Tamil and Sanskrit manuscripts. Some of them dealt with diseases of animals and even birds. Ahead of his time, Serfoji also organised a hand-painted herbarium of medicinal plants in natural colours.[14] In the eye wing of his Dhanvantri Mahal he maintained a set of ophthalmic case sheets in an album, with authentic pictures of the eye and its defects for research purposes. This is perhaps a very early example of 'methodical clinical research' under 'native' patronage, and must have induced the traditional physicians to take cognisance of the new therapies and methods.

Serfoji was not an intellectual. He was a man of resources with a genuine interest in medicine; perhaps a self-taught doctor, he is said to have learnt the art of cataract removal. In contrast, Bal Gangadhar Jambhekar was the first Indian to teach mathematics at the Elphinstone College in Bombay. He was also perhaps the first Indian to start a journal for popularising science (*Bombay Durpan* in 1831) and established the Native Education Society, which later did a commendable job of translating some European works into Marathi and Sanskrit works (like the nosology of Madhav and the anotomy of Susrut) into English. He wanted the native practitioners to improve by studying 'anatomy from the natural subject', even though touching a dead body was taboo at the time.[15] In 1837 his opinion was sought by the Bombay government on the desirability of a medical school in Bombay and the nature of medical education to be given to the natives. In a written reply Jambhekar asked for (1) the education of a limited number of natives in all branches of the science, and (2) the dissemination of the elements of medical knowledge among the vaidyas, hakims and the community of the interior in general through the means of local language.[16]

This dissemination was to be achieved through translations or writing synthetic books specifically for the purpose. Ordinary vaidyas and hakims, he felt, would respond better than the more 'learned' native practitioners, as the latter were quite convinced of their own superiority and were unlikely to compromise their status. Jambhekar wanted the government to go slowly, without ruffling feelings, and be 'as little offensive as possible'. He argued that the repugnance of the Brahmins at dissection, etc., could be overcome 'by a little perseverance'.[17] How right he was!

S. C. Chuckerbutty came from a Brahmin family. He graduated from Calcutta Medical College and was one of the first four Indian medical graduates sent to England for higher studies, in 1845. He was so much charmed by Western values and people that he even embraced Christianity before leaving for England, and put his teacher's name before his surname (he became Soorjo Coomar Goodeve Chuckerbutty). Later he pronounced 'a day in London' of more value 'than a month in Calcutta'.[18] True to his training, he lambasted indigenous practitioners: 'Every Boydo (vaidya) was a born Koberaj (physician) ... To suppose that a Boydo could not be a physician unless he passed an examination, was to question the ruling of Manu (an ancient law-giver).'[19] He was not in favour of medical education through Sanskrit or Arabic. He called it 'oriental mania'. He did not mix with the native community. As the distance grew a contemporary noted that his 'own' people could not perceive in his success (as a member of the Indian Medical Service) 'the triumph of the cause which they have so anxiously at heart'.[20] But Chuckerbutty's perceptions later changed. He came to support the vernacular medium fully and criticised Calcutta University for representing 'only European opinion and interests' and ignoring 'the national element'.[21] Long before Social Darwinism became fashionable he had attacked racialism:

> The inhabitants of the colder latitudes are white because the sun is less powerful on them ... In like manner the proteus, which dwells in caves, when exposed to the sun, becomes coloured, losing its former translucency of surface. The pride of colour, therefore, is as foolish in man as it could be in that humble creature.[22]

We have thus seen the views of a native chief, a cultural interlocutor and a 'modern' doctor. The first was action-oriented, the second persuasive, and the third served the colonial state without being servile.[23] The emerging educated class showed great aptitude for change and new knowledge. But not the traditional vaidyas. When Madhusudan Gupta dissected a dead body in 1835 a vaidya of high repute, Gangadhar Ray, is said to have left Calcutta in disgust.[24] The traditionalists were convinced that an alien government would not help them.[25] Earlier the government had abolished medical classes at the Calcutta Madarsa and the Sanskrit College. Several thousand signatures were collected in protest.[26] But nothing could stop, or even dilute, the Anglicists' victory.

In average public esteem, however, the indigenous practitioners continued to hold sway. In Calcutta Gangaprasad Sen and Neelamber Sen were extremely popular.[27] They introduced fixed consultation fees, priced medicine, the publication of sacred texts and publicity through advertisements. Gangaprasad started the first Ayurvedic journal in Bengali, *Ayurveda Sanjivani*, and even exported Ayurvedic medicines to Europe and America.[28] These were the indications that certain European practices could be internalised and turned to the advantage of practitioners of indigenous medicine. Even at the conceptual level the then reigning miasmatic theories and the humoral pathology (of the vaidyas and hakims) were not very incompatible. What the Westerners were averse to was the oriental 'process', not its substance. Almost all of them did recognise the importance of and later emphasised the use of indigenous drugs.[29] But diagnostic procedures and, of course, surgery were to remain major areas of difference for a long time to come.

Dual demands

Apart from cultivating the higher sections of Indian society, efforts were made, starting in 1800, to win popular support for Western medicine. Inoculation was the earliest mass experiment, and it involved both coercion and persuasion. Native 'tikadars' (variolators) and Brahmins were recruited for this purpose on a large scale and district collectors were asked to use their power and authority to break native resistance. Though reluctance and resistance were there, still many people, especially the propertied and educated classes, were quick to see the benefits. After all, variolation was not so dissimilar to vaccination, and was a common practice. It also gave the government an opportunity to get a tighter grip on the population, as the programme involved registering the community, gender and age details of the 'patients'.[30] By the 1840s the experiment was pretty institutionalised.

With this came demands from the Indian population of two types. One was for greater availability of Western medicine, the other for the revival and simplification of indigenous medical knowledge. In 1834 the journal *Samachar Darpan* campaigned for the publication of Western medical books in Bengali and condemned 'quacks'. In 1842 *The Bengal Spectator* felt that the country would benefit from the new Western medical institutions 'in several ways'.[31] As the Calcutta Medical College progressed the Brahmins, Vaidyas and Kayasthas responded in a big way and in its Hindustani class seventy-five out of a total of eighty-three students were Muslims.[32] This enthusiasm gradually led to greater questioning of the relevance of one system's domination. In 1864 *Somprakash* enquired why the students, after studying Western medicine, had produced 'no new invention', 'no new medicine'. 'None of them after knowing the former system of therapy (Chikitsa) have tried to examine the medicinal matters (Dravya) ... they mainly concentrate on their fees.'[33] Making money out of disease was true of the European doctors as well. In 1854 one of them described his medical practice as 'killing and curing done by contract as it were'.[34] Still, practitioners of Western medicine were making steady inroads into public opinion. In 1875 Revenshaw (the Commissioner of Orissa Division) reported that even the *pandas* (priests) of Puri, who had earlier issued a threat of excommunication to patients attending the new dispensary, were now flocking to it themselves. He wrote:

> English practice has made headway in India by pushing itself forward, by throwing open hospitals, hunting up sick folk, and demonstrating to the patients and their friends that there really is a method of treatment superior to their own, and one which can cure diseases in a manner never before seen.[35]

An influential section of Indian society was thus coming under Western medical influence. David Arnold cites the example of Jesudasen Pillai, an Indian Christian in charge of a dispensary in Madras, who in 1858 reported the diminishing influence of 'ignorant Hakims and Vitheyams'.[36]

Nonetheless, the rural masses continued to patronise the indigenous system in view of its easy availability and low cost. In the 1860s the need to extend Western medicine to the rural areas attracted some attention from the government. The cause of scientific medicine and the maintenance of a proper standard of medical practice required that only allopathic (i.e. Western medical) practitioners should be used in government-sponsored programmes. But there were not enough men or resources, nor even the political desire. In Punjab some possibilities were explored, and in 1867 the Commissioner of Sialkot, T. W. Mercer, decided to use the native hakims in the new dispensaries after giving them some training in allopathic medicine. The scheme succeeded to a large extent, and became popular. But it was strongly opposed by both the Western medical profession and the bureaucracy. They called it 'a hodgepodge exposure to Western medicine without regard to standards of training or qualifications'. Mercer himself, they said, was not interested in revitalising the *Unani-i-tibb*. His aim was 'ultimately the subversion of the system of medicine as practised by the natives'.[37] Later in 1882 the government of India examined a proposal (from the government of Bombay) for the registration of all medical practitioners. The Bill would have given practitioners of indigenous medicine who possessed university qualifications the same rights as allopathic physicians, including an equal right to sign government certificates, sue for fees, etc. This created a furore to which the government succumbed and as a result indigenous practitioners were virtually excluded from government medical service. It was considered a victory for 'scientific medicine', but the real losers were the people.

Among the Indian practitioners of Western medicine there were a few who sincerely wanted to take advantage of the indigenous system and practices. In the *Indian Medical Gazette* of 1876 an assistant surgeon of Peshawar, Chetan Shah, wrote on how 'Hakims are not so ignorant as doctors believe them to be'. In this piece Shah countered the dismissal of Yunani Hikmat by one of his colleagues, Radha Nath Roy (assistant surgeon, Aligarh), point by point, citing extensively from the *Tih-i-Akbar* (a Yunani medical text) and other traditional texts. He concluded:

> The Yunani system of medicine as contained in Persian and Arabic literature, though very inferior and in some respects absurd and ridiculous, presents several useful hints of practical suggestions which should not be lost sight of. We should not throw off the roses because they are surrounded with thorns. We can pick out and learn a few good things even from savages.[38]

But Shah obviously had few takers in an age in which the colonial arteries were hardening. In the years to come, new bacteriological researches brought about such paradigmatic changes that the indigenous practices came to look even more primitive and outdated. A new 'scientific' armoury of criticisms was added to the age-old processes of denigration and subordination. But these changes had a remarkable side effect – they sharpened debate within Indian society. Henceforth medicine became 'an active ingredient in indigenous rhetoric ... integral to an Indian drive for improvement and a redefinition of self.'[39]

Vaccines, plague, segregation, discrimination, and growing national consciousness, all criss-crossed each other, to the discomfort of the imperial government (in the form of plague riots, etc.), and to the perplexity with respect to medicine of the Indian leaders – should they adopt the new, revive of the old or attempt a synthesis of the two? Their predecessors had wanted a synthesis but could not find the way, and in the meantime the West had achieved what it wanted. Now at the turn of the century the quest for identity (which had never disappeared completely) resurfaced with fresh vigour. The manifestations were interesting.

One such development was that Indian doctors trained in modern medicine sought freedom from and even parity with the 'superior' Indian Medical Service and the Army Medical Department. They raised this issue at every session of the Indian National Congress from 1893 to 1907. The ninth session of the congress asked for the constitution of a Civil Medical Service of India, to 'raise a scientific medical profession in India by throwing open fields for medical and scientific works to the best talent available and indigenous talent in particular'.[40] Later, at its seventeenth session in 1907, a delegate complained:

> We often find a military medical officer who has spent the best portion of his professional life in doing a little of everything but being master of nothing is suddenly at the latter end of his career made a professor of a subject of which he then becomes a learner, later a teacher but never a professor. Sometimes the order is reversed. And we see a professor of surgery or midwifery transformed into a Deputy Surgeon General, or a Professor of Chemistry becoming a store keeper to Government.[41]

It would be difficult to find a more graphic description or an equally severe indictment. Chuckerbutty, whom we have discussed earlier, had himself suffered on this account.[23] Growing demand for Indianisation of the medical services signified two things: first, the internalisation of the Western medical system, and second, the initiation of a counter-hegemonic process within the system. This brought to the fore latent differences and distrust on racial grounds. In 1909 the government of India sought opinions on proposals to open more superior positions to Indians. The IMS was almost unanimous in condemnation. An IMS civil surgeon wrote that:

> Moral stamina, self-reliance and self-confidence are not yet ripe, for the Indian gentleman qualified in Europe who has passed his examination brilliantly, falls back upon the primitive prehistoric treatments, used by hakims and others, when the pinch comes.[42]

Yet the demand for greater Indianisation continued to grow, and even reputed IMS officials like Leonard Rogers and Colonel Megaw could not stem the tide. Health administration gradually came into Indian hands after the Act of 1919. It is doubtful whether the indianisation of Western medicine brought any improvement in the status of the indigenous system and its practitioners, however. The lines had been drawn in the previous century and the demarcation was almost complete. If Ayurveda had to remain in competition, then it had to 'borrow' (or imitate) and 'improve' on terms set by its epistemological 'other'. Some practitioners, of course, held out for Shuddha (pure) Ayurveda. But the changes were unmistakable. How did the indigenous practitioners cope with the changing times? To appreciate this, let us take a brief look at the two pioneers who symbolised the struggle. They worked with two different systems at two distant places, yet were very close in both substance and method.

The two pioneers

They were Hakim Ajmal Khan (1868–1927) of Delhi and Vaidya P. S. Varier (1869–1958) of Kottakal.[43] Both came from physician families of high repute. Ajmal Khan's brother had established a *Madarsah Tibbia* (school of Yunani medicine) in 1883, and the whole family was engaged in promoting Yunani medicine. In 1891 Ajmal Khan prepared a catalogue of Arabic and Persian manuscripts in medicine. In 1897 he wrote a booklet on plague in Urdu. In 1902 he started publishing a monthly medical journal, *Mujalla-i-Tibbia*. The same year P. S. Varier organised an Arya Vaidya Samajam, opened Arya Vaidyashala and started a journal, *Dhanwantari*, to promote and analyse the strength and weaknesses of the Ayurvedic system. The two seem not to have met or collaborated but were fired by similar zeal. Both had open and eclectic minds, aware of the faults of their respective systems and willing to 'improve'. The Western system was not anathema to them, and both were keen to borrow and internalise what was good and beneficial from the other systems without losing their own ground. Their works were culture-specific but not culture-blind.

This was the spirit of the age. In the areas of education and social reform similar work was being done. Indian reformers were looking to the past and their tradition in order to improve the present, simultaneously trying to take full advantage of the new developments. In Bengal this was being done by Neelamber Sen and K. C. Sen (who had established a successful pharmaceutical company in 1878). In Andhra, B. G. Devara wrote in Telugu, drawing extensively from Western explanations of the origin of disease. 'Our Telugu physicians have often been writing on the cures for the diseases, but not on the causes of their origin', he rued.[44] In Maharastra, Shankar Sastri Pade catalogued 702 medical texts and published some seventy books.[45] In Madras, Pandit Gopalchari's Ayurvedic hospital was attracting four times more patients than the local English hospitals. He organised congregations and used to conduct examinations for 'Ayurvedabhushan' which, *inter alia*, tested the knowledge of candidates in chemistry, anatomy and physiology.[46] In 1895 a native prince, Bhagvat Sinhjee, wrote a history of *Aryan Medical Science*. In his opinion, Indian medicine deserved 'preservation and investigation ... in the spirit of fairness and sympathy'.[47]

This was precisely what Ajmal Khan and P. S. Varier were doing. They were deeply engaged in the systematisation and dissemination of what may be called 'traditional knowledge in a new light' and created institutions for the purpose. To this Varier added the preparation and distribution of medicine on a commercial scale, while Ajmal Khan concentrated on education synthesising the different systems. The latter tried to bring both the hakims and the vaidyas on to one platform and in 1910 organised an All India Ayurvedic and Tibbia (Yunani) Conference which became an annual event. These activities and their growing popularity stimulated the provincial medical councils (of Western medicine) to demand an all-India Act requiring the registration of 'legally qualified medical practitioners' (by which they meant themselves). Twice before (in 1881 and 1887) similar moves had been rejected by the government of India but in 1912 such an Act was passed, excluding the indigenous system from any form of state patronage. Indigenous medical practice was now restricted to the private and voluntary sector, and discrimination was *de jure*. Ajmal Khan toured the country and lobbied extensively against the Act but to no avail. Later, in 1916, the matter was raised at the Central Legislative Council with the support of important national leaders like Surendranath Banerjee, C. Vijayraghavchariar and Madan Mohan Malviya. The government of India responded diplomatically by constituting a Drug Manufacture Committee to enquire into the utility of indigenous medicine. It also agreed to open a few Tibbia colleges. The Governor General himself laid the foundations of a Tibbia College in Delhi in 1916, and delivered a speech in defence of the indigenous system! This college had both Ayurvedic and Yunani departments, an allopathic section, a female ward, a chemical laboratory, a botanical garden and a research wing called Dar-ul-Tahqeeqat. Around the same time, in 1917, P. S. Varier opened a *pathsala* (medical school) at Calicut. It began on a humbler note than Ajmal Khan's college, nor did it include the Yunani system in its purview. But the idea was to provide a scientific education in Ayurveda with a well defined curriculum which included surgery, anatomy, chemistry and midwifery. Western and indigenous systems were to be studied side by side.

It is difficult to gauge how successful these efforts were. Conceptually they faced the same dilemma which Serfoji had faced a century before. Numerically the Tibbia College turned out a large number of students under Ajmal Khan's stewardship (over 800 Muslim and 500 Hindu between 1920 and 1927). But to what extent they could be regarded as sufficiently 'modernised' or synthesised to pose an effective challenge to Western supremacy remains a matter of conjecture, since the college later declined.

The efforts of Ajmal Khan and P. S. Varier had nevertheless aroused more awareness and presented a cultural symbol for national regeneration. Varier's journal *Dhanwantari* appeared as a powerful mouthpiece. It looked into the causes behind the decline of Ayurveda. The Raj was, of course, blamed but the vaidyas themselves were not spared. It held the half-trained vaidyas 'responsible for the present degradation'.[48] The import of expensive medicines meant a drain of hard-earned Indian money.[49] Moreover, 90 per cent of the population depended on indigenous medicine and its practitioners, which the Registration Act of 1912 was seeking to destroy. *Dhanwantari* pooh-poohed the efforts of government commissioners to enquire into the utility of Ayurveda: 'It is from the opponents of Ayurveda that these officers are taking evidence; they do not dare to enquire of the villagers who depend on the indigenous system.'[50] At the conceptual level it fully recognised the merits of the Western system and expected the latter to appreciate what was valuable in the indigenous methods and enrich them. The English doctors were requested to play a more positive role.[51] Similarly it asked the vaidyas to be more open and opposed the calls for Shuddha (pure) Ayurveda as irrational. 'It is not fair for us to think that Western medical science is full of abominations and Ayurveda alone is pure.'[52]

Similar problems were faced by Ajmal Khan when some hakims of Lucknow refused to accept anything from the vaidyas or the allopaths.[53] It was with great difficulty that he could hold a session of his All India Ayurvedic Tibbia Conference at Lucknow in 1911. Both he and Varier recognised that the future of the indigenous systems depended upon their opening up and coming together. As *Dhanwantari* once put it, 'the native medical systems should be studied historically, discriminated critically and experimented scientifically'.[54]

The strategies of both these prominent reformers were restricted by certain inherent limitations. They appealed to the landed aristocracy and enjoyed the patronage of local rulers (like the nawab of Rampur, the ruler of Bhopal and the Maharaja of Travancore). Their elitism was deliberate. To quote from *Dhanwantari* again:

> We should do our best to convince the upper class. See the development of English medicine in our country. Rather than spreading among the poor, its exponents did their best to win the confidence of the rulers and the educated. The rest would follow.[55]

A very sound logic indeed. When a judge of Madras High Court or the Maharaja of Baroda turned to the vaidyas for their ailments, it was definitely good publicity for Ayurveda.[56]

Unlike Ajmal Khan, P. S. Varier seems to have put more emphasis on the manufacture and sale of medicines than on teaching or research. He realised that Western medicines appeared more attractive to the people because they were comparatively palatable, gave quick relief and came without dietary restrictions. So Ayurveda must change accordingly. After he had made adaptations to his drug products ensuring longer shelf life and quicker transportation, sales of Varier's medicines rose from Rs 14,000 in 1902–06 to Rs 170,000 during 1914–18.[57] Sales continued to increase, and it is still a flourishing house. By contrast Ajmal Khan's educational efforts could move only up to a point (his Tibbia College is now in a moribund state). Whatever their limitations, both reformers enjoyed great esteem and a wide following. The question of indigenous medicine was not a question of medicine or medical science *per se*; it had become part of the upsurge of interest in India's cultural heritage, with all the accompanying political implications. How did the ordinary literate Indians view it? Their views are reflected best in the 'native' press, to which we turn now.

Reflections in the native press

We have seen earlier how in 1864 a Bengali journal had criticised the 'new' medical students for 'no new invention, no new medicine'.[33] The trend continued. In 1872 a Tamil journal noted that medical students in Madras were being 'complained of as incompetent and deficient'. 'In place of cramming these youths with the mysteries of a science and language foreign and distasteful, would it not be infinitely wiser, and better to encourage Native Doctors?' it asked.[58] In 1887 a Telugu weekly asked for both systems to be studied. 'Persons who are acquainted with practising English medicine and chemistry, etc. should carefully study Hindu medical works and make experiments with their medicines and write books in the vernacular languages.'[59] Despite these demands, the indigenous system was gradually losing its traditional support from even the local chiefs and rajas. In 1874 a Malayalam journal reported that the Maharaja of Travancore, 'having examined various Hindu, Jaina and Turkish works', now preferred the English doctors. It surmised that 'the time has come for the Hindu medical authorities to sink into obscurity before the English'.[60] Later it turned out to be a false prophecy. For in the last decade of the nineteenth century the revival of interest in Ayurveda was marked and widespread. Perhaps it had something to do with the emergence of the *Swadeshi* spirit (of self-reliance) and the political movements of the time.

Several outbreaks of plague, debates about the efficacy of new vaccines in combating the epidemics, the opening of bacteriological institutes (at Mukteswar, Kasauli, Bombay, Coonoor, etc.), the policy of forced segregation, and compulsory vaccination were the critical areas where suspicion (bordering on hatred) of and social opposition (resulting sometimes in riots) to Western medicine were nursed. They made the traditional alternatives more exciting and trial-worthy. In 1896 a Tamil journal asked for the introduction of the native system of medicine in government medical colleges,[61] and fourteen years later a Calcutta daily repeated this never-to-be fulfilled demand.[62]. A Telugu weekly wanted the government to spend on 'native drugs and recipes' just a tenth of what it spent on hospitals.[63] People were shifting from allopathic medicines in the wake of epidemics and forced vaccinations. Rumours were rife. One such rumour was:

> Since the germs were taken from cows, after taking it [the vaccine] one would contract small pox and after recovering, his [the patient's] face would be changed and he would have horns on his head.[64]

The European physicians were accused of 'treatment by experiments' which were injurious to those experimented upon; in some cases humans were being experimented upon first, rather than animals.[65] Even among Westerners, opinions were divided over the wisdom of opening bacteriological laboratories. Some reminded the government of the greased cartridges and the Mutiny of 1857. 'To introduce diseased animal matter into the very blood – this is sheer pollution in the eyes of thousands upon thousands of Indians.'[66] When Dr Haffkine introduced the Pasteurian system of inoculation in Bengal in 1893 the journal *Vrittanta Chintamani* was among those that welcomed it.[67] But only six years later, in the midst of a plague outbreak, the same journal criticised the authorities for preventing the native physicians from trying their medicine. 'The English doctors are too zealous and think that they have the monopoly of the knowledge of medicine', it argued.[68] Several journals pointed to the racial underpinnings of the government's policy. When British citizens were under no compulsion to accept vaccination, why should the Indian subjects be made to?[69] When an advertisement appeared asking only Europeans and Anglo-Indians to apply for some assistant surgeonships, a daily asked, 'Why should preference be given to Europeans at the cost of Indians in the country of Indians?'[70] Another raised the interesting point of the great difference between 'the Englishmen's ideas of cleanliness and ours' (the former bathing only once in eight days!), and wanted questions of sanitation to be left to the Indians themselves.[71]

Yet there were many journals (like *Swadeshmitran*, *The Hindu Satya Deepika*, etc.) that wrote appreciatively of the work of the Pasteur Institutes at Bombay, Kasauli and Coonoor.[72] Interestingly enough, some related the modern researches to their ancient texts. One found the roots of Haffkine's prophylactic in *Susruta*,[73] another related the new science of embryology to an ancient Tamil text (probably of 450 BC), *Vaidya Chintamani Tatvavidhi*.[74]

Conclusion

Western medical discourse occupied an extremely important place in the colonisation of India. It functioned in several ways: as an instrument of control which would swing between coercion and persuasion as the exigencies demanded, and as a site for interaction and often resistance. In its former role it served the state and helped ensure complete dominance. It also roused suspicions, rumours and even hostility. Both ways the scope and opportunities for interaction were rather limited. Colonial hegemonisation (which depended more on coercion than on persuasion) precluded such possibilities. And the indigenous systems felt so marginalised that they sought survival more in resistance than in collaboration. Indians accepted British law without much fuss, but not British medicine. Moreover, colonial hegemony itself was entirely different from the Gramscian hegemony based on 'spontaneous consent', in which the 'general direction' imposed by the 'dominant fundamental group' elicits consent from the masses in a 'civil' society.[75] The presence of these parameters in a colonial system is so thin that they evaporate at the slightest warmth. The colonisers did not constitute a 'fundamental group', nor did they create 'civil' society. Direction was definitely there but the consent came only when a particular 'direction' was found 'really useful'. For example, as early as 1804 the Physician General at Fort St George (Madras) reported that the natives 'have been sensible of the value of cow-pox inoculation'.[76] A century later Haffkine exulted over the massive response to his prophylactic.[77] In between there came numerous occasions of withdrawal, antipathy and resistance. It was not a unilear progress. Condemnation and appreciation moved simultaneously and in a complex relationship. And this is true of both sides.

Indigenous medical systems laboured under severe constraints.

Rampant quackery had exposed them to ridicule even by their own people. A Malayali poet, Kunjan Nambiar, wrote in a poem: 'Physicians [native] are the people who make medicines and sell them for money, send patients to hell by treating them without proper diagnosis, and camp themselves in a patient's house so as to earn food from them'.[78] Some called Ayurvedic treatment 'a crazy or criminal act'.[79] Total acceptance of the new knowledge sometimes did mean total rejection of the old. Under such pressure some of the 'old' withdrew into their own shell. But the majority favoured revival and synthesis. There were several areas in which the Western and indigenous systems could collaborate but did not. The former put emphasis on the cause of the disease, the latter on *nidana* (treatment). Microbes and microscopes constituted the new medical spectacle.[80] But the vaidyas put emphasis on the power of resistance in the human body. 'The improvement of the *Kshetra* (body of the patient) is far more important than the microbe and its destruction.'[81] The Westerners were forced to take cognisance of indigenous drugs and the vaidyas took to anatomy, ready delivery of medicines, quick relief and so forth. But the comparison ends here. As a recent critique argues, they were inclined to borrow but could not 'create a dialogue between the two epistemics'.[82] Borrowed knowledge seldom develops into organic knowledge. This was true also of the hundreds of doctors produced by the government medical colleges annually. In the melee some really good opportunities were lost. All guns were targeted at the government:

> Let the government renounce its special care for English medicines. When fought on equal fields we can see the valour of this unscientific system. Then only we can understand whether native medicine is relevant to science and how far the science of English medicine is magnificent.[83]

Such criticisms were never taken seriously by the practitioners of Western medicine. Perhaps they were too sure of their competence and superiority. They continued to ridicule the 'other'. As a professor of physiology at Lucknow wrote:

> The financing of Unani and Ayurvedic institutes by Government in the hope of finding some soul of goodness in them is precisely on a par with the same Government financing archery clubs to find out the possibilities of the bow and arrow in modern warfare.[84]

Allopathy would have established itself even without government support. 'Can it be said that physics, chemistry and other sciences or the motor car, the cinema industry and the other fruits of applied science required political support to become popular here?'[85] It was difficult to oppose the West, even more difficult to ignore it. It was readily recognised that the cross-fertilisation of age-old Indian civilisation with post-Renaissance European culture produced 'stray, bitter-sweet fruits at first, but gradually gave rise to a more satisfying and settled crop'.[86] How 'satisfying and settled' the crop was only contemporary India can answer.

Notes

I gratefully acknowledge the help received from S. Visalakshi (New Delhi), G. V. Rajmanickam (Thanjavur), Sudhakar Reddy (Guntur) and Sabu Philip (Trivandrum) in locating and translating articles from old Tamil, Telugu and Malyalam journals. To Sabu Philip I owe a deep debt. The errors, if any, are entirely mine.

1 S. C. G. Chuckerbutty, *Popular Lectures on Subjects of Indian Interest*. Calcutta, 1870: 78.

2 Deepak Kumar, *Science and the Raj, 1857–1905*. Delhi, 1995: 180–91.

3 David Arnold, *Colonizing the Body: State Medicine and Epidemic Disease in Nineteenth Century India*. Delhi, 1993: 240–89.

4 A. L. Basham, 'The practice of medicine in ancient and medieval India', in Charles Leslie (ed.) *Asian Medical Systems*, Berkeley, Cal., 1977: 40; S. H. Askari, 'Medicines and hospitals in Muslim India', *Journal of Bihar Research Society* XLIII (1–2 1957): 7–21.

5 For a catalogue see A. Rahman (ed.), *Science, Technology in Medieval India: a Bibliography of Source Materials in Sanskrit, Arabic and Persian*. New Delhi, 1982: 3–272. See also Alois Sprenger, 'Report of the researches into the Muhammadan libraries of Lucknow', *Selections from the Records of the Government of India* CCCXXXIV. Calcutta, 1896: 1–30.

6 M. N. Pearson, *Towards Superiority: European and Indian Medicine, 1500–1700*. Minneapolis, 1989: 33.

7 Variolation, for example, impressed them most. See Coult's *Account of the Diseases of Bengall* (1731) and Holwell's *Account of the Manner of Inoculating for the Smallpox in the East Indies* (1767), reprinted in Shri Dharampal (ed.), *Indian Science and Technology in the Eighteenth Century: Some Contemporary European Accounts*. Delhi, 1971: 141–63.

8 Roy MacLeod and Milton Lewis (eds), *Disease, Medicine and Empire*. London, 1988: 1–11.

9 In this 'torrid' discourse was born and reared the discipline of tropical medicine. For a critical analysis see N. Harish, 'Poisons, putrescence and the weather: a genealogy of the advent of tropical medicine'. Paper presented at Workshop on Science, Technology and Medicine in India, Delhi, March 1990.

10 For bibliographical details see Arnold, *Colonizing*, 328–38. Royle's work is missing in this otherwise extensive bibliography.

11 J. F. Royle, *An Essay on the Antiquity of Hindoo Medicine*. London, 1877: 190.

12 W. Adams, *Report on Vernacular Education*. Calcutta, 1868: 322–3.

13 S. Ganapathi Rao, 'Dhanvantari Mahal', *Journal of the Tanjore Saraswati Mahal Library* (30 1977): I–IV. Numerous books, instruments and medical case sheets survive as the Modi Raj Records at Saraswati Mahal Library, Thanjavur.

14 R. Venkatraman, 'The impact of modern science on a Tamil traditional system in the eighteenth and nineteenth centuries'. Paper sent to Seminar on Science and Empire, New Delhi, January 1985.

15 *The Bombay Durpan*, 9 January 1835: 119–20.

16 Home, Public, No. 18, K.W. Pt A, 18 July 1838, preserved at National Archive of India (NAI).

17 *Ibid.*

18 Chuckerbutty, *Popular Lectures*: 56.
19 'Lecture on the present state of the medical profession in India', in *ibid.*, dated 2 February 1864: 138.
20 *The Hindoo Patriot*, 15 March 1855.
21 'Lecture on the necessity of forming a Medical Association in Bengal', in Chuckerbutty, *Popular Lectures*, dated 27 May 1863: 135.
22 'Lecture on a defence of native education', in *ibid.*, 8 July 1858: 85.
23 Chuckerbutty may have been uncomfortable with the government. Later his professorship of *materia medica* was lumped in with medical storekeeping and his salary was temporarily stopped. General, Medical, No. 30, June 1867, West Bengal State Archive.
24 B. Gupta, 'Indigenous medicine in nineteenth and twentieth century Bengal', in Charles Leslie (ed.), *Asian Medical Systems*, California, 1977: 371.
25 G. Mukhopadhyay, *History of Indian Medicine* II, Calcutta, 1923: 18.
26 Home, Public, No. 9, 13 March 1835, and Nos. 44–5, 8 April 1835 (NAI).
27 Chuckerbutty records that one of his serious patients asked for Neelamber Sen. When the vaidya arrived people lined up to see him. The patient could not be saved but the day and hour of death foretold by the vaidya proved to be correct. Chuckerbutty, *Popular Lectures*: 139.
28 Gupta, 'Indigenous medicine': 372–3.
29 W. B. O'Shaughnessy (Professor of Chemistry, Calcutta Medical College, 1835–49) compiled a *Bengal Pharmacopoeia* to facilitate greater use of locally available drug materials and reduce expensive imports from Europe. Later Dr Waring published the *Pharmacopoeia of India* in 1868.
30 For details of the collector's role in controlling the 'bodies' see A. Murali, 'Medicine and hegemony in Colonial Andhra.' Paper presented at a workshop on Culture and Legitimacy in Colonial India, New Delhi, November 1990.
31 Benoy Ghosh (ed.), *Samajpatre Banglar Samajchitra* III, Calcutta, 1964: 184.
32 In 1849 in the English class of the Calcutta Medical College, there were fifteen Brahmins, eight vaidyas, twenty-four Kayasthas, three weavers, four barbers, two blacksmiths and five Muslims. See Report of the Medical College of Bengal, 1849–50. Calcutta, 1850: 3.
33 Benoy Ghosh, *Samajpatre* IV: 505.
34 W. Walford, *The Autobiography of an Indian Surgeon*. London, 1854: 94.
35 T. E. Ravenshaw to the Secretary to the Government of Bengal, 13 January 1875, General, Education, Nos. 1–4, February 1875 (preserved at West Bengal State Archives).
36 Arnold, *Colonizing*: 253.
37 J. H. Hume, 'Medicine in the Punjab, 1849–1911'. Ph.D. thesis, Duke University, 1977: 49–73.
38 Chetan, Shah, 'Hakims are not so ignorant as doctors believe them to be', *Indian Medical Gazette* (1 April 1876): 95–6.
39 Arnold, *Colonizing*: 241.
40 Resolution No. IV, moved by Dr K. N. Bhadurji at the Lahore session in December 1893, reprinted in A. M. and S. Zaidi (eds), *The Encyclopaedia of the Indian National Congress* II, *1891–95*, New Delhi, 1977: 406.
41 *Ibid.* IV, *1901–05*, New Delhi, 1978: 145.
42 Note by S. H. L. Abbot, Civil Surgeon, Dera Gazi Khan, dated 23 April 1908, quoted in Hume, *Medicine*: 116.
43 For details see Z. A. Nizami, *Hakim Ajmal Khan*. New Delhi, 1988; Barbara Metcalf, 'Nationalist Muslims in British India: the case of Hakim Ajmal Khan', *Modern Asian Studies* 19 (1 1985): 1–28; and K. N. Panikkar, 'Indigenous medicine and cultural hegemony: a study of the revitalization movement in Keralam', *Studies in History* 8 (2 1992): 283–307.
44 B. G. Devara, *Sukhrooga Chikitsa Sangrahmu*. Ellore, 1893, quoted in Murali, 'Medicine and hegemony'.
45 Panikkar, 'Indigenous medicine'.

46 *Dhanwantari* (Malayalam) 14 (14 June 1917): 244–6.
47 Bhagvat Singjee, *Aryan Medical Science: a Short History*. Gondal, 1895, reprinted Delhi, 1993.
48 *Dhanwantari* 2 (14 May 1905): 190–1.
49 *Ibid.* 8 (13 March 1908): 186.
50 *Ibid.* 14 (14 March 1917): 187–91.
51 *Ibid* 2 (24 June 1905): 298–311.
52 *Ibid.* 15 (11 1917): 260.
53 Nizami, *Ajmal Khan*: 33.
54 *Dhanwantari* 17 (16 November 1919): 90–1.
55 *Ibid.* 14 (15 December 1916): 211.
56 *Ibid.* 10 (16 August 1916): 256. A lower middle-class clientele was taken for granted. The rich could afford expensive European treatment, and the poor would go to free dispensaries, but the lower middle class would prefer indigenous treatment 'on account of its inexpensiveness'. *Mangalodayam* (Malyalam) IX (1923): 38.
57 *Dhanwantari* 16 (17 October 1918): 58; and 18 September 1920): 125–8.
58 *Sukirthavachani* (Tamil), 17 August 1872, from the *Native Newspaper Reports (NNR)*, Madras, January 1872–February 1874: 67.
59 *Vivekavardhani* (Telugu), August 1887, in *NNR*, Madras, 1887: 138.
60 *Paschima Taraka* (Malayalam), 30 June 1874, in *NNR*, Madras, 1874: 53.
61 *Swadeshmitran* (Tamil bi-weekly), 21 April 1896, in *NNR*, Madras, 1896: 109.
62 *Daily Hitavadi* (Calcutta), 6 July 1910, in *NNR*, 28, Bengal, 1910: 807.
63 *Rajayogi* (Telugu weekly), 1 December 1895, in *NNR*, Madras, 1895: 379.
64 K. C. V. Raja, 'Vasoorikerivekkal', *Mangalodayam* (Malayalam) II, Trichur, 1910.
65 *The Native Opinion* (Anglo-Marathi bi-weekly), 31 August 1899, in *NNR*, Bombay, 1899: 840–1. *Jayadhwaja* (Kannada weekly), 4 August 1900, reported that 'a certain doctor in charge of a hospital in Vienna is said to have in this way administered certain poison to some women that had come to him for treatment ... Is it a wonder, then, that Indians often betray a want of faith in European methods of treatment?' In *NNR*, Madras, 1900: 233.
66 *The Kathiawar News* (Anglo-Gujarati bi-weekly), 27 January 1897, in *NNR*, Bombay, 1897: 93. *The Suryodaya Prakasika* (Kannada weekly) of 1 June 1904 alleged that for the Kasauli laboratory thousands of cattle had been killed, 'to the great detriment of agriculture'. *NNR*, Madras, 1904: 209.
67 *Vrittanta chintamani* (Kannada weekly), 9 August 1893, in *NNR*, Madras, 1893: 202.
68 *Vrittanta Chintamani*, 18 January 1899, in *NNR*, Madras, 1899: 28.
69 *Hitavarta* (Calcutta), 27 July 1911, in *NNR* 31, Bengal, 1911: 95.
70 *New Times* (Karachi), 25 April 1923, in *NNR*, Bombay, April 1923, para. 6.
71 *Vijaya* (Tamil daily), 23 March 1910, in *NNR*, Madras, 1910: 580.
72 *Swadeshmitran* (Tamil daily), 23 June 1905, in *NNR*, Madras, 1905: 227; *Satya Deepika* (Kannada weekly), 30 August 1911, in *NNR*, Madras, 1911: 1308; *The Hindu* (English daily, Madras), 17 August 1911: 1229.
73 *Suryalomaku* (Telugu weekly), 5 November 1899, in *NNR*, Madras, 1899: 400.
74 *Puttuvai Kalai Magal* (Tamil), Pondicherry (4 1905): 68–70.
75 For a lively discussion see D. Engles and S. Marks, *Contesting Colonial Hegemony: State and Society in Africa and India*. London, 1994; Ranjit Guha, 'Dominance without hegemony and its historiography', *Subaltern Studies* VI, Delhi, 1989: 210–309.
76 J. Anderson, *Correspondence for the Extermination of Smallpox*. Madras, 1804: 6.
77 'The people in Dharwar not only came forward in thousands to be inoculated when the efficacy of the method was explained to them, but they paid for the inoculations'. Haffkine Papers Mss. Var. 325.78 (at the Hebrew National University Library and Archive, Jerusalem).
78 *The Malaya Rajyam Weekly* XVI (24 November 1945): 113–16.
79 *Lakshmibai* (Malayalam) 67 (29 1934): 342.
80 W. Anderson, 'Laboratory medicine as colonial discourse', *Critical Inquiry* 18 (1992): 506–29.

81 *Dhanwantari* 4 (18 February 1925): 133–5.
82 Panikkar, *Indigenous Medicine.*
83 *Dhanwantari* 18 (October 1920): 146.
84 *Indian Medical Gazette* 62 (1927): 223
85 *Srichitra Yugam* (Malayalam), 1941: 47–8.
86 *Mangalodayam* VI (1915): 76–7.

CHAPTER EIGHT

Plural traditions? Folk therapeutics and 'English' medicine in Rajasthan

Helen Lambert

This chapter utilises ethnographic and historical material to examine the contemporary character of medical pluralism in rural Rajasthan, north India. The current social organisation of rural therapeutic practice and the conceptual structuring of lay people's preferences for different forms of treatment offer some clues for an archaeological investigation of the relationships between different medical traditions since the introduction of Western medicine in Rajasthan. Historical sources that refer to a variety of these traditions provide an additional means through which to construct an account of shifts in these relationships in a former princely state. Together these approaches provide some evidence of transformations that have occurred in the putative medical system over the past 150 years, particularly in relation to the practice of certain therapeutic specialisations in which the ability or otherwise of these specialisations to professionalise and shifts in state patronage played significant parts.

In this endeavour two particular difficulties are evident, relating to the geographical locus of my enquiry – a former princely state – and to the particular types of medical tradition – folk therapies – that comprise the focus of this account. A growing body of recent work on the history of European medicine in India has provided important insights into the relationship between medicine and colonialism in the region.[1] Historical and anthropological studies of Ayurvedic medicine have also revealed the complex shaping of an indigenous medical tradition under the influences of imperial science, nationalist politics and modernisation.[2] The insights yielded by this rich body of research can, however, be applied only with caution to the present case. First, in contrast with the learned indigenous traditions, folk or popular medicine has been little considered in the history of medicine in India except in relation to the influence of religious ideas and practices on smallpox vaccination campaigns. The picture usually given of Indian medicine is that it consists, on the one hand, in the textually based traditions of classical Indian medicine – Ayurveda and Yunani – and, on the other, in religious traditions of healing found in the folk domain. To these are sometimes added the figure of the *dai*, or traditional midwife, who in most accounts – and nearly all health policy – appears as the sole indisputable representative of non-religious folk medicine.[3] A prominent analytical tendency has been to focus on Ayurveda as *the* indigenous medical tradition, in contrast with modern biomedicine, and to assume that all lay (folk, indigenous) medical conceptions and practices in Indian culture are straightforwardly derived from this textually based tradition.[4] This approach, however, assumes the ready availability of orthodox Ayurveda and a high level of resort to Ayurvedic practitioners in rural India which does not reflect either historical or contemporary reality.[5] Reliance on patronage meant that before the colonial period most learned practitioners were dependent on the patronage of royalty or wealthy merchants, while in contemporary Rajasthan the vast majority of trained practitioners in all systems of medicine are clustered in urban areas. Although the learned traditions are recognised to have been profoundly affected by the loss of royal and state patronage consequent on the introduction of European medicine, other (non-Ayurvedic) therapeutic traditions are assumed to consist mainly in either religious healing or the use of herbal medicaments and are presumed to be impervious to historical forces, including the hegemonic influence of Western biomedicine. There is scanty evidence for this view, which also ignores both the continuum between secular and religious traditions and the interpenetration of folk healing and the textually based (Brahmanic) medical and religious traditions. While there are inherent problems in any attempt to construct a historically informed account of non-literate forms of medicine, the study of popular therapeutics and medical preference in Rajasthan offers some scope for re-examining these assumptions.

Secondly, historical studies of European medicine in India have focused on epidemic disease and have relied almost exclusively on English-language sources relating to British India (areas under direct rule), while the former Rajputana was comprised mostly of princely (or native) states. As yet little is known about the processes through which European medicine became available to the Indian population in such areas. The claim that the primary motivation for the extension of European medicine in British India lay in the need to protect the health of British subjects and the military is clearly an insufficient explanation for its expansion in a region under indirect rule. The continuing power of royal patronage as a mediating influence on the imperialist mission, of which European scientific medicine became a symbol, has an important role in this context and the case of a princely state offers a useful testing ground for some of the debates that have arisen about the place of European medicine in the colonialist enterprise, although the present chapter can offer no more than a tentative beginning in this respect.

Plural traditions in contemporary northern India

In contemporary Rajasthan, ethnographic research shows that the medical domain (which I take to include the full range of practices dealing with the treatment and prevention of ill health) is highly pluralistic and not clearly systematised. There is little evidence of direct contestation or competition between practitioners of the different systems of medicine. Naturally, Western biomedicine – generally referred to in Indian English as allopathy and in Hindi/Rajasthani as *angrezi dvai*, literally 'English medicine' – occupies an important place as a form of treatment, even in remoter rural areas. Oral medication and injections are widely used in the treatment of ill health and are administered by a variety of trained and untrained practitioners. Injections in particular are in great demand and private practitioners are often preferred to the government sector primary health facilities, where free medical supplies are limited and where staff tend to change often and to have scant regard for their patients. In cases of acute illness, or major accidents, people are usually taken to a government hospital in the nearest urban centre (usually in the district or state capital).

Alongside Western biomedicine, many forms of indigenous therapy continue to be widely used. In contemporary Rajasthan I take these to include not only that administered by learned practitioners of Ayurveda and Yunani but also – and more predominantly in rural areas – the making and use of herbal remedies (*desidvai*, literally 'country medicines'), the practices of bone setting, midwifery, therapeutic massage, divination to diagnose illness, the use of mantras (sacred verbal formulas) and *jhara* (the ritual sweeping away of illness), pilgrimage, and propitiation and healing at shrines by devotees or possessed mediums of a deity.[6] To these can be added some slightly more specialised therapeutic techniques that remain in occasional use such as cautery or branding and blood cupping. Contrary to some early assumptions, biomedicine certainly has not replaced local forms of therapy. Indeed, a descriptive overview of the contemporary situation alone would suggest that, in Rajasthan at least, Western biomedicine has simply contributed a further dimension to what is conventionally described as the 'medical system' by increasing its plural character. The following exploration of the basis of choice between different types of treatment and of local understandings of Western biomedicine casts some light on the reasons for this continuing pluralism.

Categorisations of ill health and the conceptual bases of therapeutic preference

Among Rajasthani villagers, attitudes to the selection of treatment are generally highly pragmatic. The choices made by sick persons and their families are based on a variety of factors, including the knowledge available to them about the nature and cause of their illness; previous experience (personal and that of others) as to what forms of treatment are most effective for their complaint and (if outside help is required) which specialists give the most successful treatment of that type; economic constraints; the availability and accessibility of the different types; evaluation of previous therapies, both in the present and in prior episodes of illness; and, sometimes, social prestige. Despite a wealth of informal knowledge and the existence of indigenous theory about the sources of ill health and popular therapeutics which emphasises the need to ascertain the cause of a sickness in order to effect a cure, villagers construe themselves as 'hicks' (*gawar log*, 'rustic/uncivilised/ignorant people') and thus as lacking in the sort of esoteric knowledge about the nature of medicine or disease that would allow them easily to determine the cause and hence the appropriate cure in any given case of ill health. Accordingly, new forms of therapy are generally taken up with few reservations, and treatment is generally evaluated on the basis of its perceived effectiveness.

In keeping with such an approach is a general binary division of many illnesses into two categories according to the type of therapy that is considered to be appropriate and therefore effective for these complaints. People describe a range of health problems generically as *daktar/vaidya ki bimari*, literally 'physician's illness' (or as *angrezi bimari*, literally 'English illness', deriving from the term *angrezi dvai*, 'English medicine', to describe Western biomedicine). By this is meant a health problem that should be treated by a physician. A range of other illnesses are referred to as *devata ki bimari*, literally 'deity's illness' – that is, a condition for which religious rather than secular treatment is considered appropriate. Thus, in describing the evil eye a female informant stated that 'If it's a physician's illness [*dard*, pain, affliction], then physician's medicine is used. If it's the illness [affliction] of the evil eye, then physician's medicine isn't effective.'[7] Most people assert that deities treat complaints such as bodily pain and illness caused by spirits whereas doctors treat complaints like fever and stomach pain. A man of the Gujar caste described treatment preferences as follows: 'Bhomiaji [the local godling] treats people for ghosts (*bhut*), witches (*dhakan*) and things like that. He doesn't give treatment for things like fever; the doctor will treat "English illnesses" [*angrej ki bimari daktar karega*].' A Rajput woman was of the same opinion: 'For headache or fever or something people will get doctor's treatment [*daktar ki ilaj*] but for "spirit illnesses" [*upari bimari*] they'll go to some goddess-and-god's [*devi-devata*] shrine.' A woman who was talking about a previous miscarriage said that there was no treatment for the problem except from a deity (*devata*); doctor's treatment (*daktar ki ilaj*) doesn't work for it.[8] The very designation of many health problems as 'doctor's illness' or 'deity's illness' demonstrates not only that people explicitly associate the identification of cause – that is, diagnosis – with the type of therapeutic action that is considered appropriate but also that resort to biomedicine is well established as a form of treatment.

An important criterion for the classification of a particular instance of ill health in this way is the outcome of therapy itself. Initially a course of action is usually determined on the basis of the symptoms and according to circumstances such as cost and the availability and accessibility of treatment, as well as the status of the patient in the household. The outcome of initial therapy is used as a basis from which to reassess the problem if necessary.[9] If a therapy consistently fails, the patient and his/her family may conclude that it was because the initial diagnosis was incorrect and therefore inappropriate, so another form of therapy should be tried. In other cases a practitioner rediagnoses the illness and initiates a new course of action; the case of a pilgrim seen at the village shrine of the local godling, Bhomia, will illustrate the point. A woman said she had come a long way to get treatment for her sick baby, which she laid on the shrine platform. The god's possessed medium pronounced that there was an obstruction in the baby's stomach (*pet mãruk gyo*) and that the illness was not a problem of spirit affliction (*bhut-pret konahĩ*). The woman asked the deity to give treatment anyway; he replied that it would be pointless and told her to take the child to the *vaidya* at the village dispensary or to some doctor in one of the two nearest towns.

People expect healers to redirect patients or alter the diagnoses that patients have made, since diagnosis is itself a major part of the treatment process and those who treat sickness are often also the diagnosticians. Another village practitioner said that he gives ritual therapy for cases of infant pneumonia (*badala*) for two to three days. If the child is not getting better he then advises people to go to a doctor in town. A healer's (or deity's) instructions are not, though, always heeded, for other considerations and constraints also enter into the process of seeking therapy. Economic considerations are particularly important; while major religious rituals for healing can be very expensive, by and large it is considerably cheaper to take a patient to a local shrine than to seek biomedical treatment, with the costs of travel and drugs that the latter entails. Thus poor people often prefer to seek a deity's help first in the hopes that this simple action will be effective. Biomedicine carries a certain amount of social prestige, due primarily to its associations with urban life, education and modernity, so that educated and wealthier persons generally seek the help of a doctor in the first instance. Here the use of biomedicine can be seen as a sign of social distinction that, in hegemonic fashion, is spreading throughout the social hierarchy as 'alternative' modes of treatment gain acceptance among the highest (and most Westernised) social classes. But the failure of any initial treatment often leads to a different form of therapy being tried in the hope of it being more effective and the prestige value of biomedicine is generally found at the level of verbal dismissals of religiously based therapy and in the reordering of initial preference rather than in exclusive adherence in practice to that form of treatment. Nonetheless, there exists a significant gender difference, deriving from the broader social context and normative attitudes, in the utilisation of biomedicine; as an expensive and relatively prestigious form of intervention, girl children and women living in their affinal homes may be denied access to this form of medical care, while the cultural elaboration of ailments relating to women's fertility places them squarely within the realm of 'deity's illness'.[10]

The failure of biomedicine and the anger of the gods

The local interpretation of the effects of biomedical therapy offers a useful illustration of historical changes in the relationship between it and traditional medicine. One sub-set of 'deity's illness' is ill health due to *doṣ*, 'divine wrath' or 'divine blame' which results from offending a god or goddess, often by forgetting to worship him or her. If divine wrath is suspected, the specific deity who is causing the problem must be identified and is done by a traditional technique of divination known as *doṣ dekhno*, literally 'to look at the blame/censure'. People use the technique only when they already suspect that divine anger may be the cause. Certain pathological symptoms are significant; a very sudden onset of illness and, particularly, sharp and persistent pain in the eyes (known as *ghobo halno*) or persistent sharp shooting pain in the limbs may lead to the consideration of supernatural censure (*dos*) as a possible cause. However, villagers regard *an adverse reaction to biomedicine* as an especially strong indication of this cause. Following the use of Western drugs or an injection, if the illness or pain, instead of receding, significantly worsens (*dun ho javai*, literally 'doubles'), it is taken to be a sign of divine wrath; villagers say that the slighted deity is not allowing the person to recover (*nika n'aba dai*, 'does not let [him/her] [be]come well'). Thus when doctor's treatment only aggravates, rather than improves, an illness, this may prompt a re-evaluation of its cause as divine wrath. Only at that point is divination used to seek confirmation of the provisional diagnosis and to identify the wrathful being who is responsible. If the divination confirms the diagnosis, treatment consists in praying and making offerings to the offended source of the problem. In 1895, by contrast, Lieutenant Colonel T. Holbein Hendley, Residency Surgeon and Superintendent of Dispensaries at Jaipur, wrote that most Rajasthanis resort to the use of European medicine only by a process of exclusion through finding that the illness does not have a religious or supernatural cause, as would be initially presumed.[11]

This shift in interpretation clearly places Western biomedicine as the first preference on the secular side of a naturalistic/non-naturalistic categorisation of possible aetiological agents via the specification of treatment alternatives to which these are matched. The other main binary division utilised by villagers to categorise episodes of ill health refers more explicitly to aetiological notions but cross-cuts the treatment-based distinction between 'doctor's' and 'deity's' illnesses. This second classificatory mode refers to the humoral conceptions that in most accounts of Indian medicine are said to govern all indigenous medical theory and practice.[12] Common both to formal Ayurveda and to popular understanding is the concept of a continuous flow and cooking of substances and juices between and within persons and the environment, described as an 'ecological' theme by Francis Zimmerman.[13] This theme is part of a broader Hindu world view to be found both in textual sources and in popular conceptions which links proper dietary regime with climatic conditions and geographical region and emphasises equilibrium between heat and cold, the three bodily humours and the emotions.

In the predominantly rural area where I conducted fieldwork these cosmological conceptions in folk medical discourse are articulated mainly by reference to notions of 'hot' and 'cold' that relate only partially to the formal tri-humoral theory of indigenous doctrinal medicine, although a few forms of ill health – such as rheumatism and arthritis – are regarded as due to an excess of humoral 'wind' (*bay*, Hindi/Sanskrit *vayu*). Many medical conditions are categorised by villagers as illnesses of heat (*garmi ki bimari*) or of cold (*sardi ki bimari*).

The latter include colds, fever and typhoid, and all are thought to result from an excess of internal 'cold' – a term that refers not to body temperature but rather to thermal quality. This imbalance may be the result of a variety of causes, including exposure to low temperatures or the ingestion of too much 'cooling' food (food that has the effect of producing an increase in humoral coldness). Any treatment for an 'illness of cold' should include dietary modifications whereby 'heating' foods are increased and 'cooling' ones are avoided for therapeutic purposes. 'Illnesses of heat' (*garmi ki bimari*) – ranging from boils and mouth ulcers to piles and genito-urinary disorders – indicate by their nature the need for 'cooling' therapies, in the form of foods and herbal medicinal substances, and the avoidance of aggravatory 'heating' foods. While appearing 'naturalistic' in nature, however, the humoral disturbances used to characterise many health problems may still be secondary manifestations of a different ultimate cause. Thus a condition manifesting itself in an excess of heat may ultimately be the result of polluting conduct or the wrath of an afflicting deity, while an illness of cold such as infant pneumonia can be strongly linked with the malign gaze of a witch or the action of malevolent spirits. Alongside dietary modification to restore humoral balance, therefore, people may seek other treatment, including biomedicine, depending on what is appropriate to the specific illness and its presumed ultimate cause.

These forms of treatment include a wide range of ritual therapies (including *jhara*, 'sweeping', and other performative acts some of which employ *mantra*, sacred verbal formulas) in which medicinal, substantive and symbolic aspects are interwoven. While distinctions of caste, class, gender, economy and education to some extent affect the degree of utilisation of these forms of indigenous therapy, they generally comprise a prominent form of ethnomedicine among all social groups. These disparate forms of ritual therapy all have a common structure and purpose in so far as they relate not to specific aetiologies but to general characterisations of sickness as forms of inauspiciousness and are predicated on a particular, hierarchical conception of the body. They are a form of therapeutic action that I have characterised as 'prognostic' rather than aetiological, since they attempt to deal with sickness not by interventionist techniques but by ensuring an ultimately beneficial outcome, either by facilitating the natural course of the sickness through the patient's body or by removing it through transference to another vehicle.[14]

Biomedicine is understood implicitly as interference with the natural processes that are encouraged by prognostic therapeutic rituals but is not inherently incompatible with them, since they are concerned with ultimate outcome rather than short-term effect. The action of biomedicine is interpreted within the framework of the indigenous view of bodily health as arising from humoral balance. Drugs to be taken internally are considered to have a 'heating' effect on the body and thus can produce other 'illnesses of heat', so they are taken with caution and sometimes along with 'cooling' foods to counteract their heating effects. Local practitioners often recommend pills to be taken with milk (a 'cooling' substance) to counteract the effects. Villagers regard the therapeutic use of diet and other naturally occurring medicinal substances as a way of dealing with the imbalances in the body that are the 'root causes' of illness. In contrast both lay people and medical practitioners assert that 'English medicine', although extremely popular because it is 'strong' and works rapidly, treats only the symptoms of illness and not the causes, which may take longer to correct. Thus while it is frequently selected over indigenous forms of therapy as a preferred mode of treating ill health owing to the rapid alleviation of symptoms that it effects, it is not considered inherently superior by nature, and the scientific principles that underlie its action are without significance to its users. On the contrary, English medicine is regarded – unlike any form of indigenous therapy – as iatrogenic in many respects, such that episodes of ill health regarded as 'heat'-related are sometimes attributed to heating doses of English medicine that were taken months or years previously. The clear implication behind such views, while rarely explicitly asserted, is that English medicine, though functionally effective, is essentially maladaptive to the environmental conditions of local life. A student who helped me as an interpreter on visits to the shop of an indigenous pharmacist (*pansari*) during the first months of my fieldwork in Jaipur city interpreted my interest in Ayurvedic and Yunani medicaments as being for practical purposes. She finally expressed her puzzlement at its relevance to application elsewhere as follows: 'The climate in England is very different from the climate in Rajasthan. What is the significance of your study?'

These underlying attitudes are in striking contrast to Western assumptions about the superior efficacy of Western medicine, both past and present. Expectations among international health experts up till the early 1980s that biomedicine would naturally come to supplant indigenous medical traditions altogether owing to its superior efficacy only duplicated British attitudes to Indian medicine during the colonial period, in which support for indigenous systems was just one means of preparing for its eventual displacement by its superior rival, a medicine based on Western scientific principles.[15]

Contemporary practitioners and the structure of folk medicine

A particular feature of the contemporary provision of medical treatment in rural areas is that each form of therapy tends to be administered by different specialist practitioners. While expertise in any given therapeutic mode depends to varying degrees on the acquisition of some specialist knowledge, the ethnomedical concepts which underlie all therapeutic traditions locally constitute 'ordinary' knowledge that is shared by individuals from all castes and social groups. A model of medical systems developed for the purposes of comparative anthropological analysis categorises health care into three overlapping sectors – popular, folk and professional.[16] Professional practitioners are deemed to be those who administer therapy as an occupation and practise a comprehensive form of medicine based on a bounded system of textually based knowledge and whose theoretical understanding of illness and medicine is not fully shared by the patients. Folk practitioners are those who do not necessarily administer therapy as a full-time occupation, who practise a form of therapy based on an unbounded field of medical knowledge that does not necessarily constitute an internally coherent theoretical system, and whose conceptual understanding of sickness and medicine is substantially shared by the patients who are treated. Popular medicine refers to lay health care, including domestic treatment and self-treatment.

In urban areas of India, as elsewhere, this may be a useful means of characterising different types of health care. Resort to therapy outside the home necessarily entails moving outside the context of kin and community, and the urban milieu tends to bring about the institutionalisation of all folk practice. In Jaipur, the capital of Rajasthan State, for example, 'folk' practitioners from bone setters to traditional midwives and religious healers usually operate in an institutional setting separate from the domestic context and administer therapies which are functionally distinct to some extent from the forms of therapy administered in the home. They tend to be professional in that they accept payment for treatment and that their therapeutic role is their primary or sole occupation.

In rural Rajasthan, by contrast, no easy demarcation line can be drawn between the 'popular' and the 'folk' spheres of health care and medical treatment. While the same therapeutic specialisations exist as in urban areas (though with a wider geographical spread), they are variously provided either by lay persons (who would be part of the 'popular' domain) or by folk practitioners. There is thus a continuum between 'popular' and 'folk' treatment for any given therapeutic specialisation. At one extreme is found the lay person who through observation and experience has acquired a very limited familiarity with a form of therapy (scarcely greater than that known to all other adults) and who occasionally practises it, of necessity, in a completely informal way for family and neighbours. At the other extreme is found the folk practitioner who through inherited or acquired knowledge and personal experience has developed a more extensive and esoteric understanding of and skill in that same therapeutic specialisation, and who practises it semi-professionally for a large clientele, many of whom are not personally known to him. In both cases no *direct* remuneration is accepted and medical practice is not the person's primary occupation.

The specialisations of bone setting and massage provide examples of this kind of differentiation. In Jaipur a few traditional hereditary practitioners known as *pahalvan* (literally, 'wrestler') treat fractures, dislocations, sprains, swellings and bruises, and utilise a number of inherited medicinal remedies in treatment. The *pahalvan* possesses considerable specialised knowledge of anatomy and therapy, although the principles according to which he administers treatment are, unlike those of practitioners of learned systems of medicine, broadly shared by his clients. Thus the *pahalvan* also practises a form of therapeutic specialisation described not as massage but as 'stomach rubbing' (*pet sonthno*), 'seating the vessel' (*nas bithano*) or 'seating the navel pulse' (*dharn bithano*) that is underpinned by folk physiological conceptions. Indigenous conceptions of body physiology posit a system of internal vessels or channels (*nasa*), akin to veins or nerves, that carry both blood and air around the body. 'Massage' techniques are predicated on the concept that certain of these internal vessels (*nas*) are subject to displacement, particularly that which runs medially through the abdomen and inside which the umbilical pulse beats. Abdominal pain accompanied by a range of symptoms is usually attributed to such displacement and is treated by manipulating the vessel, directly or indirectly, through massage and, if necessary, vacuum cupping, to move it and the pulse back into place in the umbilicus.

Although the *pahalvan* offers this form of folk therapy his practice is in other respects professional, in that he operates within an institutional context (a small shop), charges fees for treatment, and practises therapy as a primary occupation. In rural areas, in the absence of such professionals, both bone setting and 'navel massage' are carried out as exclusive specialisations by folk practitioners. They have usually acquired their role out of initial necessity and the subsequent development of skill through practice rather than through inheritance, although informal apprenticeship often plays a role. Such practitioners usually have another occupation and do not charge for their services. They also range from the lay to the semi-professional, that is, from those who (in the case of bone setting) occasionally treat others within their immediate family or kin group for minor problems such as sprains, to those who are highly reputed within a particular region and whose aid is invariably sought by local people for major fractures, usually in both people and livestock. Treatment for major dislocations is also carried out by more expert practitioners using particular procedures of physical manipulation, while a domestic procedure is often used for minor dislocations and injuries to toe, knee or elbow joints.

Rural bone setters at any point on this spectrum, however, do not perform abdominal massage; rather, that is undertaken by different lay specialists of both sexes who are known locally as experts in this type of therapy, although same-gender practitioners are generally preferred. In some cases women who act as midwives are skilled in this form of massage; in others, the client–patron (*jajmani*) relationship that exists with respect to other types of work is replicated when a client with expertise in abdominal massage administers it on members of the patron's household. In other cases, again, a sufferer simply seeks help from an older woman or another individual in the residential area who is known to be able to treat people for abdominal discomfort, and such services are rendered without direct remuneration.

Similarly, therapeutic rituals including *jhara* ('sweeping') and other performative acts that often employ *mantra* (sacred verbal formulas) are performed in their more exoteric variants by locally famed folk healers and priests and in their more popular esoteric ones by mothers, agricultural workers or anyone else who has knowledge of a particular formulation. While some expert practitioners are known to have knowledge of a range of ritual techniques for treating a variety of health problems, and derive some indirect remuneration from their practice, the help of many lay specialists is sought for one specific type of complaint only, for such individuals have no other medical expertise. Local or country medicine, *desidvai*, is another form of therapy which exists primarily in the popular sphere. All adults have some familiarity with the allopathic principles by which ingested substances act on internal bodily state, and all know at least some simple remedies for complaints such as minor injuries, colds, spots and diarrhoea. More extensive knowledge of medicinal substances and herbal remedies is usually confined to women. Particular specialist knowledge is often associated with midwifery, both being learned from female relatives, although some women who do not practise midwifery except in the home (particularly those from higher castes) have quite extensive medicinal knowledge. Thus home remedies that employ household substances or readily available medicinal plant substances are commonly used and in most villages there are two or three people with more extensive knowledge of herbal remedies whose advice may be sought. There is not, however, a specialised folk tradition of herbalism in Rajasthan such as is found in Himalayan communities, and medicinal knowledge is not locally regarded as a distinct form of therapeutic speciality, although those who are ill or their relatives certainly employ such knowledge for treatment and refer to individuals who possess more extensive knowledge than themselves. This tradition thus exists purely in the popular domain of home-based treatment.

All the indigenous medical traditions I have so far described are still widely used despite the availability of biomedicine; indeed, the 'prognostic' domain of therapeutic ritual in particular is remarkably similar to the range of practices referred to in Victorian accounts of north Indian folklore.[17] From an ethnographic perspective it would thus be easy to conclude that, overall, Western medicine has simply contributed a further dimension to what is conventionally described as the 'medical system', by increasing its plural character. Contrary to some early assumptions, Western medicine certainly has not entirely replaced local forms of therapy. This view of biomedicine as complementary to indigenous traditions has been widely held, and its assumptions about traditions of folk medicine contrast with historians' and Indologists' views of the impact of biomedicine on the classical medical traditions. A comparison between the contemporary division of medical labour and its organisation in the past suggests a need to revise this view. I have described how, in the main, secular therapies such as bone setting, the use of herbal medicines and abdominal massage in rural areas are today mainly in the hands of lay, non-professional practitioners rather than folk specialists. Healers possessing any degree of esoteric medical knowledge, apart from a few religious specialists, seem to be rare in this region. It was not always the case, as becomes clear on examining those accounts of popular medicine in India that are to be found in the writings of early European travellers and later of British medical officers.

The apparent resemblance in these writers' descriptions of folk healers to contemporary folk medicine is only partial. I suggest that the spread of European medicine in Rajasthan has in fact had profound effects on folk therapeutic traditions, although these effects are difficult to trace because they relate mainly – though not exclusively – to a specific level of indigenous medicine comprising particular, non-religious therapeutic specialisations which are now rare or extinct and which were rarely recorded when they did exist. Accounts of medicine in Rajputana from the mid-nineteenth century onwards refer not only to vaids, hakims, priests and 'wise women', but repeatedly to Muslim and Hindu barber-surgeons, to inoculators and also to itinerant lithotomists who cut for stone and travelling hereditary oculists who performed cataract operations.[18] It seems that the specialisations which were most profoundly affected by the introduction of European medicine under the British were those that were themselves complementary to indigenous learned medicine – particularly surgical traditions – and it is possible to trace their decline indirectly.

The development of European medicine in Rajputana

British supremacy in Rajputana was established in 1818 through treaties concluded with all the native states of the province, and 1821 saw the founding of the Jeypore Political Agency. A Residency Hospital was immediately started, and the appointment of the first British Medical Officer to this facility signalled the first major introduction of European medicine to the region. As a native state, Rajputana probably saw the development of European medical facilities take a different route from areas of India under direct administration. One significant factor would have been the absence of large numbers of Europeans, for whom, in British territories, medical provision was mainly intended, so that the Indian population became the focus of European medicine at a comparatively early stage. The first medical dispensary for the public along European lines was opened in Jaipur city in 1844, ordered and funded by the Regency Council which managed Jaipur State during the minority of Maharaja Ram Singh. Support of public medical facilities was a continuation of royal charitable traditions; prior to indirect rule, medical provision outside the royal courts was supported by thakurs or minor princely landholders, and wealthy banias or merchants, who used to employ hakims who would treat the public free of charge with medicines supplied by their patrons.

During the late 1850s the British Agency surgeon in Jaipur established a school to train local youths in European medicine, and once they were qualified several district dispensaries were opened, starting with three in 1870. In the same year the foundation stone of Jaipur's Mayo Hospital was laid, and under Maharaja Ram Singh dispensaries were established in most of the towns in Jaipur State and in several wards of the capital itself. Ram Singh also ordered the building of drains, a piped purified water supply and other sanitary measures, roads and gas street lighting in Jaipur. Given his equal enthusiasm for the establishment of educational and other public institutions, it is hardly surprising that the Maharaja was regarded as 'one of the most enlightened of Indian Potentates'.[19] During the same decade, the Rajas of a number of the Jaipur court's feudatory states began to open public charitably run dispensaries, no doubt under the influence of their enthusiastically modernising sovereign. Some of the other native states of Rajputana province also established dispensaries, particularly those to the east such as Bharatpur and Alwar which bordered on areas under direct rule. The Rajputana medical report for 1872–73 mentions opposition to the new medical facilities by vaidyas and hakims, and the establishment of European medicine as the privileged recipient of royal charitable benevolence may have been a factor in the decline of royal patronage for the classical medical traditions.[20]

The second half of the nineteenth century saw a continuing expansion of medical facilities. Undoubtedly, though, the adequacy of medical facilities for the rural population and their quality depended in large measure on the enthusiasm for European medicine of the local ruler, the size of his court and his coffers, and on the commitment of local IMS officers to public medicine. British officers were well aware of the role of the durbars, and in a late nineteenth-century report the advance of Western medicine in Rajputana is explicitly attributed to the native princes. In many areas of the province, though, they were apparently reluctant to finance the provision of Western medical facilities in rural areas. Hendley noted that:

> The smaller States seem indifferent in many cases to the extension of dispensaries in the districts, while their rulers are most anxious to keep up such institutions at the Capital. It's not understood by many as yet why Hospital Assistants should require so much more pay than the indigenous *baids* and *hakims*, and this may be one reason for the dislike to greater expenditure, but the chief one no doubt is the comparatively heavy cost which attends the keeping up of a small court.[21]

Dispensary and administrative reports from Rajputana indicate that, as elsewhere, British attitudes towards indigenous practitioners also changed during the course of the nineteenth century.[22] Until the 1840s or so, although the Ayurvedic and Yunani pharmacopoeias were considered to be of value, their practitioners, as elsewhere in India, were generally despised. British attitudes towards non-learned practitioners, in contrast, appear to have been more positive, a number of medical officers' reports commenting favourably on the skills of indigenous surgeons and couchers. Until the late nineteenth century British medical officers also took some interest in non-learned or folk practitioners and saw them as having potential in the extension of European medicine, suggestions being made for their employment in European-style medical facilities.

By the turn of the nineteenth century, however, a rather different picture of medicine in Rajputana and of views towards indigenous practice emerges. No further mention is made of enlisting native practitioners in the expansion of European medicine. Rather, this is replaced by an attitude of competition in which European medicine, practised exclusively by British medical officers and British-trained native doctors, is expected to gradually replace indigenous medical practice. The preoccupation with malarial fevers, cholera and, above all, smallpox control that featured in many British medical reports and accounts earlier in the nineteenth century began to be superseded by increasing emphasis on forms of surgical intervention. Despite some awareness of its potential in earlier years, it was not until the 1880s that surgery started to be a feature of European-style dispensary treatment to any degree, presumably because of understandable pre-antisepsis reluctance to perform surgery at all. In 1872–73, when the first combined dispensary returns were made for the whole province, few major operations were being performed, and the majority were carried out at Jaipur. Of minor operations, the types which indigenous practitioners also carried out, such as lens extraction for cataract, lithotomy, and excision for the fungal disease, mycetoma, were reported only in tiny numbers. Within the next two decades, however, substantial increases in the number of surgical operations are recorded and the majority were on the eye, although operations on anal fistula and internal haemorrhoids, refracture for badly united bones, reconstructions of the nose, amputations for mycetoma and some other surgical procedures were also performed. Such increases indicate a rapid uptake of the superior new facilities for surgical intervention, and in 1900 T. Holbein Hendley, the Chief Medical Officer, suggested that it was success in the field of surgery that 'impresses the native public and most popularizes our institutions ...'[23]

These successes were indeed in marked contrast to the indigenous response to European medicine in general, the vaccination campaign making slow progress and the dispensaries continuing to record low levels of attendance. In seems that the hereditary itinerant professionals who traditionally performed these types of surgery were increasingly made redundant by the spread of modern surgery in Rajasthan. Hendley noted that frequency of attendance at dispensaries varied with religious affiliation. Moslems apparently resorted to European medicine more than Hindus, and Hendley attributed this to pollution avoidance of European drugs. Surgery was, for the most part, in the hands of Muslim practitioners and, if initially Muslims turned to allopathy in cases of illness more readily than Hindus, that too may have had some effect on the practice of various indigenous forms of surgery, including that of the *jarraha*, barber-surgeon. Indigenous inoculators, of course, also disappeared some time after the introduction of European medicine and the implementation of smallpox vaccination campaigns which in general were imposed in disregard of indigenous approaches to prevention.

Conclusion

In subtle respects, then, the spread of European medicine in Rajasthan did have consequences for indigenous practice and for the rural provision of therapy. While religious healing traditions and certain other local therapeutic practices such as vessel manipulation and the use of domestic herbal remedies may have remained relatively little affected, these originally constituted only a part of folk medical tradition. It seems likely that a proportion of sickness was always treated by hereditary specialists, many of whom were itinerant and provided medical and surgical services to the rural population. British influence and the spread of an exclusively European medicine probably led to the closure of such avenues of resort, particularly for the rural population. While ethnographic reports of such folk practitioners are scarce, it seems likely that they possessed considerable therapeutic knowledge in specialised fields. *Jarrahas*, or barber-surgeons, with technical skills and familiarity with specific local complaints such as mycetoma still exist in Rajasthan, but they are rare today compared with the position they were reported to hold around the turn of the century.

While the decline of surgical specialisations can be directly related to competition from Western medicine, the case of another type of indigenous specialist provides an illustration of the indirect effects of the withdrawal of royal patronage. The specialisation in bone setting and massage practised by the *pahalvan*, literally 'wrestler', is a therapeutic tradition associated with the sporting tradition of wrestling which was formerly patronised by the royal houses under Mughal influence, and one of the few hereditary pahalvans still practising in Jaipur claims former familial associations with the Jaipur court. A direct analogue with the pahalwan's therapeutic speciality is the hereditary specialisation in massage and bone setting practised professionally by the Kurup caste of Kerala State, south India. Kurups acted as fencing masters to the dominant martial Nayar caste and developed their therapeutic specialisation in relation to this role.[24] In Kerala, though, this specialisation is accorded official state recognition as Marma, a registered system of indigenous medicine, whereas no such status is accorded the Rajasthani pahalvan, whose hereditary skills appear now to be rare. In the absence of government recognition and professional accreditation such a hereditary, esoteric medical specialisation seems barely to have survived the loss of traditional patronage. The 'indigenisation' of Western biomedicine began at a relatively early stage, at least in Jaipur State, and was in large part due to the acceptance among the educated ruling classes of European medicine as one of the hallmarks of modern civilisation. Moreover, in Rajputana European medicine was less tied to the financial constraints and political rigidities that existed within British India[25] and the direct transfer of patronage from indigenous traditions to European medicine probably had a significant effect on the former.

In Rajasthan today, with a few exceptions, folk medicine is confined to popular, exoteric traditions of therapy which do not involve such specialised therapeutic knowledge. The demonstration of superior efficacy in the case of surgical intervention and the withdrawal of financial support in the case of certain other hereditary specialisations have combined to narrow the range of medical pluralism somewhat, while biomedicine has gradually increased in popularity. The fact that Rajasthani villagers regard an adverse reaction to Western-style medical treatment as indicating a non-natural cause shows how preferences for different kinds of treatment have shifted since Western medicine first became available, despite the continuing interpretation of illness within a broader Hindu cosmology. The current levels of utilisation of biomedicine in Rajasthan thus provide a clear example of the general principle that conceptual disjunctions do not necessarily index resistance to introduced forms of treatment, because people's behaviour is rarely governed in a deterministic fashion by their system of beliefs. The data presented in this chapter suggest that, contrary to the common claim in international health circles that in non-Western settings indigenous health beliefs constitute 'cultural barriers' to the use of modern medicine, 'traditional culture' is very receptive to innovations that are readily available, observably efficacious and have prestige value. The conceptual systems that underlie health-related ideas, however, are much more gradually restructured to accommodate the changing realities of practice. Moreover, introduced practices have themselves been indigenised to a significant degree by adaptation to local needs and expectations, so that biomedicine is utilised selectively. An injection administered by a conveniently located and personally known, albeit unqualified, practitioner is generally preferred to a time-consuming visit to a government clinic and a lengthy and expensive antibiotic course prescribed by a trained but (at best) indifferent doctor. Resistance to biomedicine and its underlying scientific knowledge is articulated not by refusal to utilise a form of treatment that often has dramatically beneficial effects and demonstrates the social status of its user but through reinterpretation of its underlying principles and, most radically, through popular dismissal of the expert claim to its inherent and general superiority over indigenous medicine.

Notes

The ethnographic material presented in this chapter derives from field research conducted in 1984–86 mainly in Jaipur city and in a village of Tonk District, Rajasthan (together with short visits in 1987 and 1993). I acknowledge the support of the Social Science Research Council (now the Economic and Social Research Council) in funding the original research as part of a D.Phil.

1 See, for example, David Arnold, *Colonizing the Body: State Medicine and Epidemic Disease in Nineteenth-century India*, Berkeley, Cal.: University of California Press, 1993; I. J. Catanach, 'Plague and the tensions of empire: India, 1896–1918', pp. 149–71, and D. Arnold, 'Smallpox and colonial medicine in nineteenth-century India', pp. 45–65, in D. Arnold (ed.), *Imperial Medicine and Indigenous Societies*, Manchester University Press, 1988; Radhika Ramasubban, 'Imperial health in British India, 1857–1900', in R. MacLeod and M. Lewis (eds), *Disease, Medicine and Empire: Perspectives on Western Medicine and the Experience of European Expansion*, London: Routledge, 1988, pp. 38–60; Mark Harrison, *Public Health in British India: Anglo-Indian Preventive Medicine, 1859–1914*, Cambridge University Press, 1994.

2 See C. Leslie, *Asian Medical Systems: a Comparative Study*, Berkeley, Cal.: University of California Press, 1976; C. Leslie, 'Interpretations of illness: syncretism in modern Ayurveda', pp. 177–208 in C. Leslie and A. Young (eds), *Paths to Asian Medical Knowledge*, Berkeley, Cal.: University of California, 1992.

3 See R. Jeffery, *The Politics of Health in India*, Berkeley, Cal.: University of California Press, 1988, pp. 42–4, 49–50. Jeffery also asserts (p. 43) that Leslie's claim of a complex reality which included bone-setters, midwives and shamans is supported by no evidence and that (p. 58), given the dearth of material about folk medical practice before the mid-twentieth century, the impact of colonial rule on folk healers is impossible to assess. This chapter constitutes a small beginning in this regard.

4 See, for example, G. Obeyesekere, in Leslie's *Asian Medical Systems*; M. Opler, 'The cultural definition of illness in village India', *Human Organization* 22: 32–5, 1963; and Charles Leslie's introduction to his influential edited volume *Asian Medical Systems: a Comparative Study*. Berkeley, Cal.: University of California Press, 1976.

5 Cf. C. E. Taylor, 'The place of indigenous medical practitioners in the modernization of health services', in Leslie, *Asian Medical Systems*, pp. 285–99; and M. Nichter, *Anthropology and International Health: South Asian Case Studies*. Dordrecht: Kluwer, 1989, p. 190.

6 In the rural area where fieldwork was undertaken there were no vaidyas or hakims offering traditional treatment within the Ayurvedic or Yunani systems of medicine, with the exception of the vaidya at the government Ayurvedic dispensary, whose Ayurvedic medicines were regarded as useless and who primarily offered biomedical treatment on a private basis. Locals recalled one *nari vaidya* (literally, 'pulse physician', referring to the traditional method of Ayurvedic diagnosis) who used to practise in a nearby village, but the most popular vaidya, located in the nearest town, offered exclusively Western-style biomedical treatment. In other rural areas visited during the course of fieldwork the use of classical indigenous medicine in treatment was found to be similarly rare, with most trained practitioners of all types practising Western biomedicine.

7 The verb *lagno* in this context can also mean 'does not take', 'is not efficacious' as

well as 'is not applied, used'.

8 Miscarriage is colloquially called, literally, 'illness of kicking', because it is generally thought to result from a barren or malevolent woman having stepped on the foot of the pregnant woman. It may be remedied if the offending party touches the pregnant woman's foot and then her own forehead, a common abbreviated gesture of respect. Otherwise miscarriage, once having occurred, is liable to recur until remedied by religious healing. A male foetus is considered more likely to abort from such a 'kick' than a female one, reflecting the predominant value inequality between boys and girls.

9 Arthur Kleinman designates 'the management of therapeutic outcomes' as one of the five 'core clinical functions' of health care systems. A. Kleinman, *Patients and Healers in the Context of Culture: an Exploration of the Borderland between Anthropology, Medicine, and Psychiatry*, Comparative Studies of Health Systems and Medical Care No. 3. Berkeley, Cal.: University of California Press, 1980, pp. 71–2, 82–3.

10 See H. Lambert, 'Of bonesetters and barber-surgeons', pp. 92–111 in N. K. Singhi and R. Joshi (eds), *Folk, Faith and Feudalism*, Jaipur: Rawat Publications, 1995, p. 109.

11 T. Holbein Hendley, *A Medico-topographical Account of Jeypore*, Calcutta: Calcutta Central Press, 1895.

12 G. Foster, 'Disease etiologies in non-Western medical systems', *American Anthropologist* 78: 773–82, 1976.

13 Francis Zimmerman, *The Jungle and the Aroma of Meats: an Ecological Theme in Hindu Medicine*, Berkeley, Cal.: University of California Press, 1987; 'The Jungle and the aroma of meats: an ecological theme in Hindu medicine', *Social Science and Medicine* 27, 3: 197–215, 1988.

14 See H. Lambert, 'The cultural logic of Indian medicine: prognosis and etiology in Rajasthani popular therapeutics', *Social Science and Medicine* 34 (10, pp. 1069–76, 1992.

15 Cf. Arnold, *Colonizing the Body*, pp. 55–6.

16 See Arthur Kleinman, 'Concepts and model for the comparison of medical systems as cultural systems', *Social Science and Medicine* 1980, 12B: 85–95.

17 See, for example, W. Crooke, *Religion and Folklore of Northern India*, London: Oxford University Press, 1926, and *Natives of Northern India*, London: Constable, 1907.

18 See, for example, A. H. E. Boileau, *Personal Narrative of a Tour through the Western States of Rajwara, in 1835*, Calcutta: Baptist Mission Press, 1837; Hendley, *A Medico-topographical Account of Jeypore*, and *General Medical History of Rajputana*, Calcutta: Office of the Superintendent of Government Printing, 1900; R. H. Irvine, *Some Account of the General and Medical Topography of Ajmeer*, Calcutta: Thacker; W. Moore, *Native Practice in Rajputana*, 1871; P. D. Pank, *A Medico-topographical Account of Ajmere, Rajputana*, Calcutta: Office of the Superintendent of Government Printing, 1900; also A. K. Roy, *History of the Jaipur City*, New Delhi: Manohar, 1978.

19 W. H. Russell, *The Prince of Wales' Tour: a Diary of India*, 1877, II, p. 357 (cited in Jadunath Sarkar, *A History of Jaipur* c. *1503–1938*, New Delhi: Orient Longman, 1984, p. 361).

20 The year 1872 was the first when joint returns for dispensary attendances were made from all Rajputana dispensaries to the government of India in the annual Rajpootana Dispensary, Vaccination, Jail and Sanitary Reports, while 1874 saw the first annual report of the Jaipur Medical and Metereological Institutions. By this time British political agencies had been established in every major state of the province and it seems that the patterns of medical provision roughly followed the lead of Jaipur.

21 Hendley, *General Medical History of Rajputana*, p. 28.

22 Government of India, *Rajpootana Dispensary, Vaccination, Jail, and Sanitary Report for 1872–73* (Sections from the Records of the Government of India, Foreign Department, No. CXX), Calcutta: Foreign Department, 1873; Government of India,

Rajpootana Dispensary, Vaccination, Jail, and Sanitary Report for 1874 (Selections from the Records of the Government of India, Foreign Department, No. CXX), Calcutta: Foreign Department, 1875; Government of India, *Report of the Political Administration of the Rajpootana States, 1874–75* (Selections from the Records of the Government of India, Foreign Department, No. CXXII), Calcutta: Foreign Department, 1875. On the withdrawal of initially favourable support for indigenous medicine by British administrations see T. J. Patterson, 'The relationship of Indian and European practitioners of medicine from the sixteenth century', in G. Jan Meulenbeld and D. Wujastyk (eds), *Studies on Indian Medical History*, London: Wellcome Foundation, 1987.

23 Hendley, *General Medical History of Rajputana*, p. 96.

24 See Francis Zimmerman, 'From classic texts to learned practice: methodological remarks on the study of Indian medicine', *Social Science and Medicine* 12, 1978, pp. 97–103.

25 Cf. Arnold, *Colonizing the Body*, p. 60.

CHAPTER NINE

The reduction of personhood to brain and rationality? Japanese contestation of medical high technology

Emiko Ohnuki-Tierney

That science is not culture-free but embedded in its cultural tradition has been accepted in some scholarly circles but not in others. Before Kuhn articulated that science and its paradigms are constructs of culture at a particular historical period, Marx observed that Darwin saw a representation of English society in the behaviour of beasts and plants, that is, *nature*. Darwin's *science*, therefore, embodied *culture*, i.e. English society. Sahlins, too, has chided sociobiology as 'scientific totemism'.[1] Medical science is no exception. In fact medicine, which involves humans – with their body, birth and death, and health and illness – in a more direct way than other sciences, is deeply embedded in the Western cultural tradition. Yet this so-called biomedicine has been introduced to every corner of the world as a culture-free objective medical *science*. Even more important, it has been willingly accepted by the people themselves as science and as a mark of progress of human wisdom. In order to understand this process, we must first understand medicine as an expression of Western culture, or, more specifically, of the Enlightenment tradition of the high culture of the West. We must also be aware of what I have called 'cultural imperialism', by which I refer to the 'non-Western' peoples' *willing* acceptance of the Western premise that Western civilisation, with science and technology at its core, is more advanced and higher than other civilisations.[2] Cultural colonisation is far more widespread and has become part of the attitude and view of the 'non-Western' peoples, including those who have never been politically colonised. This is so even though most peoples have consciously or unconsciously 'contested' Western medicine, or even Western civilisation in general. In order to understand the power inequality – political, economic and cultural – involved in the global flow of knowledge, 'contested knowledge' must be examined within a broader context of both contestation of knowledge and its absence.

The major part of this chapter deals with the new medical high technology of organ transplantation. Despite the mounting pressure from outside and some from within the medical profession, the Japanese have shown remarkable resistance to the notions of brain death and organ transplantation. I argue that the new medical technology is an outgrowth of Enlightenment philosophy and thus it is based on the assumption that rationality is the defining feature of humans – a definition not shared by other peoples who contest brain death as a person's death and organ transplantation as a new medical miracle. The specific cultural context of the Japanese reluctance to accept the new technology is discussed. The chapter also points to serious political and ethical implications of the world-wide delivery of this technology in the context of apparent power inequality among the nations.

The reluctance of the Japanese to accept the notion of brain death as a person's death, and subsequent organ transplantation, is then placed in the broader context of other types of contestation of Western medicine, especially their retention of *kampō*, their own medical system with its Chinese origin, whose theoretical premisses depart radically from those of Western medicine.

For the purposes of this chapter, I engage in bold interpretations and make global comparisons. I use terms such as 'the Japanese', 'the West/Western' and even 'non-Western', realising that there are serious problems with such blanket terms. Augé and Cohn pointed out long ago the basic issues involved in lumping 'the rest' of the world into a residual category of 'the non-West'.[3] By the term 'Western culture' I refer primarily to the 'high culture' of the intellectuals of France, Germany, the United Kingdom, a few other countries, primarily in western Europe, and the United States. I commit all the grave sins of totalising and essentialising, as postmodernists would say, but anthropologists interested in larger socio-cultural themes cannot avoid generalisations altogether.

The new high technology: organ transplants and brain death

In the United States and a few other Western countries, multiple transplants of human organs and experimental transplants using non-human primate organs are receiving much media attention, while implants have been so 'naturalised', as Foucault, Bourdieu and Barthes would say, that they are taken for granted and are thus no longer newsworthy.[4] However, Israel, Denmark (until 1991) and Japan remain resistant to this new medical 'high technology'. Note that Denmark, a Western country, parted company with the West until 1991 in this regard, while Israel, if it may be called 'Western', and Orthodox Jews in the United States continue to reject this medical technology. Furthermore, there are many individuals who do not subscribe to the tradition of acceptance even in the countries where organ transplantation is most developed. Conversely, there are many individuals in 'non-Western' countries and cultural traditions who advocate the new technology. The refusal or reluctance to pursue this new medical technology in these so-called advanced countries, which possess both the financial and the technical capacity to adopt it, invites anthropological enquiry as to the reasons.

Under influence from abroad, the Japanese Medical Association and Japanese physicians and lawyers have pressed the Japanese government to pass legislation accepting brain death as the death of a person. The government created a special task force, chaired by Takeuchi Kazuo, to present the standards for brain death, known as 'the Takeuchi standards'. Following the United States and Canada (but not the United Kingdom), this 1985 report advocated defining brain death as the non-functioning of the entire brain and specified six conditions.[5] It was signed by thirteen members of the committee and three participants.[6] However, the report included a minority opinion signed by two committee members and two participants who opposed the legal sanctioning of brain death. Umehara Takeshi, one of the opponents, subsequently edited a book in which fifteen authors explained their reasons for opposition.[7] Six opposed such legislation from a medical perspective, five opposed it from a legal perspective, and four offered philosophical or religious reasons. While the passage of legislation to equate brain death with the death of an individual is likely to occur, and public opinion is increasingly in support of the idea of brain death as death and that of organ transplantation (see Appendix 9.1), in 1995 it remains uncertain whether the public will in fact adopt it fully. At any rate, the situation with Japan indeed contrasts with that in some Western countries (see Appendix 9.2). Not only the Japanese remain reluctant to transplant organs from the brain-dead. The figures in Table 9.1 demonstrate the Japanese situation in contrast to that in the United States. Japanese are also reticent about using organs from cadavers. Thus, while 80 per cent of kidney transplants in the United States are from cadavers, only 30.8 per cent of kidney transplants and only 22 per cent of liver transplants in Japan are from cadavers.

Needless to say, the issue of brain death and organ transplantation is enormously complex, involving economic, political, legal and other dimensions. The purpose of this chapter excludes more subtle and complex arguments about the entire issue of organ transplantation and brain death, including: benefits from this new technology in many cases; the legal implications; the cost of keeping the brain-dead alive; the negative impact of the media on medical professionals to choose ethically and financially questionable cases of transplants that are nonetheless 'dramatic' and hence newsworthy; and inequality of access to the new technology both within a society and across societies whereby the more powerful and the rich in the wealthier countries are more likely to receive its benefits.[8]

Table 9.1 *Transplants in the United States and Japan*

	United States		
Organ	*1983*	*1991*	*Japan*
Kidney[a]	6,112	10,051	6,951[b]
Heart	172	2,126	1[c]
Heart–lung	20	51	0[c]
Liver	164	2,953	50[d]
Pancreas	61	533	12[d]
Lung	–	403	0[c]

Note

[a] Approximately 20 per cent from living relatives.

[b] By 1989.

[c] By 1994.

[d] By 1992.

Sources The US figures are from Myron Genel, 'Regulation of Organ and Tissue Transplantation.' Paper read at a conference on *Organ Transplantation and Human Rights: Cross-Cultural Perspectives* (The Orville H. Schell, Jr. Center for International Human Rights, Yale Law School, April 15–17, 1993): n.p.; Further statistical information is presented in Ohnuki-Tierney, 'Brain death'.

My focus here is on conceptual issues. Let me first briefly discuss how the new technology represents the concepts of life and death, the body, personhood, etc., that are deeply embedded in a dominant Western intellectual tradition, the Enlightenment tradition.

Brain death as a new cultural institution

Although it is framed as if it were the most scientific and thus most culture-free notion, the notion of brain death is as much a cultural construct as a religion. As each society now struggles to define this new concept of death, it faces the choice of part(s) of brain. Today there are two types of brain death: (1) 'death' or non-function of the cerebrum – brain death in the United Kingdom; (2) non-function of the entire brain, including the cerebrum and the brain stem – brain death in the United States and Japan. The non-functioning of the cerebrum leads to a 'persistent vegetative state'. In other words, brain death is a new phenomenon determined by social agents in each culture; culture, instead of nature, plays the dominant role in its construction.

For the Japanese and for many other peoples, before the notion of 'brain death' emerged, the inactive 'brain' represented a prolongation of life rather than a prolongation of the process of dying, as people in some Western countries have come to view it. Previously, even medical doctors did not equate brain death with biological death. Brain death is therefore an entirely new concept of death.[9]

The notion of brain death constitutes a radical transgression of traditional notions of death in most societies in that it represents an altogether different death. While the culturally defined person is not dead, i.e. the body is still warm and the heart is still beating, the person may be 'killed', in the traditional sense, through the removal of organs for transplantation.

The brain and rationality in Western tradition

The conceptual bedrock of brain death is the cherished principle of Western high culture, especially the Enlightenment philosophy espoused by intellectuals since the seventeenth century primarily in France, England, Germany and the United States, in which rationality is the most important criterion of what constitutes humans. As a corollary, the brain – the seat of rational thought – occupies the most prominent place among the body parts. In this dominant 'Western' philosophical perspective – *Cogito ergo sum* – a 'person' ceases to exist when the functions located in the cerebrum are 'irreversibly' lost. The brain-dead are, naturally, dead persons.

In spite of this logic, Fox and Swazey emphasise that medical professionals continue to find it difficult to identify the brain-dead as a 'corpse', and are bewildered by having to treat 'dead' patients during and after the removal of organs.[10] Younger *et al.* similarly point to this ambivalence, referring to labels for brain-dead organ donors, such as 'beating-heart cadaver' or 'neomort', which have yet to become either emotionally or culturally acceptable even in the United States. Yet they report, 'Most would agree that these donors are no longer "persons".'[11]

The heart too is an important organ in Western cultures. Its significance is expressed in the enormous importance placed on love, which has occupied a central place in many Western cultures since the time of chivalry. Today, in the United States, commercial establishments rampantly exploit the notion of love with iconographic representations of the heart to promote gift-giving on Valentine's Day, Mothers' Day, etc.

Note, however, that while in Western culture the heart is associated with emotions, the brain is associated with rationality and consciousness. To push the symbolic association further: at least in the past, males represented rationality, while women represented emotionality, as is evident in the familiar Freudian schema. The brain, then, represented the essence of humans, as *Man* represented Humans. In this symbolic construct the brain is arguably the most important part of the human anatomy. It is the seat of 'the mind', while the heart indicates the presence of mere biological life.

Since classical times, through Descartes, Kant, Rousseau and others, and even more vigorously since the rise of modern science, rationality as the essence of humanity in the Western intellectual tradition has been expressed in numerous ways. For example, ethology in the West has focused on the question of whether non-human primates possess language – the tool of rationality – or whether it is unique to humans. In anthropology itself, the question of rationality has occupied a central stage of enquiry, whether in its relationship to magic and religion, or 'the primitive mentality', since the time of Lévy-Bruhl, and has been discussed by almost all major figures in anthropology since then. On the other hand, equation of the rationalist tradition with the entirety of Western intellectual tradition is an enormous oversimplification. Even within the high culture of the 'West', a far more complex picture of the notion of rationality must be recognised. The relationships between rationality and empiricism, and between rationality and discursive logic, are but two of many complex dimensions of the question of rationality.[12]

As Keith Thomas points out, 'a "rationalist" attitude had existed long before the work of Galileo or Newton', and Aristotle and Cicero are but two examples of the rationalist authors of classical antiquity. In his explanation of the decline of 'magic', Thomas argues that 'What the scientific revolution did was to supersede this type of reasoning and to buttress up the old rationalist attitude with a more stable intellectual foundation, based on the mechanical philosophy.'[13] I am arguing that the new medical technology and its widespread acceptance in certain Western societies is evidence not only of the success of the scientific revolution but, more important, that the rationalist tradition has deep roots in the thoughts of ordinary people, and not just intellectuals, in these Western societies.

It is no accident that biomedicine has focused on the brain as the crucial organ in determining whether 'the person' is alive or dead. The readiness with which brain death is recognised as signalling the death *of and as* a human is simply a corollary. Without a functioning cerebrum, the human becomes a thing: a non-person and non-human. Brain death is the opposite of the ideal model – 'an independent individual making rational decisions'.

Hybrid monster as human

If the new culturalised nature, i.e. the human body, represents the pre-eminence of the brain, with the heart as a replaceable organ, then it reinforces the argument that rationality, located in the brain, rather than emotionality, located in the heart, is the only critical part of the anatomy for defining the self. If so, the new medical technology signals the ultimate triumph of rationality and represents a new solution to the Cartesian dualism – this technological revolution will accomplish what the Enlightenment strove for with only partial success.

The triumph is so revolutionary that it overturns most received wisdom and poses a threat to human culture and most cultures. Thus transplant technology implies the alarming possibility of creating a new human, if it takes the 'rationality' model to its logical conclusion. The new human would have a number of organs – some artificial, others from non-human animals, and still others from other humans – with only the cerebrum remaining from the original body. In short, a hybrid monster.

Transgression of the animate–inanimate distinction

Artificial organs and tissues, or 'implants', have become so common that most Americans do not give much thought to this curious combination of the inanimate (implants) with the animate (the human body). Note that the artificial heart has been arguably the most important type of implant. Transgression of the boundary line between the animal and the inanimate, then, is no longer consciously recognised.

Transgression of the human–non-human distinction

Transplant surgeons have long experimented with organs from various animals, including such 'lowly' animals as pigs. For a long time they have regularly replaced diseased heart valves with heart valves taken from pigs.[14] At present, the mass media eagerly await another 'breakthrough' in organ transplantation – successful transplantation of organs from baboons and other non-human primates into humans.

The enthusiastic welcoming of the new ape man sheds light on the relationship between religion and science in the West. In the biblical tradition the ape man would be the most blasphemous transgression. In Genesis, God created the binary division of humans and non-human animals, just as He created night and day, land and water, etc. The line dividing humans from non-human animals is therefore not just important but sacred. Its transgression is a sacred taboo. In western fairy tales, such as those of Aesop, a true metamorphosis between humans and non-human animals does not take place – animals simply don human attire.

On the other hand, this tradition has been challenged since the nineteenth century by Darwinian evolutionism, which has been a powerful force not only among the intellectual elites but also among the folk. Through Darwinism the evolutionary proximity of an affinity between humans and apes became a scientific 'truth'. The current welcoming attitude to the new, literal ape man, then, signals the ultimate triumph of Darwinism and scientific rationality in general over religion in the West.

In the cosmologies of many peoples, including the Japanese, many deities are animals. Thus, human metamorphosis into animals is transcendental. The notion of transmigration in East Asian religions also denies a hard-and-fast line between humans and non-human animals. Despite the continuum which the Japanese and many other peoples see between humans and non-animals, these people nevertheless establish a delicate demarcation line between the two categories of beings. It is for this reason, as I have explicated elsewhere,[15] that the monkey in Japanese culture poses a threat to humans, who must ensure human superiority over the monkey by not allowing the monkey to transgress the demarcation line. The cosmologies of peoples to whom scientific rationality has not yet become hegemonic may insist on a sensitive line between humans and non-human animals.

Transgression of self and other

For the self-identify of individuals in all cultures, the body holds intense emotional power. The existential seat of the personhood is the body. 'I' is experienced through 'my body', in relationship to the other and his/her body. Organ or tissue transplantation creates a human body in which 'my brain' co-exists with 'his, her, or even its heart'. Self/other distinction is transgressed in a most immediate and psychologically powerful way.

If body parts are freely replaceable, then 'I' or 'me', which is existentially represented in every culture by the body, loses its identity and permanency. 'I' with a part of his/her/its body no longer represents the unique person. Given that the self is unique from the perspective of the person in every culture, the new potential hybrid self offered by Western biomedicine threatens the personhood experienced through the body by each individual.

This translates in actual cases into how the gift of self – the most inalienable gift of all – may in fact be rejected. Hosaka describes a Japanese man who received a kidney from a living donor. He regained bodily 'health' but lost his mind – he was ready to knife his doctor because 'my body is no longer mine'.[16] An additional factor involved in such rejection is the notion of impurity, which is almost universally assigned to the dead body. The transplanted organ in one's body is not only 'not mine' but also impure, a defiling body part of a dead person.

Transgression of nature and culture

In the Western tradition the human body has occupied an ambivalent position in the symbolic dyad of nature and culture. It represents human-ness and human culture, on the one hand, but it is also the seat of the 'Beast in Every Body' – the uncontrollable sexuality and animality of humans – representing 'nature', on the other hand.

The new technology – the epitome of culture – has created a new vision of personhood, which is located in the brain, thereby eliminating the ambivalent or dual nature of humans expressed through the body. The new body, synthesised by the new technology, has become the natural body which has been purged and become, I am tempted to add, 'pure reason'. It has eliminated the beast, although, ironically, allowing parts of literal beasts, e.g. baboon hearts, to enter the human body. The new human body represents another round of cultural construction of nature.

The idea of rationality as the hallmark of humanity and the pre-eminence of brain is not universally shared. A cursory review of cultural valuations of body parts reveals that the brain, and the heart, for that matter, do not enjoy similar pre-eminence in other cultures. Even in the so-called West we find variations. For example, in the Orthodox Jewish tradition the heart, not the brain, is considered to be the seat of life, leading to Orthodox Jewish opposition to the notion of brain death.[17]

Japanese resistance to medical high technology

In the Japanese folk concepts of *ningen* (human beings) and personhood, rationality, as defined above, does not always occupy an important place. Nor does the brain claim pre-eminence as a body part. It is not that the Japanese are non-rational. Japanese folk religiosity has an enormously pragmatic side, and its practices and beliefs are 'logical'.[18] If we take the minimal definition of rationality as 'logical consistency', the Japanese too espouse rationality, but of an altogether different kind.[19]

With regard to the high culture of Japan, many sophisticated debates have taken place on the emphasis on the reason and reasoning. Scholarly debates have focused on metaphysical *v.* phenomenological, discursive *v.* non-discursive logic, dualistic *v.* non-dualistic cosmology and a host of other finely tuned considerations to understand the Japanese intellectual tradition.[20] None, however, ever claimed that there is a 'rationalist' tradition in the Western sense, until some intellectuals started to adopt the latter. The debate over the intellectual tradition on this issue is succinctly summarised by Eisenstadt:

> This rationality was characterized by a continuous extension of the arenas in which instrumental rationality, *Zweckrationalitaet*, could develop without the development of a discourse of *Wertrationalitaet*, of critical reflexivity about the sphere of ultimate values rooted in some type of transcendent orientation. Accordingly, the development of instrumental rationality did not become interwoven with such reflexivity.[21]

The soul (tamashii) as the hallmark of the beings of the universe

Instead of rationality, the ownership of the *tamashii* is of crucial importance to personhood. Note, however, that its ownership is not unique to humans. Deities, ancestors, animals and other beings of the universe all own the soul. Thus ownership of the soul contrasts with the Western notion of rationality whose distinctive role is to distinguish humans from animals. For the Japanese, that the soul is of paramount importance for defining humanity and personhood is not in contradiction with the notion that all other beings too own the soul.

Sharing the soul with non-humans, the Japanese reserve for humans a special capacity which is not exactly affectivity or emotionality, as expressed in these English terms, which are thoroughly embedded in the dualism of rationality and emotionality.[22]

Given the importance of the soul, the Japanese have chosen it as a distinguishing characteristic in relation to other peoples, as seen in such expressions as *wakon kansai* (Japanese soul and Chinese brilliance) or *wakon yôsai* (Japanese soul and Western brilliance) – two phrases used to identify the Japanese self in its encounter with the other. When the Japanese encountered a highly developed Chinese civilisation during the fifth and sixth centuries, and when the Japanese encountered Western civilisation at the end of the nineteenth century, they eagerly embraced these foreign civilisations. But, in an effort to protect Japanese identity and pride, they identified themselves with the Japanese soul, and credited the Chinese and the Westerners with *sai*, i.e. brilliance, rationality, etc. In this way they achieved 'the best of both worlds'.[23]

The soul and the body parts

In the well known interpretation by Orikuchi of the belief in the soul in ancient Japan, there is no mention of the precise location within the body where the soul was believed to reside.[24] Since the late medieval period the soul has been thought to be located in the general and broadly defined area called *hara*, the stomach, which is the most important part of the body. The *seppuku* suicide of warriors derives from the hunter's tradition of taking the slain animal's intestines.[25] Medieval warriors threw their intestines at the enemy when they committed *seppuku*, thereby releasing their soul from the body. Elsewhere I have extensively discussed the importance of the stomach in the past as well as at present when no Japanese believes that the soul is located in the stomach.[26]

In the past, upon death the soul was thought to leave the stomach via the neck through the nostrils or the ears, establishing the custom of covering one's ears to prevent one's soul from being lured away at the time of the death of someone close (called *mimifusagi* or *tomobiki*). Note also that *onryô*, the soul of the deceased who has remorse or vengeance, was believed to stay at the neck. The neck, then, is an enormously important part of the body, next to or equal to the stomach.[27]

A crucial piece of ethnographic evidence for the importance of the neck comes from a funeral practice, which continues to the present day, of saving the last vertebra and placing it in an urn after cremation. Although it is part of the *kubi* (neck), because of its visual resemblance to the adam's apple, which the Japanese think of as resembling the praying Buddha in his sitting position, the bone is referred to as *nodo botoke* (adam's apple; 'buddha in the throat'). In other words, it is the 'neck' that represents the body of the deceased. I think it is for this reason that the enemy's 'head' is always referred to as the neck, *kubi*.

With the neck and the stomach claiming crucial importance as the abode of the soul, we see little evidence for either the head or the brain, which became important only among intellectuals after the introduction of the Western rationalist tradition.

The relation of the body to the soul

That the welfare of the body is essential to the welfare of the soul is clearly expressed in the two most important and interrelated characteristics of the Japanese concept of the body: the intactness of the body (*gotai*) and non-violence to the body. Together these notions lead to the Japanese emphasis on the 'natural' state of the body or the 'natural' course of life.

At birth one receives a body with all its weaknesses, including one's *taishitsu* – inborn constitution – and *jibyô* – a chronic illness one is born with and which one 'nurses' throughout life. One nurtures this body given at birth, rather than drastically conquering or altering it, while constantly monitoring minute fluctuations of the body. Even with the spread of jogging and other health care practices from the United States, perfect health is seen as ephemeral and ordinary health is a condition that fluctuates.

Above all, the Japanese emphasise the intactness of the body, expressed as *gotai* – 'the five body parts' – meaning the entire body, which they attempt to keep intact not only throughout life but also at death. The number five is a basic number in Japanese numerology. The concept of *gotai* derives from Confucianism, although most contemporary Japanese would not recognise its origin in Confucianism (which may have simply institutionalised a folk concept). It held that if a person dies with his/her body intact, then his/her soul will be transmitted to a descendant and live in his/her body.[28]

When a baby is born the parents are anxious to ascertain that the baby's *gotai* is intact. Conversely, those whose *gotai* is missing or deformed, termed *gotai fugu*, encounter considerable cultural and social discrimination. This was especially so in the past. For example, the crippled were thought to embody religious impurity.[29]

The *gotai* notion lies also at the basis of Japanese repugnance towards implants. To date, no pacemaker implant has been manufactured in Japan, although a model was once presented at an international conference by a large watch and clock manufacturer, which chose not to market it for fear that a malfunction might lead to deaths of patients.[30] The technology of enteroproctia (artificial anus) is also most highly developed in the United States and Japanese patients use products made in the United States. The patients who use it are extremely conscious of it, and Watari, a popular actor, dreaded its use more than the colon cancer which had been removed.[31] In the view of these Japanese, implants are not absorbed by one's body but remain permanently foreign elements, and the body therefore ceases to be intact.

The *gotai* notion is closely related to the Japanese taboo against any violence to the body which might cause imbalance in it. When the Japanese adopted religions, technology, town planning, a legal system, imperial accession rituals and many other socio-cultural institutions from China during the fifth and sixth centuries, they did not adopt ear-piercing, foot binding for women or castration to produce eunuchs. It is only recently that young Japanese have started to pierce their ears and undergo plastic surgery to make their eyes more Western-looking – a conspicuous case of symbolic violence in Bourdieu's sense.

The Japanese have long been aware that the Chinese practise ear-piercing and yet they did not adopt it from them. Some Japanese even used it as a point of distinction between us, the Japanese, and them, the Chinese. Even today older Japanese still regard it as 'impurity'. When they pierce their ears, however, the young often do so against their parents' wishes or purposely do not consult them beforehand. Newspapers reported that one of the qualifications of a prospective bride for Crown Prince Naruhito was that she should not have pierced ears – a qualification met by Owada Masako, who married the prince on 6 June 1993. Many other types of body mutilation for aesthetic purposes are practised in other cultures of the world but, except ear-piercing and plastic surgery today, virtually none has been performed by the Japanese. Traditionally, bodily transformations for aesthetic purposes are confined to tattooing, which is confined to some members of marginalised social groups. Note also the almost complete absence of the ritual sacrifice of animals, which is widely practised in many cultures.

By the same token, and despite eager adoption of Western medical technology, the Japanese have been cautious about surgery. Arguably surgery is the most important 'healing' technique in biomedicine. Organ transplantation is predicated upon the notion of surgery, and both share the basic premiss of modern Western medicine – the notion of causation, which defines disease as located in an organ attacked by pathogenic agents.[32] Surgery that removes a diseased organ and replaces it is a logical solution. This view of disease in biomedicine has been quite powerful in recent times but is relatively new in Western medicine, arising around 1800 in Paris and accepted in the United States some fifty years later.[33]

Although surgery as a medical technique is so naturalised in the contemporary world, it is by no means a universal means of restoring health. Anthropological studies of humoral medicines in various parts of the world have introduced us to the notion of the equation of the bodily balance with health and of imbalance with illness.[34] Similarly, traditional Chinese medicine is based on what Porkert has called 'a system of correspondence', rather than on 'a system of causation'.[35] For the Japanese traditional medicine of *kampō*, derived from Chinese medicine, the basic premiss of medical treatment is the restoration of the balance of the body, which will then remove aetiological conditions and therefore pathogens as well. Thus treatment is not aimed directly at removing the pathogen. In this system of medical thought, surgery is the polar opposite of the notion of treatment and is actually seen to aggravate the body's imbalance. Therefore, despite the prestige accorded to biomedicine in Japan, the Japanese have been quite cautious and selective about adopting surgery.[36] Although Japanese surgeons too enjoy considerable prestige and power, in this respect they are a pale shadow of US surgeons, who, especially the brain and heart specialists, are at the apex of both professional and popular acclaim.[37] Note, however, that in the United States the large number of unnecessary surgical operations has attracted sharp criticisms in recent years.

For the Japanese, who avoid going outside after taking a bath in order not to give the body a shock from the cold air, and who have never practised bodily mutilation for aesthetic purposes, surgery is an extreme form of violence to the body, although its popularity has rapidly increased in the last couple of decades.

The body and the soul of the deceased

Death in the Japanese view is marked by the departure of the soul, which is signalled by the cessation of breathing. The word *iki* means both breath and life. Expressions such as *iki o hikitoru* (to withdraw one's breath) or *iki ga kireta* (the breathing stopped) are common expressions for death. They do not take loss of consciousness (*ishiki ga nakunaru,* one loses consciousness) as the criterion for death, since the same happens when one faints.

But the relationship between the body and the soul continues to be of crucial importance after death. The body must be treated properly for the welfare of the departing and departed soul. For the Japanese, the *gotai manzoku* (intactness of the five body parts) is important not only to the living but also to the dead. A dignified death requires the body to be intact. The ideal death is *daiôjô,* the grand way of dying, in which a person fulfils his/her life given at birth and dies without pain after a natural life course. This belief, I think, is fairly consistent throughout history.

Yanagita suggests that the custom of barring dogs from some islands used as cemeteries is based on dogs' 'abominable habit' of digging up the bones of the dead, thereby depriving the dead of *gotai*. He also calls attention to the frequency in the records left by court officials in Kyoto to references to a crow dropping a baby's hand and a *tengu* (mythical creature) carrying a bone. The references reveal an extreme fear of missing body parts of the dead.[38]

Although I have emphasised the Japanese aversion to violence to the body, 'cultural explanations' are not always 'logical' from a cross-cultural perspective. For example, *seppuku* or *harakiri* (suicide by cutting the abdomen open to release one's soul) involves 'violence'.[39] Conversely, Japanese warriors took the enemy's neck (*kubi*), that is, 'head' in English. This act, in my view, constituted the ultimate killing because it prevented the enemy's *gotai* from remaining intact, thus preventing the enemy's rebirth.

While the official explanation of cremation in Buddhism proclaims that cremation establishes the abandonment of the attachment to the body, Buddhism preached the *mujô* (impermanence) of this world and detachment from one's body, which epitomised humans' earthly desires. In their preaching, Buddhists visualised the dead as *hakkotsu* (bleached bones) and endorsed cremation to express the abandonment of the attachment to one's body. Cremation was in practice before the eighth century and became common among the elites during the Nara (646–794) and the Heian (794–1185) periods. The cremation and subsequent scattering of the ashes of the Junna emperor in 840 (Jôwa 7) are well known, although at that time the prototypical burial was still *dosô* (interment in the ground). When the government began to collect statistics on cremation in 1925 (Taishô 14) cremation constituted only 43·2 per cent of funerals. Between 1935 and 1945 cremation became more common than interment. Although the rate of cremation dropped just after World War Two, in 1990, 97·5 per cent of all burials were cremation.[40] Some consider that cremation became the prevalent mode of burial among the people in part because it guaranteed the intactness of the dead body until the moment of cremation, thus eliminating the precarious stage of deterioration during which the body may lose its intactness.

A series of mortuary rituals is testimony to the Japanese belief in the soul after death. Nowhere is the belief more explicitly expressed than in the custom of the *shijû-ku-nichi*, forty-nine days after the death of a person (counting from the day before the death), during which the soul of the dead is considered to hover around the house, especially the rooftop, and during which survivors make sure the dead will accomplish *jôbutsu*, that is, the achievement of the status of a *hotoke*, a Buddha, or, more accurately from the folk perspective, the status of an ancestor. This is done through the continuous burning of incense, candle light, and the offering of tea, water and rice. The food offering is made because during this process the deceased is considered to breathe and eat, like a living person, while gradually abandoning such worldly behaviour and achieving the status of a pure soul. The organs, then, are vital during this period.

A human being is gradually created in the womb, where the soul becomes united with the body. At death the soul becomes gradually detached from the body during the *shijû-ku-nichi*. Again, this is the natural course. To shorten the length of the mourning period is considered to shorten the life cycle of the dead. The removal of organs from the brain-dead is tantamount to depriving the deceased of a cultural and social death.

The following story, therefore, does not have persuasive power for everyone. The story, entitled 'The Story of Brian,' is part of a package provided by the Elliot Hospital in Manchester, New Hampshire, and by University Hospitals and Clinics in Madison, Wisconsin, to patients before they undergo any surgery so that they may will their organs for donation in the event that they die. In the story, the enormous altruism of 'The Gift of Life,' consented to by Brian's parents, is praised in terms of the use of his organs and tissues for others:

> Brian's heart went to a 35-year-old father of two. The liver forestalled death in a 20-year-old college student. One of Brian's kidneys went to a teacher who had been on dialysis for five years; the other kidney went to a young wife and mother of three youngsters. Brian's eyes were removed so that his corneas could restore sight to two blind people. His donated skin helped save the life of a severely burned baby. Bone from Brian's legs and hips were removed so that a 14-year-old boy would not have to undergo amputation of a leg due to bone cancer and so that another child's severely deformed face could be reconstructed by a plastic surgeon. From this single tragedy sprung new life, new health, and new hope for nine of Brian's fellow humans and nine American families.

In other words, virtually nothing is left of Brian, whose body is hollow inside. But note also that in 'Renewing Life through Organ and Tissue Donation', a brochure for potential donors provided by the University of Wisconsin Hospitals and Clinics, they add: 'The funeral will not be delayed, the body will not be disfigured, and they can hold a viewing.' This statement unwittingly acknowledges the importance of the body of the deceased to a 'proper' death.

From the perspective of many Japanese facing death, foremost in their minds is often the care of their soul and the family ancestral alcove after their death, even though most contemporary Japanese have practically no vision of what the after-life is about. For this reason, sometimes the will has a special provision for the offspring who is responsible for the care of the family tombs and the ancestral alcove.

The modern Japanese, who only visit a shrine at New Year, if at all, and who proclaim 'deities exist only when you need them' (*kommata toki no kamidayori*), offer tea, water and rice every day to the ancestral alcove and pay homage to the family grave on *obon* and at other prescribed times. Note also that when a guest comes to the house, he/she often first prays at the ancestral alcove, offering fruit or whatever gift he/she may have brought. In fact mortuary ritual and so-called 'ancestor worship' are at the symbolic core of Japanese culture even today.

There are signs that the Japanese will come to accept the notion of brain death, and that organ transplantation may also become more accepted in the near future. But, even so, the medical technology introduced and practised in Japan will be transformed on Japanese soil, just as biomedical delivery in general has undergone profound changes since its introduction to Japan.[41]

Plural system of medicine in contemporary Japan

The Japanese attitude to medical high technology, discussed above, follows the pattern of Japanese selective adoption of biomedicine and the retention of traditional medical systems. In contemporary Japan there is more than one system of health care, and most Japanese use more than one simultaneously or sequentially. The most powerful is biomedicine, developed in the West since the late nineteenth century, when it was also imported into Japan, replacing the earlier form of Western medicine introduced to Japan by the Dutch in the late eighteenth century. Other important medical systems include: *kampō*, a medical system originated in China but which had been introduced to Japan by the sixth century; religious institutions, such as Buddhist temples and Shinto shrines, which continue to play an important role in the health care of contemporary Japanese; a number of powerful new religious sects whose major focus is on health care; shamanistic medical practices, which declined significantly after World War Two; and home care, usually administered by women.

Unlike in other spheres of activity, in which the Japanese have shown extraordinary eagerness to copy and emulate aspects of Western civilisation, they have domesticated biomedical delivery by remoulding it as a Japanese medical system.[42] Furthermore, they have kept other systems of medicine quite actively. Here I briefly introduce the *kampō* practice.

In contemporary Japan *kampō* comes in all shades, from orthodox practice to mass-produced and pre-packaged extracts of herbs, to a street-corner computer diagnosis. The orthodox *kampō* practice today is a medicinal system developed in Japan which therefore differs considerably from the Chinese medicine originally introduced from China and the medicine practised in contemporary China. Its treatment consists of moxibustion, acupuncture, and herbal and animal medicine. In a radical departure from biomedicine, *kampō* does not recognise categories of illness. Each departure from health is diagnosed on the basis of the combined total of symptoms which the patient experiences and those which the *kampō* doctor detects. The sum total, called *shôkôgun*, is carefully evaluated against the sex, age and constitution of the patient, and the climate in which the patient resides, in order to reach a proper prescription for treatment. A *kampō* doctor, using the auditory, tactile, olfactory and visual faculties in reading the patient's conditions, prescribes a specific treatment. In the case of herbs, it is a mixture consisting of a dozen or so herbs, which the patient brews in an earthen kettle for a long time and then drinks. Every patient therefore has a unique illness and therefore requires a unique set of treatments. Diagnosis does not consist of labelling the illness. In fact the whole effort is focused on cure – the prescription of a certain combination of herbs, and/or moxibustion or acupuncture on certain points of the body, depending upon the nature of the affliction.

The conceptual basis of *kampō* is that an illness is caused by a bodily imbalance and thus the restoration of bodily balance is the basic premiss of the cure. It emphatically denies the merit of surgery, even in the case of cancer.

This premiss contrasts sharply with biomedicine, which defines 'disease' in terms of a particular set of symptoms or syndrome; its usual practice is to identify the patient's problem within the biomedical classificatory schema so that a proper treatment for that disease category can be prescribed. Any symptoms which do not constitute a part of the defining symptoms are often not considered important enough for treatment. Thus there is often a situation whereby a patient feels an 'illness,' but a doctor tells her/him that she/he does not have a 'disease', a term I use referring to the departures from health as defined in biomedicine.

While the contrast has been put here in an overly simplistic way, it is reasonable to conclude that the premiss of *kampō* is closer to the way lay people understand and experience their departures from health. It is perhaps for this reason that Japanese lay people have supported *kampō* practice even though it has twice been suppressed by the government. First, during the late nineteenth century the Japanese government instituted a rule that one must receive biomedical training in order to practise *kampō*. It did so in order to 'modernise' Japanese medicine. Second, the US occupation forces prohibited moxibustion and acupuncture after the end of the World War Two. In contemporary Japan, *kampō* has become enormously popular, not only among lay people but also with the government, which has rendered aid to this system of medicine by financially supporting research in *kampō* and gradually adding *kampō* treatments to health insurance. *Kampō* now exists in a symbiotic mode with biomedicine in that it specialises in chronic illnesses, especially those accompanied by chronic pain, and new types of illness, including those caused by environmental pollution and traffic accidents, for none of which biomedicine has been successful.

There are other reasons for the increased popularity of *kampō*. Reaction to the negative sides of biomedicines is in part responsible for the phenomenal come-back of *kampō*. Biomedicine has demonstrated its devastatingly negative effects, tarnishing its almighty image. Nor has it been able to cope with changes in the epidemiological pattern. It has not been effective in treating chronic illnesses or various kinds of pain.

The increased popularity both of *kampō* and religious healing may also have something to do with the changing self image of the Japanese *vis-à-vis* the Other, which in the recent past has been represented by the West. To the Japanese, Westerners have represented the Other with dual power, both positive and negative – as the source and model of scientific and technological achievements and as the destructive power epitomised in the atomic bombs at Hiroshima and Nagasaki. With the country's 'conquest' of world markets in high technology, the motor industry and other fields, however, the image the Japanese have of the Other has changed, and this change has in turn transformed their self-image. It is less their economic success as such that has affected the Japanese concept of the collective self; it is more its symbolic nature. By overtaking the science and technology of the West, many Japanese no longer feel inferior to the Other. The Japanese no longer have to hold biomedicine in awe, but are comfortable in using their own medicine, be it religious healing or *kampō*. If so, Japan's case also illustrates how cultural imperialism plays a significant role in the acceptance of biomedicine in various countries of the world.

Discussion: medical high technology in cross-cultural perspective – organs as 'the gift of life'?

'The gift of life' has become virtually the definition of organ and tissue donations in the United States.[43] Yet organs are not and cannot be the gift of self, because organ donation lacks the most critical elements of gift giving and exchange. Not only are organs given without return – the essential feature of gift giving as a means of establishing social relations[44] – but current practice, understandably in many ways, conceals the identity of the donor; it seals off any of the human relationships involved in most social transactions. It is for this reason that 'the gift of life' has not been widely accepted in Japanese society, where gift giving is a central social, economic and political institution.

Although, in practice, social transactions are never quite clear-cut, I present the following schematic distinctions between gift, commodity and charity as three modes of exchange:

1 *Gift exchange*

Inalienable objects (gifts).
Interdependent transactors.
Creation of social bonds.

2 *Commodity exchange*

Alienable objects.
Independent transactors.
Absence of social relations.

3 *Charity*

Quasi-alienable objects.
Quasi-independent transactors.
Quasi-absence of social relations.

Gift-giving practice is an exchange of quasi-inalienable objects ('part of the self') to maintain or establish interdependence; commodity transactions involve alienable objects between independent actors, and charity involves alienable objects between actors whose are only indirectly interdependent.

Organ donation, then, is none of these, since the object, which is as inalienable as an object can be, is given to a total stranger with whom no social relationship is established. The absence of a social relationship between donor and receiver is the very reason that leads organ donation to commercialisation. Without the social context in which real social agents engage in transaction, the organ – or any object, for that matter – becomes a candidate for commodification. That is, without a social agent an object in itself has no meaning. No restriction is placed upon the way in which the 'meaning' or the value of the organ is interpreted by the recipient. The most inalienable of all inalienable gifts thus easily turns into a commodity.

Ethical issues in technology delivery

This commodification is what is happening in the 'organ market'. Terms such as 'organ farms' and 'harvesting of organs' are commonly used, signalling the increasing impersonalistion of the organ donation process and decreasing resistance to commodification on the part of donors and recipients. Thus the *gift of self* is in imminent danger of being transformed into the *sale of self*.

In cross-cultural perspective, we are witnessing a rapid development of the black market in human organs, possibly involving children.[45] For example, in India, Bombay has become the international centre for the black market in organs, one in ten of which is HIV-infected.[46] Even 'donors' themselves are willing to sell organs. The cover story of the July 1990 issue of *India Today*, by Raj Chengappa, is replete with stories of Indians selling their organs in order to build a brick house, etc. The magazine cover graphically portrays the sale prices of various body parts: a 'live' eye for Rs80,000, a kidney for Rs27,000 and skin for Rs300 per square inch. The author concludes by warning that 'the nightmare of "human organ farms" may soon become reality'. A similar dehumanisation of the human body is involved in the removal of organs from executed criminals in the People's Republic of China.[47]

The present state of the world-wide supply of organs suggests that this medical technology may ultimately victimise the poor in poor countries where people sell their organs to rich individuals, usually from rich countries, including Japan. Yet the 'gift of life' is the moral framework within which this practice is introduced to other peoples. Organ and tissue donation is the ultimate expression of Judaeo-Christian values or, in less religious terms, an expression of the ultimate virtue of altruism. When the Japanese and other peoples are presented with this new medical technology, their acceptance or refusal often involves this broader context of symbolic inequality. Japanese who advocate its adoption, thus, put the argument in such a way as to suggest that if their compatriots do not adopt the transplant technology they are 'backward' – that Japan lags behind other industrial countries not only in advanced medical technology but in morality, which prevents them from embracing rationality and a more advanced Western ethics of altruism. Those Japanese who refuse the technology often counter the charge by stressing their own cultural and moral superiority.

It is, then, in fact, too dangerous to cloak organ donation in the guise of gift giving, not only because it misrepresents the practice, as indeed it does, but also because the morality of this gift giving further restricts the freedom of choice of people to whom the technology is introduced. To put it another way, when the new medical technology is introduced to other countries, it is not a neutral item – it represents for recipient peoples not only the technical expertise but the morality of Western civilisation. Because biomedicine previously wrought miracles such as the eradication of epidemics and dreaded diseases, the new technology is seen as yet another miracle epitomising the superiority of Western civilization. Furthermore, it is presented as an altruistic practice, an expression of Christian love – the superior morality of the West. One must be quite cautious, lest Western 'science' be allowed a free rein in symbolic violence (in Bourdieu's sense) – the gentle force exercising its power before people realise its hegemony.

Personhood in cross-cultural perspective

The question of when life ends and when death starts is enormously complex. Anthropologists have long emphasised that 'death' is always a cultural phenomenon, that is, it is culturally defined, although it may be expressed in biological terms. Culturally identified signs of death – such as the cessation of the heartbeat and the gradual decrease of the body temperature – allow survivors to observe the 'process', and not the instant happening, of death, so that they can feel the passing of the deceased. The concept of brain death has created an altogether different sort of death. Death is executed by medical professionals who alone make death happen, not allowing survivors to experience it as a gradual process of 'dying'. The important process of passing is surrendered to the professionals.

In all cultures the welfare of the soul of the departed depends upon the proper treatment of the body, and not just its parts but the entire body. Universally, the body is essential to life and death of a person and personhood.[48] It is for this reason that the symbolic construction and destruction of a person are both predicated upon a ritual enactment, positive and negative, on the body. Therefore, for many cultures of the world today, the removal of organs from the brain-dead person constitutes an act of transgression – it deprives the deceased of the final process that enables them to leave this world with dignity and as a person. It deprives them of a social and cultural death. From this perspective, the removal of organs from the brain-dead is analogous to what happens in the scene in the film *Zorba the Greek* where the islanders begin to grab a prostitute's possessions while she is dying.

Personhood in Japanese culture, as in many cultures, should not and cannot be reduced to 'rationality' and the rest of the body to an afterthought of the brain. The basic premiss of the new technology, which is a product of the rationalist tradition in the West, remains alien to the concepts of life and death, the human, personhood and the body as felt and experienced by many individuals both in 'Western' and in 'non-Western' societies.

Appendix 9.1 Public opinion poll on brain death and organ transplantation

Opinion polls, published in the *Yomiuri* newspaper on 11 December 1992 and summarised below, show a steady increase among the general public in support for the brain-death criteria and organ transplantation. The figures represent percentages.

Question 1. At present in Japan some believe that when the brain is dead the person is dead, while others hold that, even if the brain is dead, the person should not be pronounced dead until the heart stops. What is your opinion?

	October 1982	*November 1992*
Brain death should be judged as death	15·2	32·4
Brain death is death, if we must decide	13·4	19·8
Hard to say	23·4	22·4
Inclined not to equate brain death with death	14·7	10·7
Brain death should not be judged as death	24·8	11·9
No answer	8·5	2·8

Question 2. When a person is pronounced brain-dead, some doctors ask surviving relatives for the deceased's organs. Choose one of the following choices that most clearly represents your feelings:

	October 1982	*November 1992*
Would agree to give organs	13·2	21·8
Would agree if the recipients are close relatives or friends	12·8	7·0
Would agree only if the deceased had agreed	15·1	28·2
Would continue care until the heart stops	–	4·6
Would reject the request	8·7	11·2
Cannot tell until one faces it	47·0	25·7
No answer	3·2	1·5

Question 3. If you were told that your life might be saved by transplanting someone's organ, would you request the transplant? Choose one of the following responses that most closely represents your feelings:

	October 1982	*November 1992*
Would accept anybody's organ	13·3	23·9
Would accept organs only from parents, siblings, friends, or others close to me	25·9	12·3
Would absolutely refuse	19·9	19·3
Cannot tell until the time comes	37·9	43·0
No answer	30	1·5

Question 4. Unlike the kidney, the heart and the liver must be transplanted from the brain-dead. Do you think Japan should continue to move towards performing heart transplantation?

	November 1985	*November 1992*
Yes	63·1	73·8
No	16·4	14·0
No answer	20·5	12·2

Question 5. Should Japan move towards liver transplantation?

	November 1987	*November 1992*
Yes	72·4	76·4
No	13·0	11·7
No answer	14·6	11·9

Question 6. Opinion among scholars and specialists on the definition of death is divided. The standards for brain death vary among medical institutions. Do you favour legislation of the brain-death criteria?

	November 1992
Agree	64·5
Oppose	18·6
Other	1·1
No answer	15·7

Although nearly two-thirds (64·5 per cent) of respondents supported legalisation of the criteria, there was considerable regional variation, ranging from 59·9 per cent in Kyūshū to 69·0 per cent in Chūbu.[49]

As of July 1993, legislation establishing brain death as the death of a person had not been passed. A survey of 116 hospitals and other medical institutions during January 1993 revealed the following reasons for not performing organ transplantation from the brain-dead:[50]

Reason	*No. of hospitals*
No legislation	89
No consensus of public opinion	82
Police investigation	45
Poor development of network	27
Underdevelopment of network	10
Lack of government effort	10
Lack of interest by emergency doctors	9
Effect of the Wada incident	6
Lack of effort by transplant surgeons	5
Other (lack of trust in doctors, etc.)	27

The responses point to the absence of consensus of public opinion being almost as important as the absence of legislation as the reason for not performing organ transplantation from the brain-dead. This is important in revealing the split in public opinion, as perceived by the medical institutions, while the answers to the previous questions show an increasingly positive attitude towards transplantation from the brain-dead.

The 'Police investigation' column refers to the rule requiring an autopsy on traffic accident victims in order to certify that the victim was not the victim of a crime.[51]

Not covered in the survey but important is the present insurance system (*shakai hoshō*), which covers the cost of life support for the brain-dead until the heart stops, making it easy not to declare brain death as the death of a human.[52]

Interpretation of the surveys

The answers to the survey clearly indicate that, during the past decade, the Japanese, as represented in this survey, have become more accepting of brain death as the criterion of human death and of organ transplantation from the brain-dead.

The answers to question 2 in 1982 and 1992 indicate that by 1992 survivors were more willing to offer organs from the deceased relative to non-relatives, people were more willing to honour the wishes of the deceased, and people were more willing to confront the issue rather than postponing their decision until they face the problem.

The general trend towards approval of these specific issues is probably a result of public debates over the issue in newspapers, television and other mass media. The media also provide information about the situation in the United States and other countries where organ transplantation is far more frequent.

Some recent episodes in Japan have also helped to create a more positive attitude towards organ transplantations involving the brain-dead. For example, a fifty-three-year-old woman potter, Akiko Ogawa, had a living will to donate her eyes and kidneys. On 16 October 1992 she went into a coma after being stung by a bee, and her kidneys were transplanted to two individuals.[53] Her case was widely reported by the mass media and she was heralded as an unselfish individual by supporters of euthanasia and of organ transplantation involving brain death.

Japanese attitudes may eventually change to accommodate this new medical technology, just as they did with regard to blood donation. From stubborn resistance to blood donation, Japan now has one of the highest rates of blood donation in the world,[54] and cornea transplantation has made significant inroads, with 24,784 transplants between 1963 and 1992.[55] On the other hand, it should be noted that in 1992 only 32·4 per cent of respondents were decisive in equating brain death with death (question 1); only 21·8 per cent would unconditionally donate organs of a deceased relative; only 23·9 per cent would accept anybody's organ.

Appendix 9.2 A brief history of organ transplantation

Kidney transplantation. Kidney transplants were the first transplants in Japan and are the most common kind. The first kidney transplant, which used a pig's kidney, took place in 1956. The first successful transplantation of a kidney from a live human donor occurred in 1964, and the first successful *cadaveric* transplant was in 1969.[56]

In 1979 the Diet passed an Act concerning the Transplantation of Cornea and Kidney, which led to an increase in the number of kidney transplants.

During 1989, 757 were performed, of which 233 (30·8 per cent) involved kidneys from cadavers. By 1989 a total of 6,951 kidney transplants had been performed in Japan. In 1992, 187,000 persons were registered with the kidney bank to donate their kidneys after death.[57]

Liver transplantation. The first liver transplant which involved a father and his son, was performed in 1989.[58] By 1992, fifty liver transplants had been performed, and, of these fifty livers, thirty-nine were from living donors.[59] Some Japanese seek transplants abroad. For example, parents sometimes take an infant with congenital biliary atresia to another country for liver transplantation. In the meantime Japan carries out more kidney dialyses than any other industrial country.[60]

Pancreas transplantation. The first pancreas transplantation was a pancreas–kidney double transplant in 1984. This operation involved a brain-dead person and raised considerable controversy, including a murder charge. No more pancreas transplants were performed until 1990, but between 1990 and 1992 eleven cadaveric transplants were done. Only five cases – all performed at the Medical School of Tokyo Women's College – were successful.[61]

Heart transplantation. Heart transplantation in Japan began in 1968 with an unfortunate incident. Toshirō Wada, a professor at Sapporo Medical School, transplanted the heart of a victim of drowning, Yoshimasa Yamaguchi, to Nobuo Miyazaki, who had a chronic cardiac problem. Initially the transplant was celebrated in the media and applauded by the people. Wada and the transplant team became celebrities. However, Miyazaki died after eighty-three days and questions about the procedure surfaced in newspapers. Critics became convinced that the donor was not really brain-dead at the time his heart was removed, and that the recipient's heart condition was not serious enough to warrant a heart transplant. Critics claimed that Wada had committed a double murder in order to perform his 'medical miracle'. Owing to 'lack of evidence', however, Wada was never convicted in court.[62] This incident became a deterrent for the Japanese, who were already sceptical of organ transplants. No other transplantation has been performed in Japan, but by 1992 about twenty Japanese had received hearts overseas, usually in Canada, England or the United States.[63] In contrast to Americans and other Western peoples the rate of heart problems among the Japanese is quite low, although the complete absence of heart transplantation is still remarkable.

Cross-cultural comparison. The history of organ transplantation in Japan contrasts sharply with that in the United Kingdom, France, and the United States. The figures for heart transplants in 1986 were: 176 heart transplants in the United Kingdom (127 liver, 149 kidney); 300 heart transplants in France; and 1,368 heart transplants in the United States.[64] The United States is the leading country not only in heart but also in other organ transplants. The following are the number of transplants of different organs in two different years, 1983 and 1991, in the United States:[65]

	1983	*1991*
Kidney	6,112	10,051
Heart	172	2,126
Heart–lung	20	51
Liver	164	2,953
Pancreas	61	533
Lung	–	403

Although more kidneys are transplanted in Japan than other organs, Japan and the United States differ dramatically as regards the number and types of organ transplants. The use of the organs of brain-dead persons in the United States is the most important factor giving rise to these differences. Kidney transplantation is relatively easy because it involves taking only one of a live donor's two kidneys, and only part of a liver can be used for transplant purposes. The success rate for transplants of other organs is low if the organ is removed only after cardiac death. It is for this reason that brain death became a crucial issue – the heart and other organs of brain death are kept 'alive' until their transplantation, increasing the success rate dramatically.

Notes

1 Thomas S. Kuhn, *The Structure of Scientific Revolutions*. Chicago: University of Chicago Press, 1962; Karl Marx and F. Engels, *Selected Correspondence*. Moscow: Foreign Languages Publishing House [Follows the Russian edition (Gospolitizdat, 1953)], n.d.: 156–7; *id.*, *The German Ideology*. London: Lawrence & Wishart, 1965: 531; Marshall Sahlins, *The Use and Abuse of Biology: an Anthropological Critique of Sociobiology*. Ann Arbor, Mich.: University of Michigan Press, 1976: 106.

2 Compare Emiko Ohnuki-Tierney, 'The ambivalent self of the contemporary Japanese', *Cultural Anthropology* 5, 1990: 196–215.

3 Marc Augé, *The Anthropological Circle: Symbol, Function, History*. Cambridge University Press, 1982 [1979]: 10–11; Bernard S. Cohn, 'History and anthropology: the state of play', *Comparative Studies in Society and History* 12, 1980: 198–221 at 211.

4 See, for example, Pierre Bourdieu, *Outline of a Theory of Practice*. Cambridge University Press. 1977 (1972): 164.

5 Yasamasu Hosaka, *Zôki Ishoku to Nihonjin* (Organ transplantation and the Japanese). Tokyo: Asahi Sonorama, 1992: 6–8.

6 Nihon Ishokugakkai Shakai Mondai Kentô Tokubetsu Iinkai, ed., *Zôki Ishoku eno Apurôchi* (An approach to organ transplantation). No. V. Osaka: Medika Publisher, 1991: 4.

7 Takeshi Umehara, ed., *'Nôshi' to Zôki Ishoku* (Brain death and organ transplantation). Tokyo: Asahi Shinbunsha, 1992.

8 For a fine exposition of the problem in the United States see David Rothman, *Strangers at the Bedside: a History of How Law and Bioethics Transformed Medical Decision Making*. New York: Basic Books, 1991.

9 There are other important factors, such as the technology that allows the maintenance of other 'vital functions' after the death of the brain, that are responsible for the creation of the notion of brain death (Robert Levine, personal communication).

10 René C. Fox and Judith P. Swazey, *Spare Parts: Organ Replacement in American Society*. Oxford University Press, 1992: 62–3. See also Takao Saitô, 'Nôshi no hito no shi to shite yoika' (Should brain death be equated with the death of a human?), in T. Umehara, ed., *'Nôshi' to Zôki Ishoku* (Brain death and organ transplantation),

15–29. Tokyo: Asahi Shinbunsha, 1992: 15.

11 S. J. Younger, M. Allen, E. T. Barlett *et al.*, 'Psychological and ethical implications of organ retrieval', *New England Journal of Medicine* 313 1985: 321–4 at 323.

12 See, for example, Ernest Gellner, *Reason and Culture*. Oxford: Blackwell, 1992; S. J. Tambiah, *Magic, Science, Religion, and the Scope of Rationality*. Cambridge University Press, 1990; Bryan R. Wilson, ed. *Rationality*. Oxford: Blackwell, 1970.

13 Thomas, Keith. *Religion and the Decline of Magic*. New York: Scribner, 1971: 646.

14 Levine, personal communication.

15 For details see Emiko Ohnuki-Tierney, *The Monkey as Mirror: Symbolic Transformations in Japanese History and Ritual*. Princeton University Press, 1987.

16 Hosaka, *Zôki Ishoku to Nihonjin*: 28.

17 Rothman, 'Strangers': 164.

18 Emiko Ohnuki-Tierney, 'Brain death and organ transplantation: cultural bases of medical technology', *Current Anthropology* 35 (3), 1994: 233–54.

19 Tambiah, *Scope of Rationality*: 117.

20 Ohnuki-Tierney, 'Brain death'.

21 S. N. Eisenstadt, *Japanese Civilization: A Comparative View*. University of Chicago Press, 1996: 424.

22 For details see Ohnuki-Tierney, *Monkey as Mirror*; Ohnuki-Tierney, 'Brain death'.

23 Emiko Ohnuki-Tierney, *Rice as Self: Japanese Identities through Time*. Princeton University Press, 1993; see also David Pollack, *The Fracture of Meaning: Japan's Synthesis of China from the Eighth through the Eighteenth Centuries*. Princeton University Press, 1986.

24 Shinobu Orikuchi, 'Ônamesai no hongi' (The meaning of the *Ônamesai*). *Orikuchi Shinobu Zenshû* (Collected works of Orikuchi Shinobu). III. Tokyo: Chûôkôronsha. 1975 (1928): 174–240.

25 Miyata personal communication; see also Tokuji Chiba, *Seppuku no hanashi* (Essays on seppuku). Tokyo: Kôdansha. 1981 (1973).

26 Emiko Ohnuki-Tierney, *Illness and Culture in Contemporary Japan: an Anthropological View*. Cambridge University Press, 1984.

27 Miyata, personal communication.

28 Hosaka, *Zôki Ishoku to Nihonjin*: 156.

29 Kunio Yanagita, 'Katame no sakana' (The one-eyed fish). *Teihon Yanagita Kunio Zenshû* 30 1982 (1917): 136–47 at 137; Kunio Yanagita, 'Imi to monoimi no hanashi' (On taboos). *Teihon Yanagita Kunio Zenshû* 27 1982 (1933): 312–25 at 317.

30 Jurô Wada and Kazuo Miwa, 'Minshushugi to Yû Na no kyôda' (Cowardice called democracy). *Shokun!* 24 (6) 1992: 62–73.

31 Tetsuya Watari, 'Gan senkoku, watakushi no bawai (Cancer verdict, in my case). *Bungei Shunjû* 70 (2) 1992: 370–85 at 384.

32 Compare Howard F. Stein, 'Commentary on Kleinman's "Lessons from a clinical approach to medical anthropological research".' *Medical Anthropology Newsletter* 8 (4), 1977: 15–16.

33 Levine, personal communication.

34 Richard Currier, 'The hot–cold syndrome and symbolic balance in Mexico and Spanish-American folk medicine'. *Ethnology* 5 (3) 1966: 251–63; George Foster, 'Relationship between Spanish and Spanish-American folk medicine'. *Journal of American Folklore* 66 1953: 201–17.

35 Manfred Porkert, *The Theoretical Foundations of Chinese Medicine: Systems of Correspondence*. Cambridge, Mass.: MIT Press, 1974.

36 For details see Ohnuki-Tierney, *Illness and Culture*.

37 See, for instance, Robert Bazell, 'Hearts of gold'. *New Republic* 2 1985: 17–20.

38 Kunio Yanagita, 'Niko no shima' (The islands of cats). *Teihon Yanagita Kunio Zenshû* 22 1982 (1939): 390–8; Kunio Yanagita, 'Sôsei no engaku ni tsuite' (A brief history of mortuary customs). *Teihon Yanagita Kunio Zenshû*, 15 1982 (1929): 499–520 at 507.

39 For the history of *seppuku* and interpretations of it, see Chiba, *Seppuku no hanashi*.

40 Masao Fujii, 'Nôshi to zôki ishoku – seikatsu Bukkyô no tachiba kara' (Brain death

and organ transplantation – from the perspective of day-to-day Buddhism), in Umehara, *Brain Death*: 284–304 at 292–5.

41 Ohnuki-Tierney, *Illness and Culture*.

42 *Ibid.* for details.

43 Compare Fox and Swazey, *Spare Parts*: 39–40.

44 Marcel Mauss, *The Gift: Forms and Functions of Exchange in Archaic Societies*. (Original publication in French in 1925) London: Cohen & West, 1966.

45 Vitit Muntarbhorn, 'The Black Market in Organs.' Paper presented at a conference, 'Organ Transplantation and Human Rights: Cross-cultural Perspectives'. Yale Law School, 15–17 April 1993.

46 A. S. Daar, 'Ethical issues – a Middle East perspective.' *Transplantation Proceedings* 21 (1 1989): 1402–4.

47 *South China Morning Post*, 11 May 1991.

48 For a study of this in the case of the Ainu see Emiko Ohnuki-Tierney, *Illness and Healing among the Sakhalin Ainu: a Symbolic Interpretation*. Cambridge University Press, 1981.

49 *Yomiuri Shinbun*, 11 December 1992.

50 *Yomiuri Shinbun*, 23 January 1993.

51 *Yomiuri Shinbun*, 11 December 1992.

52 Hosaka, *Zōki Ishoku to Nihonjin*: 342.

53 *Yomiuri Shinbun*, 18 October 1993.

54 Rihito Kimura, 'Japan's dilemma with the definition of death', *Kennedy Institute of Ethics Journal*, June 1991: 123–31.

55 Kōseishō (Ministry of Health and Education), ed., *Kōsei Hakusho* (Report of the Ministry of Health and Education), Tokyo: Gyōsei, 1993: 301.

56 Hosaka, *Zōki Ishoku to Nihonjin*: 23, 24.

57 Hosaka, *Zōki Ishoku to Nihonjin*: 24, 710.

58 Teruhisa Nakamura *et al.*, *Ketsudan-seitai kan-ishoku no kisoku* (The decision history of the live liver transplant case), Tokyo: Jiji Tsûshinsha, 1990.

59 Hosaka, *Zōki Ishoku to Nihonjin*: 29–39.

60 Takashi Tachibana, *'Nôshi' to zôki ishoku* (Brain death and organ transplantation), Tokyo: Chûôkôronsha, 1991.

61 *Yomiuri Shinbun*, 4 October 1992.

62 Tachibana, *'Nôshi' to zôki ishoku*: 298–318.

63 Hosaka, *Zoki ishoku to Nihonjin*: 52.

64 Hosaka, *Zoki ishoku to Nihonjin*: 60.

65 Myron Genel, 'Regulation of Organ and Tissue Transplantation.' Paper presented at a conference, 'Organ Transplantation and Human Rights: Cross-cultural Perspectives', Yale Law School, 15–17 April 1993.

CHAPTER TEN

Rumoured power: Hong Kong, 1894 and Cape Town, 1901

Mary Preston Sutphen

> Many rumours of an alarmist character [wrote the editor of the *Hong Kong Daily Press* in May 1894] were in circulation yesterday. We heard that forty deaths from the disease, as described from Canton, had occurred in Taipingshan during forty-eight hours, that in Tank Lane one whole family had died suddenly from fever and dysentery, and that many houses had been abandoned by people, who had left for their native villages.[1]

The disease from Canton, according to the Hong Kong Assistant Principal Medical Officer, was bubonic plague. A few days later, the Governor notified the Colonial Office in London that many Chinese pupils in the schools had panicked, incited by rumours going around in the schools. One rumour, he reported, claimed that government agents were seizing young children from their classrooms and incising their livers for bile, an alleged remedy for the plague. Any child with a pimple or boil, went another rumour, was to be sent to a European hospital ship, the *Hygeia*, anchored in the harbour.[2] Plague broke out in this period in other British colonial cities, and, as in Hong Kong, rumours surfaced in newspapers and in accounts to the Colonial Office. In 1901 in Cape Town, at a meeting of the city's local advisory board on plague control, one member asked Dr A. J. Gregory, one of the board's doctors 'in connection to inoculation, whether the rumour that had been current that several people who had been inoculated had to have their arms amputated was true'.[3]

Common to the accounts from Hong Kong and Cape Town were vivid images: amputated arms, sudden death and excised livers, as well as a lack of information about the sources of the rumours. They were, as one folklorist has defined rumour, 'short, non-narrative expressions of belief'.[4] While those who passed the stories may or may not have 'believed' them, by giving them currency they gave them legitimacy.

And those who referred to the stories as rumours were denigrating them.

Rumours were contested knowledge from the underground. In both cities rumours brought to the surface fears about individuals or groups who might upset carefully honed relations between Europeans and other ethnic and racial groups. In Cape Town outside experts were seen by some, certainly not all, as a danger to the racial and class hierarchies firmly entrenched in colonial society. In Hong Kong, Chinese English-speakers were perceived by many British residents to threaten the colonial order.

Although they must be interpreted with much caution, rumours provide an index for assessing the reception by the European community in Cape Town of laboratory medicine, and in Hong Kong for how some of the Chinese community reacted to the imposition of Western technology and medicine on Chinese society. Often attached to reports of rumours were references to debates current in both cities which were deeply troubling to members of the English-speaking communities. Once a rumour had been reported in the lay press in Cape Town or Hong Kong, letters to the editors and editorials discussed in much detail who was to blame for them and why they spread. In Cape Town, for example, rumours about inoculation against plague revealed deep rifts within the English-speaking community over the value of outside advisers and ideas brought by outsiders. The historian Elizabeth Van Heyningen has argued cogently that rumours were a form of resistance to inoculation, one of the 'foreign' anti-plague measures the colonial authorities imposed on the city's residents.[5] This chapter examines what was at stake in rejecting inoculation. In Hong Kong the British blamed a small minority of influential Chinese – those who were English-speaking and Western-educated – for many of the rumours. Historians have discussed the emergence of this elite, but there has been less interest in British reactions to it.[6] A study of one community and not the other skews the interpretation of both. While the British claimed that these Chinese were not foreigners – the British referred to themselves as the foreigners – they were both insiders and outsiders. The rumours in Hong Kong reveal ambivalence on the part of the British about the role of Western-educated English-speaking Chinese in the government of the colony.

At first glance a comparison between Hong Kong and Cape Town may seem forced and inappropriate. The make-up of the populations was entirely different, with Chinese in the majority in Hong Kong, and black Africans and coloureds in Cape Town. At the Colonial Office the two cities fell under the jurisdiction of two different departments, one which dealt with Africa and another with Asia. Finally plague broke out in one of the cities, Cape Town, during a colonial war, the second Anglo-Boer war. Nonetheless the two cities had much in common. When plague broke out both had a large number of transients. As a result of the troops sent to fight and refugees fleeting the war in the Transvaal, Cape Town had an abnormally high immigrant population.[7] In its normal course, Hong Kong was a gathering point for thousands of Chinese travelling overseas to labour in Australia, Singapore and the United States. Although the two colonial cities were the responsibility of different departments, by the time of the outbreak in Cape Town, reports were routinely given to a small, informal group at the Colonial Office who dealt with all outbreaks of plague in the British empire. According to colonial officials in Hong Kong and Cape Town the outbreaks were supposedly the first of their kind in each city. Last of all, in both cities a minority of practitioners argued that research from laboratory medicine would provide methods of controlling and curing epidemic diseases, including plague.

Rumours are compelling historical sources. Historians have taken a number of approaches to them, as have sociologists, psychologists, anthropologists and folklorists.[8] One historian, Elizabeth Sinn, in her analysis of the plague epidemic in Hong Kong in 1894, analysed the origins of some of the rumours allegedly current in the Chinese community as a means of assessing Anglo-Chinese relations.[9] Elizabeth van Heyningen, in her analysis of the 1901 plague epidemic in Cape Town, saw rumours differently, finding in them a tool of resistance to plague inoculation, one of the anti-plague measures colonial authorities had put in place.[10] She viewed rumours as responsible for galvanising the public of Cape Town to oppose inoculation. In her study of political unrest in Natal at the turn of the twentieth century Shula Marks claims that the presence of rumours constituted 'a highly sensitive barometer of group tension'.[11] Another approach is that taken by Anand A. Yang, who has recently argued that rumours are a valuable historical source for examining the popular mentalities of societies where few read or wrote.[12] Pule Phoofolo viewed rumours recorded during a rinderpest epidemic in South Africa in the 1890s as 'nothing less than the spoken thoughts of an otherwise silent majority'.[13] It is hard, however, to say whether rumours were the 'spoken thoughts' of a majority, since they may have been recorded by individuals for purposes other than to relate the precise wording of the accounts. It is very difficult to determine whether the recorder of a rumour altered it. In his analysis of rumours reported in India during the outbreak of plague at the turn of the twentieth century David Arnold provides a valuable analysis of the uses of rumours as historical sources on popular discourses.[14] He points out many of the ways in which they were 'far from being uncontaminated sources'.[15] In his view they were often recorded as evidence of Indian absurdity.[16] Having enumerated many of the problems with using them, he provides examples of different types, with some analysis of their content in order to reveal the many meanings attached to them by Indians. The rumours, he argues, provide explanations for many seemingly unrelated aspects of the plague epidemics, and they reveal anxiety on the part of Indians over the efforts of the British to preserve their power on the subcontinent.[17] Rajnarayan Chandavarkar also discussed the uses of rumours reported during the Indian plague epidemic, as well as why they are problematic sources.[18] He maintains that many used rumours as a means of mediating wretched circumstances. He holds that individuals of all classes, creeds and caste divisions used them to express anger and to sustain hope.[19] Thus rumours have been studied as a means to: analyse popular discourses; examine the level of group tensions; and investigate the limits of colonial power.

As Arnold and Chandavarkar have pointed out, the interpretation of rumours in colonial societies presents many methodological problems. Rumours are, at best, difficult sources. They were usually unattributed, and their provenance was vague. Jean-Noel Kapferer has argued that, in the construction of rumours, those who pass the rumours on and those who listen to them each contribute to their content.[20] While tellers and retellers probably contributed to the construction of rumours in Cape Town and Hong Kong, those who recorded them may have done so too. Without a number of examples of the same rumour from many different sources it is difficult to determine whether those who recorded the rumours substantially remade them. Despite the methodological difficulties rumours bring with them, they offer one approach to analysing the ways in which knowledge was contested in the colonial context.

Plague in Hong Kong

By the time plague broke out in Hong Kong the colony was one of the world's largest entrepots. Much of the trade was with China: in 1890, for example, 55 per cent of China's imports and 37 per cent of its exports passed through Hong Kong.[21] The majority of the population, around 180,000 out of 200,000, were Chinese men, mostly from the region around Canton.[22] They migrated for short periods when they worked on the docks or in the factories. A relatively small number of Chinese had settled in Hong Kong for decades, and there existed a small, powerful Chinese elite. The European community, whose size was about 10,000–12,000, consisted primarily of British traders or government officials who spent a few years in the colony and then moved on.

In May 1894, Dr J. A. Lowson, a government doctor, travelled from Hong Kong to Canton to learn more about an epidemic disease reported in one of the English-language dailies in Hong Kong, the *Hong Kong Daily Press* as causing panic among the Chinese.[23] While in Canton he supposedly learned how to diagnose the disease, which he and others held was bubonic plague, and on 8 May, the day after his return to Hong Kong, he diagnosed several cases.[24]

The measures the colonial government put in place included the following: burying the dead in a separate cemetery; flushing and disinfecting house drains; sanitary inspectors making house-to-house visits; disinfecting all houses containing plague patients; and removing all plague patients from the Tung Wah hospital – a hospital established by the Chinese community which treated patients with Chinese medicine – and sending them to the *Hygeia*, a European hospital ship anchored in the harbour.[25] In theory most of the measures were applicable to all Chinese but in practice all but one – taking patients from the Tung Wah to the *Hygeia* – applied only to the working class. In her recent history of the Tung Wah hospital Sinn has shown that, until the plague broke out, members of the Tung Wah Committee were among the most powerful of Hong Kong's Chinese elite. The removal of Chinese patients from the Tung Wah to the European hospital ship seemed to signal a loss of the elite's power in the Chinese community who were no longer able to protect ill Chinese from being treated with Western medicine.[26]

Reports in the *Hong Kong Daily Press* on plague in Canton painted a grim picture, with one claiming that the city's stock of coffins was almost gone. In Hong Kong the paper reported, there were many rumours 'of an alarmist character' abroad, including the rumour already mentioned which claimed that forty people had died in Taipingshan, a working-class quarter of the city. The paper claimed that it had enquired at the office of the Registrar General – a colonial official responsible for liaison between the Chinese and British communities – and reassured its readers that no suspicious deaths had occurred.[27] This account illustrates some of the biases held by the paper's editor: members of the Chinese community were liable to exaggerate, as they allegedly did with this rumour, making the situation appear to be worse than British officials considered it to be. It also indicated the ways in which the paper would treat rumours over the next few months. The *Hong Kong Daily Press* reported on the presence of rumours but seldom on their content. When the paper related the substance of the rumours it generally debunked them, by, for example, citing something like the Registrar General's report. While the rumours from the Chinese community provided glimpses of current belief, the editor of the paper chose to keep them on a tight rein. The Chinese rumours were in the foreground if they could be represented as untrue.[28]

From the Chinese perspective, if the content of the rumours was related more or less accurately, some indication would be given of the methods that individual Chinese used to cope with an unsettling situation. Those who passed the rumours on may have considered the information from 'official' sources as too little too late or as simply untrue.[29] Perhaps, by postulating a frightening scenario, the rumours served to underscore to those who heard them that they were lucky but that they should be cautious about the disease. Many came from Canton and may have feared for their families' lives, as well as for their own. The rumours may also have been a means of reassuring the middle and upper strata of Chinese Hong Kong society: the working-class Chinese in Taipingshan needed to worry about the disease, but not 'us'.

Over the following weeks many Chinese registered their objection to the anti-plague measures by leaving the colony, and by exhibiting fierce resistance to the measures colonial officials put in place. The *Hong Kong Daily Press* claimed that efforts by colonial authorities to inspect and disinfect parts of the city were being frustrated by 'a certain section of the Chinese' who 'assert aggressively the ignorance and stupidity which peculiarly belong to the multitude of the natives'.[30] According to the account in the newspaper, the Chinese objected to being forced to abandon the Tung Wah and go to the *Hygeia*, where they would be treated by 'Western skill and science'. The editorial claimed that several members of the Tung Wah hospital 'imbued with anti-foreign feeling' influenced the 'native population' and created staunch opposition to the measures.[31]

As the number of reported cases increased, the number of rumours mentioned in the *Hong Kong Daily Press* and in accounts the Governor sent to the Colonial Office also increased. One rumour, with several variations, was that government officials or plague doctors were forcing Chinese patients into the plague hospital when they obviously did not have the disease. The *Hong Kong Daily Press*, for example, reported that there was no foundation to the story that a pregnant woman was sent to the *Hygeia* having been mistaken for a plague patient.[32] One way to interpret the pregnant-woman rumour is that many Chinese considered the British unable to diagnose the disease correctly. Interpreted this way, Chinese practitioners were far superior to the ignorant British, who drew no distinction between a normal pregnancy and plague. The editor, however, had a different interpretation of the purpose of the rumour. 'This fable,' he claimed, 'is only one of many, some even more preposterous, which some ignorant and malignant-minded Chinese are disseminating among the coolies for the very evident purpose of stirring up bitter feelings against the European medical practitioners.'[33] The editor may have seen the 'bitter feelings' against the European medical practitioners as a direct threat to the government of Hong Kong.

An editorial in the 25 May issue of the *Hong Kong Daily Press* expanded on the theme of 'ignorant coolies' being duped by 'malignant' Chinese. It claimed that in the Chinese community there was 'a dangerous spirit abroad' where 'the coolie class are blindly led by busybodies among their countrymen occupying higher stations in life. It is men in good positions with anti-foreign proclivities who disseminate wild stories to bring the Government and its officers into detestation.'[34] The colony's working class, claimed one editorial, was ready to 'credit any foul slander' on the British, 'as shown by the absurd and disgusting reports which have found credence respecting the treatment of plague patients'.[35] The paper suggested that once the busybodies were identified they should be deported at once. If those who had been spreading the 'baseless and mischievous rumours' were British citizens, and thus not able to be deported, the government should in future be cautious about allowing Chinese citizens to be naturalised.[36]

A letter to the editor from one Tse Tsantai took umbrage with the accusations.[37] Tse claimed instead that the rumours:

> have been caused by the ignorant coolie classes, male and female, whose friends, kinsmen, or children, being plague stricken, may have been forcibly removed from their houses, it being lawful, and conveyed against their will to the hospital ship *Hygeia*. Here, unfortunately, through their ignorance all trace is lost of them ... These ignorant people cannot understand such stringent proceedings, and without a knowledge, or satisfactory explanation of the proclamations, notices, and sanitary by-laws, are consequently through their ignorance terrified and alarmed.[38]

There they become frightened, which 'naturally leads to the spread of evil, absurd, and malicious rumours'.[39] The letter asked what grounds the author of the editorial had for making the 'defamatory assault upon the Chinese community in Hongkong?'[40] Tse speculated that perhaps the author 'has the anti-missionary riots on the brain', referring to a series of recent assaults in China on Western missionaries.[41] One, for example, had been reported in the *Hong Kong Daily Press* on 15 May where a mission in Shenhsi was nearly burned. Tse's letter prompted one response from 'Peakite' – an individual who presumably lived on the Peak, an exclusively European residential neighbourhood – who continued to denigrate the Chinese community and blamed 'our Chinese neighbours' for having malicious tactics during the plague.[42] 'By the way', wrote Peakite, 'what has become of the Hon. [*sic*] Dr Ho Kai? This is just the time when one would have expected him to the front, but from all one can hear he has been effectively hiding his light under a bushel?'[43] Ho Kai was prominent in the Chinese community as well as in the British community, in part because he was a member of the colony's local committee on public health, the Sanitary Board. He qualified in medicine at Aberdeen in 1897, and the same year he was admitted into Lincoln's Inn.[44]

Tse's tone in blaming the 'ignorant coolie classes' differed from the one the editor of the *Hong Kong Daily Press* took. Reporting that many Europeans at the Peak were greatly inconvenienced because the Chinese would not work in 'cloudland' any more, the editor claimed that the exodus was due to:

> some Chinese placards posted and distributed … urging the Chinese to leave because the Peak tramway was the cause of the plague! As soon as the authorities heard of these leaflets they took steps to remove them … No arrests, however, have been made.[45]

The villains in the paper's account were not the 'coolies' who, judging from the use of the exclamation point, were silly to believe that there was a connection between the plague and the tramway. The villains of the rumour, according to the *Hong Kong Daily Press*, were the authors and distributors of the placards.

The report highlighted one of the ways in which rumours in Hong Kong were supposedly passed on: placards with warnings were posted in the streets. In her study of plague in China Carol Benedict claims that placards were common in communities and were full of advice – either medical or moral – on how to cope with the disease.[46] The placards in Hong Kong had meaning only to those who read Chinese script, hence they catered to the literate portion of the Chinese community. The British were perhaps disturbed by them because they were written in a language unintelligible to many of them and hung in the midst of what was supposed to be a European enclave. The account in the paper contained a strong streak of fear that the enemy was 'among us' and able to communicate openly under the noses of British citizens.

One interpretation of the content of the rumour was that the tramway was the instrument which made habitable the part of the island where Europeans were constructing a segregated settlement, where Chinese were allowed to work but not live. This was perhaps more disturbing to a new and small Chinese elite which emerged during the 1880s and 1890s.[47] Sinn has argued that a small group of Chinese, fluent in English, wanted to distance themselves from the older elites, such as the Tung Wah Hospital Committee.[48] They may have had little or no interest in living on the Peak, but they may have resented the *de facto* segregation.

The editor of the *Hong Kong Daily Press*, 'Peakite', and Tse offered divergent explanations of who was responsible for the rumours and what the stories were supposedly doing to colonial society. Most of the editorials and 'Peakite' blamed a clique of educated Chinese for using rumours to undermine the authority of Western practitioners treating plague patients. In their eyes, working-class Chinese were 'dupes' to listen to the stories. The real danger for the editor and for 'Peakite' lay in the educated elite who supposedly concocted the stories. In their view malice and desire to subvert the colonial government were at the heart of the rumours, and the stories took on a sinister cast, with 'evil' Chinese trying to obstruct the efforts of the government to stamp out plague. For Tse, the rumours were harmless, simply the result of ignorance and fear on the part of working-class Chinese. The villains, in Tse's view, were Europeans who cast aspersions on the Chinese community, and who put in place anti-plague measures which frightened working-class Chinese.

In the middle of June, after a report that two women missionaries had been attacked in China, the editor claimed that the attack indicated 'the volcanic nature of Chinese sentiment towards foreigners at the present time'.[49] As evidence of the tension between British and Chinese, the editorial cited the rumour that the shadow of a battleaxe had appeared on pictures of the God of War hanging in shop windows. Some believed, the paper claimed, the battleaxe was a portent that there would be fighting between Chinese and foreigners.[50] The editor reassured the paper's readers that 'any native rising could be speedily dealt with'.[51] As further evidence of antipathy on the part of Chinese towards 'foreigners' the editor noted that there was a rumour about the burning of Taipingshan. Colonial authorities had begun to discuss what to do with Taipingshan, which they claimed was rife with plague, in mid June. One suggestion the Governor made to the Legislative Council was that the area should be burned down and rebuilt according to European sanitary principles.[52] The paper claimed that the burning was supposedly to allow the colonial authorities the chance to 'give the poorer classes of Chinese ... superior dwellings'.[53] According to the editorial, 'evil intentioned agitators, who are now busily at work', made the suggestion seem an 'act of oppression and cruelty towards the native community'.[54] Again, according to the editor, most of the Chinese did not comprehend the reasons, based on

Western 'scientific knowledge', for burning the area down, and a few capitalised on the 'ignorance' of the many. The editorial concluded that there was 'a dangerous feeling abroad' where rumours 'of a more or less wild character are sure to prevail'.[55]

In a letter to the paper 'Indignant' explained who was responsible for the 'demonstrations, more or less thinly disguised, of bitter anti-foreign feeling on the part of certain members of the Chinese community'.[56] The letter claimed that 'certain English-speaking natives' had 'ridiculed and indignantly rejected' Western medicine and treated other Chinese 'on the barbarous and ridiculous principles of the Chinese pharmacopeia'.[57] They, the author maintained, were probably educated at great public expense at Victoria College and 'inculcated into all that is the best of European civilization'.[58] According to 'Indignant', though, the college – where students were instructed in Chinese – was a 'hot-bed, the birth-bed indeed of rabid anti-foreign sentiments'.[59] Teach Chinese students in English, claimed the author, 'and perhaps one day we may leaven a portion of the ignorant whole'.[60] Perhaps what bothered the writer most was that Chinese students should have 'known' better. In his or her view a graduate of Victoria College, having been 'inculcated into the best of European civilization', should have been more responsive to Western practices. The idea that Chinese doctors were still treating Chinese patients with Chinese medicine was perhaps, in his or her eyes, 'proof' that graduates of Victoria College did not appreciate the education they were given.

One reason for European hostility to Western-educated Chinese may have been that they were part of a new order. By blaming them for rumours, Europeans 'put them in their place', a position subordinate to Europeans despite their having supposedly been uplifted by a European education. The matter, however, was not straightforward. For example, the *Hong Kong Daily Press* published a long editorial on the value of teaching Chinese medical students Western medicine in English, an education such as the graduates of the Hong Kong College of Medicine for the Chinese received. The college trained practitioners solely in Western medicine, and they were to promote it in the Chinese community.[61]

> It is not [the editorial proclaimed] by driving patients into foreign hospitals at the point of the bayonet in a time of crisis that the immemorial traditions of the Chinese can be broken down … but by continuous gentle persuasion the native community will in course of time be led to look upon foreign medicine in a different light from what they do now.[62]

While some of the editorials in the *Hong Kong Daily Press* accused educated Chinese of being malignant and evil, ready to cause trouble at any turn, this one considered that Chinese doctors trained in Western medicine might be of use for convincing Chinese patients of the value of Western medicine.

Rumours in Hong Kong during the plague epidemic revealed some of the tensions in the British and Chinese communities over colonial rule. One editorial claimed that a reason for the presence of rumours in Hong Kong was that the British 'to our shame ... are not now and never have been ... in touch with the native mind, that the Briton and the Chinaman each lives his separate life, having no common ground to meet upon'.[63] Those Chinese who had a Western education from one of the government schools, the small number of Chinese fluent in English and the equally small number of English fluent in Chinese came closest to bridging the separate lives of the communities.[64] The bridges, though, were narrow and rickety. Changes in either community affected how each viewed the other, and there were major changes afoot in the Chinese community.[65] Sinn argued that Ho Kai was 'the archetype of a new generation in Hong Kong', Western-educated, sought after by the government for advice on Chinese matters, and he advocated reforms for China.[66] In 1894 he and several British residents petitioned the Colonial Office, asking it to change the structure of government in Hong Kong. They wanted more representatives on the local governing council to be freely elected by citizens of British nationality.[67] Tse was another of the new breed, one of the founders of Furen Wenshe, a local society devoted to reform and revolution in China.[68] Individuals such as Ho Kai and Tse were changing the nature of the Chinese elite. As Sinn argued about the Tung Wah, traditionally its leaders were wealthy merchants who also held Chinese degrees.[69] Unlike Tse and Ho Kai they may not have been Western-educated. The blame for rumours apportioned to Western-educated Chinese was perhaps a signal of the uncertainty British residents felt toward the Western-educated elite.

According to several British residents, rumours in Hong Kong were a powerful force, capable of inciting large numbers of Chinese to leave their jobs and reject Western medicine. In Cape Town many perceived them as equally powerful.

Plague in Cape Town

Cape Town in 1901 was a more heterogeneous community than Hong Kong in 1894.[70] Besides the small population of Europeans there were coloureds, Malays, and black and white Africans. Most of the black population, though certainly not all, were Xhosa-speaking men who came to the city for short stints of work and returned to their families in the Transkei and Ciskei. For the most part whites living in Cape Town came originally from Europe, with a number who considered themselves to be British, though their ancestors may have emigrated decades earlier. Others considered themselves Afrikaner, having a separate language (Afrikaans) and cultural identity, while still others came from Germany or eastern Europe.

In early February the Acting Medical Officer of Health for the Cape Colony, Dr A. J. Gregory, claimed that plague was present in the city.[71] Soon after he had reported this to the Governor of the Cape, Sir Hely Hutchinson, the colony decided to consult a British doctor, William Simpson, who was studying enteric fever in troops stationed in the Transvaal. Simpson had written a number of articles on plague, as well as a circular on the disease which the Colonial Office had sent to all colonies.[72] Well regarded by Dr Patrick Manson, the London medical adviser to the Colonial Office, Simpson was to give T. L. Graham, the Colonial Secretary, advice on the control of the disease.[73] Simpson worked with the Plague Advisory Board, the committee which the local authorities appointed to advise them on controlling the disease.[74] As in Hong Kong, the city undertook a massive campaign to clean up areas local physicians claimed were filthy, as well as to isolate plague patients and those who had been in contact with plague patients.

One anti-plague measure not available in Hong Kong in 1894 but available in Cape Town was Haffkine's prophylactic, a series of injections to inoculate against plague. Simpson was a strong supporter of the method. In 1897, while editor of the *Indian Medical Gazette*, he had promoted it, claiming that it would 'rob the plague of its terrors'.[75] At that point, although he endorsed the prophylactic in print, he had no experience with it in practice. Unlike Simpson, Gregory had actually used the prophylactic before, during a small-scale epidemic of plague in King William's Town.[76]

Free inoculations were given to all who wanted them.[77] In the middle of March, in response to what they claimed was an increase in the number of cases of plague, Simpson and Gregory started to put into effect compulsory inoculation for the black African population. On 20 March the *Cape Times* announced that 3,000 'kafirs' had been inoculated.[78] At a meeting of the Plague Board one doctor asked Gregory about inoculating the public at large, and Gregory argued that it should be done.[79]

The editor of the *Cape Times* endorsed inoculation, claiming that 'the advisability of the process appears to be very generally recognized'.[80] Not all agreed with the editor. 'The present may be an opportune time,' claimed the editor a few days after endorsing the process, 'to refer to the many rumours that have been current during the past week regarding, not only the value of the precaution against the disease, but as to the danger liable to supervene upon the operation.'[81] The editor claimed that, 'happily', Simpson had been able to clear away all the doubts when he answered a question on inoculation at a meeting of the Plague Advisory Board which the paper published.[82] As with the approach to rumours of the editor of the *Hong Kong Daily Press* in 1894, the editor of the *Cape Times* also reported on the presence of rumours, but the paper contained only the scantiest details of their contents. The lack of detail in the *Cape Times* may have been a result of the editor not wanting to give the rumours currency, since publishing details of them might give inoculation a bad name. The editor did not indicate in which sections of Cape Town's highly stratified community the rumours were supposedly current. Although it is hard to tell from the accounts of meetings of the Plague Advisory Board and from the newspaper articles, it is most likely that the rumours were present among the British community, and perhaps among the coloured also.

Not all agreed with the editor, Gregory, and Simpson about inoculation. At the end of March an article appeared 'By A Doctor of Medicine' which claimed that many people were 'exercised' about the value of inoculation and were asking their doctors about it.[83] The opinion of doctors, the piece argued, 'may or may not be well informed, but doctors are supposed to know ... So that generally a doctor's opinion is the end of all controversy.'[84] The author included long extracts from a paper by F. S. Arnold on inoculation in India which quoted criticism of it by the Indian Plague Commission, a committee of British doctors who had compiled a four-volume report on plague in India, with one volume dedicated to reporting on the value of Haffkine's prophylactic. 'A Doctor of Medicine' also cited research by Professor Gujjar, which 'showed that whenever inoculations have been introduced, the results have been most disastrous on the uninoculated'.[85] The author concluded that there was 'fairly strong evidence' that inoculation 'temporarily lessens the liability of plague and the cases of mortality among the inoculated'.[86] The author claimed that the inoculated were a danger to the community, since they might pass the disease to others. Inoculation, he or she wrote, 'is distinctly bad, and nowhere can the method claim a triumph like that gained by the Sanitary Department in Egypt by reliance on well devised and strictly enforced sanitary measures'.[87]

The letter prompted a stream of other letters. Simpson replied to the allegations about inoculation, claiming that the author had selected only parts of the criticisms of the Indian Plague Commission and used them out of context.[88] One from 'Layman' highlighted the question of evidence and inoculation, a question which would resurface often over the next months. He or she claimed that 'A Doctor of Medicine' had not been convincing in the evidence brought to bear on inoculation: 'instead of solid, definite facts ... we have only the opinions of some native doctors and one European, who have nothing more tangible to offer than vague suspicion and hypothesis'.[89] 'Layman' dismissed the views of one European doctor and several Indian doctors as insufficient grounds to reject inoculation.

Over the next months more questions about inoculation were raised at subsequent meetings of the Plague Advisory Board, especially about the death rate among those who had been inoculated.[90] At the same time, a series of articles on the procedure appeared in the *Cape Times* which were unabashedly pro-inoculation. The editor had made clear the position the paper would take, and the articles may have been a direct response to the rumours mentioned in the Plague Advisory Board meetings, such as the one about several people being inoculated and then having their arms amputated as a result. The articles set out in much detail research from the Indian Plague Commission. 'As there is a good deal of misconception,' claimed the article, 'about ... the nature of the process, and as it has been rumoured on more than one occasion that inoculation has resulted in infecting the individual operated on with plague', the author undertook to explain the production of the prophylactic.[91] He or she also used a number of statistical examples to 'prove' that inoculation was efficacious. The author claimed that, in one military encampment of 1,830 persons, 671 had volunteered for inoculation, and since they were 'acting under strict military discipline ... [this] makes the accuracy of the figures unquestionable'.[92] Out of the 671 inoculated, 32 cases of plague occurred, while out of the 830 uninoculated, 143 cases occurred. The author reasoned that if the 671 inoculated had refused the procedure, then 112 cases would have occurred and 77 deaths. 'As a matter of fact', the author concluded, 'inoculation produced a reduction in the death rate of 80 per cent.'[93] Another article claimed that it was 'almost a public duty to submit to the operation'.[94] Thus statistics and descriptions of scientific practice were supposed to quell the rumours.

Neither the public duty argument nor the statistical evidence appeared to convince many of the value of inoculation. The procedure came under even more fire in April when two of the nurses who had been working on the plague ward, and had been inoculated, died of plague. At a meeting in late April the death of one of the plague nurses was discussed.[95] Gregory argued that the value of inoculation should not be judged on the basis of one case. Instead it should be evaluated on the basis of a number of cases.[96]

In a letter to the editor of the *Cape Times* signed 'Cleanliness' the author brought up the case of the nurses, as well as the advisability of the procedure for others in Cape Town. 'These two sad cases,' wrote 'Cleanliness', 'together with other deaths through, or shortly after inoculation, ... are apt to shake one's faith in experts' advice or opinions.'[97] Although the author did not single him out, the most visible expert on plague in Cape Town at the time was Simpson. The author of the letter was little impressed with the evidence which Gregory marshalled at meetings of the Plague Advisory Board. Statistics, in the view of 'Cleanliness', were especially suspect, since 'figures can be made to prove anything'.[98] The author concluded that inoculation should be of little concern anyway to the 'better-class people, that is those who are scrupulously clean in their person and habits' because they did not need it.[99] 'Cleanliness' was not arguing that inoculation was useless, simply that it was not necessary for all classes. Since by far the majority of the middle and upper classes were whites, though there were small minorities of middle-class black Africans, coloureds and Malays, the author was arguing that, in effect, inoculation was of value only for certain races. In his view, class, race and cleanliness were directly linked. Gregory's suggestion in March that inoculation was of value to all nullified the hierarchy the author implied.[100]

In summing up the anti-plague campaign in a memorandum to the Colonial Office, Gregory claimed that 'only 15,798' had been inoculated out of a population of around 60,000, and most of those, around 7,000, were 'natives' many of whom had been forced to undergo the procedure.[101] In his summing-up of the campaign Simpson related that the government had 'by every means in their power endeavoured to bring into prominence the advantages of inoculation'.[102] He judged, however, that the efforts were to little avail. During periods 'when the inhabitants were in a state of alarm', he related, 'inoculation was readily accepted, but at a later period, in consequence of certain unfounded and sinister rumours concerning the dangerous effects of the inoculations, volunteers for the treatment rapidly decreased.'[103] He also argued that compulsory inoculation would be of value to those he considered at risk, 'the poorer classes', including whites, coloureds, black Africans and Malays.[104] In Simpson's view the problem was not with the evidence he, Gregory, and others had marshalled to 'prove' the efficacy of plague inoculation, it was the rumours, which, in their perceptions, were ephemeral but powerful forces in Cape Town. Rumours were the villain and the scapegoat in the story he told the Colonial Office.

As in Hong Kong, rumours in Cape Town highlighted tensions in the English-speaking community over advice on how to control plague, especially advice from 'outsiders'. On the one hand were those, like Gregory, who welcomed Simpson's advice and considered the research results from India to be credible. The editor of the *Cape Times* took a similar view. He published a series of articles on plague precautions which argued that the Cape Town public should welcome a 'handy little' book by W. G. King, Sanitary Commissioner of Madras.[105] If King's ideas 'can be applied successfully in India, with her teeming millions, it should be capable of no less application in South Africa, where the population is so very much smaller'.[106] On the other hand many in South Africa considered the country to have a unique environment which demanded unique methods of controlling disease. One physician wrote, before the outbreak of plague, 'we have a semi-barbarous native population to deal with, and we shall have a long wait before we can hope to find among our coloured brethren an enlightened public opinion, or a due sense of responsibility, in sanitary matters'.[107] Medical practices and sanitary measures had to be tailored to a unique environment in South Africa. In the case of the letter from 'Cleanliness' only certain classes needed to be inoculated, though in theory inoculation was supposedly of value to all, regardless of race. Simpson's support for inoculation and his letter to the editor of the *Times* denouncing the letter by 'A Doctor of Medicine' may have been seen by some as advice from someone who did not understand South Africa.

The Anglo-Boer war may also have played an important role in the reaction to inoculation Simpson and others recorded. Whether English-speaking or not, the residents of Cape Town were living in a city where thousands of refugees and troops came and went. To the British, either by birth or culturally, many of the refugees from the Transvaal would be 'outsiders', either the enemy Afrikaners or immigrants from Europe. Other 'outsiders', as Saul Dubow has argued, included black Africans, who were perceived as belonging not in the country's cities but on the land.[108] The suggestion that inoculation was of value to all may not have appealed because, in a sense, it unified the residents of a city striving to remain divided.

Even though it is difficult to tell how or whether the editors of the *Cape Times* and the *Hong Kong Daily Press*, or colonial officials writing their reports, changed the rumours they recorded – and not knowing this is one of the thorniest problems with using rumours as a historical source – their existence forced into the open discussion of who 'knew best' how to control or cure plague. In Hong Kong many of the Chinese contested the imposition of Western medicine, while the graduates of the Hong Kong College of Medicine not only accepted

Western medicine but practised it. The accounts in the *Hong Kong Daily Press* of rumours circulating among the Chinese community signalled a deep mistrust on the part of some Europeans of most Chinese, even those who were educated at a government school, Victoria College. Those Chinese who were awarded a modicum of trust were graduates of the Hong Kong College of Medicine, because they might serve to educate the rest of the community. As evidenced by the rumours, though, even these Chinese may have been suspect to some of the British community. At issue in Cape Town was, obviously, not Western medicine in general but a method of plague control developed in a foreign laboratory by outsiders unfamiliar with the make-up of South African society.

In both cities rumours acted as a catalyst to discussion of the complicated ties between Europeans and other ethnic and racial groups. Outsiders, particularly experts, were seen by some in Cape Town as a threat to the city's racial and class hierarchies. Likewise in Hong Kong the 'outsiders' who were 'insiders' – Chinese who spoke English – were perceived by many British residents as undermining the colonial order.

Notes

I would like to thank Patricia Matthews and Marybeth Hamilton for sharing with me their knowledge of sources on rumours; John Carson, Bridie Andrews and Andrew Cunningham gave me much valuable editorial advice. I am grateful to the Wellcome Trust for financial support.

1 'The plague at Canton', *Hong Kong Daily Press*, 10 May 1894, p. 2.
2 CO 129/263/10935, Despatch from the Governor to the Secretary of State, 23 May 1894.
3 'Plague Board', *Cape Times*, 4 April 1901, p. 6.
4 Patricia A. Turner, *I Heard it through the Grapevine: Rumor in African-American Culture* (Berkeley, Cal.: University of California Press, 1994): 5. Gordon W. Allport and Leo Postman forty years ago defined rumours as beliefs passed by word of mouth 'without secure standards of evidence being present'. *The Psychology of Rumor* (New York: Holt, 1947), p. ix. Jean-Noel Kapferer, in a recent and comprehensive analysis of the field, used a similar definition, claiming that rumours represented '… the emergence and circulation in society of information that is either not yet publicly confirmed by official sources or denied by them'. *Rumors, Uses, Interpretations, and Images* (New Brunswick, N.J.: Transaction, 1990, originally published in 1987 as *Rumeurs: la plus vieux média du monde*, by Editons du Seuil, Paris. Revised edition published in English. Translated by Bruce Fink), p. 13. Turner's definition is more flexible than that used by other researchers, covering the types of accounts, which were often short stories, sometimes only a line or two, buried in an editorial or colonial report.
5 Elizabeth van Heyningen, 'Cape Town and the plague of 1901', *Studies in the History of Cape Town* (1984): 101.
6 Carl T. Smith, *Chinese Christian: Elites, Middlemen, and the Church in Hong Kong* (Hong Kong: Oxford University Press, 1985); Elizabeth Sinn, *Power and Charity: the Early History of the Tung Wah Hospital, Hong Kong* (Hong Kong: Oxford University Press, 1989); and Jung-Fang Tsai, *Hong Kong in Chinese History: Community and*

Social Unrest in the British Colony, 1842–1913 (New York: Columbia University Press, 1993).

7 On refugees see Elizabeth van Heyningen, 'Refugees and relief in Cape Town, 1899–1902', *Studies in the History of Cape Town* 3 (1984): 64–113. On immigration see M. Shain, 'Diamonds, pogroms and undesirables: anti-alienism and legislation in the Cape Colony, 1898–1910', *South African Historical Journal* 12 (1980): 13–28.

8 The anthropologist Peter Lienhardt contended that psychologists and sociologists have investigated the therapeutic value of rumours for society, whereas historians have treated them as symptomatic of a society's approach to coping with a stressful situation. Peter Lienhardt, 'The interpretation of rumour', in J. H. M. Beattie and R. G. Lienhardt (eds), *Studies in Social Anthropology: Essays in Memory of E. E. Evans-Pritchard by his former Oxford Colleagues* (Oxford: Clarendon Press, 1975), p. 123. The following is a sampling of studies on rumour which illustrates the range of approaches researchers have taken. P. Carroll, 'Alligators in the sewer, dragons in the well and Freud in the toilet', *Sociological Review* 32 (1984): 57–74; T. Shibutani, *Improvised News: a Sociological Study of Rumor* (Indianapolis, Ind.: Bobbs-Merrill, 1966); G. Boyes, 'Belief and disbelief: an examination of reactions to the presentation of rumor legends', in P. Smith (ed.), *Perspectives on Contemporary Legend* (Sheffield: Sheffield Academic Press, 1984), p. 64–78; G. A. Fine, 'Redemption rumors: mercantile legends and corporate beneficence', *Journal of American Folklore* 99 (1986): 208–22; P. B. Mullen, 'Modern legend and rumor theory', *Journal of the Folklore Institute* 9 (1972): 95–109; Gary Alan Fine, 'Rumors of Apartheid: the ecotypicafication of contemporary legends in the new South Africa', *Journal of Folklore Research* 29 (1992): 53–71. Rumours during World War Two were the subject of one of the earliest studies by psychologists Allport and Postman, p. viii. See also Leon Festinger, *A Theory of Cognitive Dissonance* (Stanford University Press, 1962); R. Knapp, 'A psychology of rumor', *Public Opinion Quarterly* 8 (1): 22–37; M. Jaeger and R. L. Rosnow, 'Who hears what from whom and with what effect: a study of rumor', *Personality and Social Psychology Bulletin* 6 (3): 473–8; I. D. and M. B. London, 'Rumor as a footnote to Chinese national character', *Psychological Reports* 37 (1975): 343–49; R. L. Rosnow and G. A. Fine, *Rumor and Gossip: the Social Psychology of Hearsay* (New York: Elsevier, 1976); R. L. Rosnow, 'Psychology of rumor reconsidered', *Psychological Bulletin* 87 (1980): 578–91. R. L. Rosnow, 'Inside rumor: a personal journey', *American Psychologist* 46 (1991): 484–96.

9 Sinn, *Power and Charity*, pp. 162, 164, 171–2.

10 Van Heyningen, 'Cape Town and the plague of 1901', p. 101.

11 Shula Marks, *Reluctant Rebellion: the 1906–08 Disturbances in Natal* (Oxford: Clarendon Press, 1970), p. 144.

12 Anand A. Yang, 'A conversation of rumours: the language of popular *mentalités* in late nineteenth-century India', *Journal of Social History* 20 (1987): 486.

13 Pule Phoofolo, 'Epidemics and revolutions: the rinderpest epidemic in late nineteenth-century southern Africa', *Past and Present* 138 (1993): 134.

14 David Arnold, *Colonizing the Body: State Medicine and Epidemic Disease in Nineteenth-century India* (Berkeley, Cal.: University of California Press, 1994), pp. 218–26. See also David Arnold, 'Touching the body: perspectives on Indian plague, 1896–1900', in R. Guha (ed.), *Subaltern Studies* V. *Writings on South Asian History and Society* (Delhi: Oxford University Press, 1987), p. 55–90.

15 Arnold, *Colonizing the Body*, p. 218.

16 *Ibid.*

17 *Ibid.*, p. 224.

18 Rajnarayan Chandavarkar, 'Plague panic and epidemic politics in India, 1896–1914', in Terence Ranger and Paul Slack (eds), *Epidemics and Ideas: Essays in the Historical Perception of Pestilence* (Cambridge University Press, 1992), pp. 223–6.

19 *Ibid.*, p. 225.

20 Kapferer, *Rumors, Uses, Interpretations*, p. 8.

21 G. B. Endacott *A History of Hong Kong* (London: Oxford University Press, 1958), p. 253.

22 *Ibid.*, p. 252.
23 CO 129/263/10928, Despatch from the Governor of Hong Kong to the Secretary of State, 17 May 1894. Lowson wrote a report on his trip, dated 16 May 1894, which was included in the despatch to the Colonial Office. Lowson had an M.B. from Edinburgh as well as a C.M.
24 *Ibid.* For a longer discussion of Lowson's trip to Canton and the basis of his diagnosis of plague see Mary Preston Sutphen, 'Imperial Hygiene in Calcutta, Cape Town, and Hong Kong: the early Career of Sir William John Ritchie Simpson (1955–1931)', Ph.D. dissertation, Yale University, 1995, pp. 126–8.
25 CO 129/263/12777, Despatch from the Governor of Hong Kong to the Secretary of State, 17 May 1894. See also Sinn, *Power and Charity*, pp. 162–3.
26 Sinn, *Power and Charity*, p. 183.
27 'The plague at Canton', *Hong Kong Daily Press*, 10 May 1894, p. 2.
28 I would like to thank John Carson especially for discussing these ideas with me.
29 Allport and Postman (*Psychology of Rumor*, p. 2) argued that rumours surface when important events occur and news is lacking or 'subjectively ambiguous'. Kapferer (*Rumors, Uses, Interpretations*, p. 46) has argued that rumours were 'a socially acceptable safety valve for repressed aggressiveness'. In general outline Kapferer agrees with Allport and Postman that rumours are often evident when information has not been 'publicly confirmed by official sources or denied by them', (*ibid.*, p. 13).
30 'The plague', *Hong Kong Daily Press*, 21 May 1894, p. 2.
31 *Ibid.*
32 'The plague', *Hong Kong Daily Press*, 24 May 1894, p. 2.
33 *Ibid.*
34 *Hong Kong Daily Press*, 25 May 1894, p. 2. Sinn (*Power and Charity*, p. 181) also discusses the perception in European newspapers that the elite Chinese were to blame for the trouble.
35 *Hong Kong Daily Press*, 25 May 1894, p. 2.
36 *Ibid.*
37 Sinn also discussed this letter briefly, see *Power and Charity*, p. 169. According to Sinn, Tse Tsan Tai was a government clerk, who later became a social reformer and revolutionary. *Power and Charity*, p. 169 and note 58, p. 258.
38 Tse Tsantai, 'A Chinese protest', *Hong Kong Daily Press*, 30 May 1893, p. 2.
39 *Ibid.*
40 *Ibid.*
41 *Ibid.*
42 Peakite, 'A reply to Tse Tsantai', *Hong Kong Daily Press*, 31 May 1894, p. 2.
43 *Ibid.*
44 G. H. Choa, *The Life and Times of Sir Kai Ho Kai, a Prominent Figure in Nineteenth-century Hong Kong* (Hong Kong: Chinese University Press, 1981), p. 16.
45 'The plague', *Hong Kong Daily Press*, 8 June 1894, p. 2.
46 Carol Benedict, 'Bubonic plague in nineteenth-century China', Ph.D. dissertation, Stanford University, 1992, p. 298.
47 Jung-fang Tsai provides a valuable analysis of the changes in structure and membership of Chinese elites in Hong Kong at the turn of the twentieth century, see *Hong Kong in Chinese History*, pp. 92–6.
48 Sinn, *Power and Charity*, p. 183.
49 *Hong Kong Daily Press*, 14 June 1894, p. 2. See also 'Disturbances in Canton', *Hong Kong Daily Press*, 13 June 1894, p. 2.
50 *Hong Kong Daily Press*, 14 June 1894, p. 2.
51 *Ibid.*
52 CO 129/12777, Despatch from the Governor of Hong Kong to the Secretary of State, 20 June 1894.
53 *Hong Kong Daily Press*, 14 June 1894, p. 2.
54 *Ibid.*
55 *Ibid.*

56 'Indignant', 'Victoria College and anti-foreign feeling', *Hong Kong Daily Press*, 16 June 1894, p. 2.
57 *Ibid.*
58 *Ibid.*
59 *Ibid.*
60 *Ibid.*
61 *Hong Kong Daily Press*, 22 June 1894, p. 2.
62 *Ibid.*
63 *Hong Kong Daily Press*, 29 June 1894, p. 2.
64 For an account of many of these individuals see Smith, *Chinese Christian*, chapter 7, especially pp. 167–71 and Tsai, *Hong Kong in Chinese History*, chapter 3.
65 Later in the year defeat at the hands of the Japanese during the Sino-Japanese war galvanised many Chinese into developing a strong sense of nationalism. Chan Lau Kit-ching, *China, Britain and Hong Kong, 1895–1945* (Hong Kong: Chinese University Press, 1990), p. 2; Sinn, *Power and Charity*, pp. 154–5.
66 Sinn, *Power and Charity*, pp. 153–4, and Tsai, *Hong Kong in Chinese History*, pp. 97–9.
67 Endacott, *History of Hong Kong*, p. 224.
68 Sinn, *Power and Charity*, p. 155 and note 179, p. 256. Chan Lau Kit-ching, *China, Britain and Hong Kong*, pp. 21–2.
69 Sinn, *Power and Charity*, pp. 84–5.
70 On Cape Town see John Vivian Bickford-Smith, 'Commerce, Class and Ethnicity in Cape Town, 1875 to 1902', Ph.D. dissertation, University of Cambridge, 1988; Elizabeth Boudina van Heyningen, 'Public Health and Society in Cape Town, 1880–1910', Ph.D. dissertation, University of Cape Town, 1989. I would like to thank Hilary Sapire, who has given me much valuable information about the make-up of Cape society.
71 T. Harrison Butler, *Bubonic Plague, with Special Reference to the Epidemic in South Africa in 1901: a Thesis for the Degree of Doctor of Medicine of the University of Oxford, 1902* (London: Operative Jewish Converts' Institution, 1902), p. 41.
72 CO 854/36, W. J. Simpson, 'Memorandum on the Influence of Rats in the Dissemination of Plague', 7 June 1900.
73 On Graham's powers see CO 48/551/11519, Despatch from the Governor of the Cape to the Secretary of State, 13 March 1901. On Simpson's responsibilities see van Heyningen, 'Public Health and Society in Cape Town', p. 80, and Sutphen, 'Imperial Hygiene', chapter 4.
74 For the membership of the Cape Advisory Boards see *Cape of Good Hope Report and Proceedings, with Annexures, of the Cape Peninsula Plague Advisory Board, Appointed to Advise the Government on Matters connected with the Suppression of Bubonic Plague* (Cape Town: Richards, 1901), p. 2.
75 'M. Haffkine', *Indian Medical Gazette* (1897), p. 103.
76 MH/19/261/4225, Milner to the Secretary of State, 7 December 1900. The despatch included a minute by J. Gordon Sprigg which recorded Gregory's actions.
77 See for example, an advertisement for free inoculations at the Free Dispensary, *Cape Times*, 22 March 1901, p. 2.
78 'The plague. On the down grade. Satisfactory bulletin. Five cases', *Cape Times*, 20 March 1901, p. 7.
79 'Plague Board', *Cape Times*, 21 March 1901, p. 5.
80 'The plague. On the down grade. Satisfactory bulletin. Five cases', *Cape Times*, 20 March 1901, p. 7.
81 *Cape Times*, 22 March 1901, p. 4.
82 *Ibid.*
83 'By a Doctor of Medicine', 'Inoculation. The case for and against', *Cape Times*, 30 March 1901, p. 10.
84 *Ibid.*
85 *Ibid.*
86 *Ibid.*

87 *Ibid.*
88 W. J. Simpson, 'Inoculation', *Cape Times*, 3 April 1901, p. 3.
89 'Layman', 'Inoculation', *Cape Times*, 2 April 1901, p. 2.
90 For example, see *Cape Advisory Board*, p. 99.
91 'Inoculation. Plague preventive. The evidence of facts. Extracts from Indian official reports', *Cape Times*, 25 April 1901, p. 5.
92 *Ibid.*
93 *Ibid.* See also the next day's account, 'Inoculation. Plague preventive. The evidence of facts. Extracts from Indian official reports', *Cape Times*, 26 April 1901, p. 5.
94 'Inoculation. Plague preventive. The evidence of facts. Extracts from Indian official reports', *Cape Times*, 29 April 1901, p. 5.
95 'Plague Board', *Cape Times*, 25 April 1901, p. 7.
96 *Ibid.*
97 'Cleanliness', 'Inoculation', *Cape Times*, 9 May 1901, p. 5.
98 *Ibid.*
99 *Ibid.*
100 For a valuable discussion of race, class and ethnic hierarchies in South Africa see Shula Marks and Stanley Trapido, 'The politics of race, class, and nationalism', in Marks and Trapido (eds), *The Politics of Race, Class and Nationalism in Twentieth Century South Africa* (London: Longman, 1987), pp. 1–70.
101 CO/48/551/19672, Despatch from the Governor of the Cape Colony to the Secretary of State, 22 May 1901. The despatch contained a report entitled 'A Memorandum by Acting Medical Officer of Health, Cape Colony'.
102 CO/48/551/19672, Despatch from the Governor of the Cape Colony to the Secretary of State, 22 May 1901. Included in the despatch was a report entitled, 'A Memorandum by Professor Simpson'.
103 *Ibid.*
104 *Ibid.*
105 'Plague precaution. Lessons from India. Travelling restrictions, their merits and defects', *Cape Times*, 30 May 1901, p. 6.
106 *Ibid.*
107 Herbert Caiger, 'Johannesburg as a typhoid-distribution centre', *South African Medical Journal* (1899): 264.
108 Saul Dubow, 'Race, civilisation and culture: the elaboration of segregationist discourse in the inter-war years', in Marks and Trapido, *The Politics of Race*, p. 75.

CHAPTER ELEVEN

Drug-resistant malaria: a global problem and the Thai response

Helen Power

> I think there's a genuine prospect of untreatable malaria unless there is considerable incentive to develop new drugs, and that the spectre of untreatable malaria will rise within the relatively near future. We could have untreatable malaria as we go into the next century.[1]

The world is facing a problem which modern medicine considered it had solved – the chemotherapy of malaria. In particular, treatment of the potentially lethal *falciparum* malaria. Strains of this parasite have become resistant to both synthesised drugs and quinine.[2]

After the end of World War Two cheap, easily administered synthetic antimalarials promised to back up the use of DDT in eradicating malaria on a global scale.[3] The development of parasite resistance to these drugs was initially accorded only passing attention; if anti-mosquito measures could be stepped up, the need for curative medicines would decline.[4] As the technical, administrative and operational problems associated with eradication gradually overcame the gains made in malaria control, the need for efficient chemotherapy increased. In South East Asia warfare sharpened the perceived need. The US army embarked upon the biggest drug screening project in the history of malaria chemotherapy, and interest grew in the possibility of a malaria vaccine. When the US arsenal was exhausted, and American interest numbed by withdrawal of troops from Vietnam, from nowhere it seemed Chinese researchers presented the West with qinghaosu. A paper in the *Chinese Medical Journal* in 1979 presented a detailed report from the Qinghaosu Antimalarial Co-ordinating Research Group.[5] Just as the West followed a concerted policy aimed at developing drugs for the treatment of malaria, so too had the Chinese. However, their project used different resources, both pharmacological and ideological. Far from the West accepting the validity of the Chinese work, qinghaosu appears to have become the central prop in a play where the extras are those who live in malarious regions of the world and are exposed to parasites resistant to existing drugs.

Enter Thailand: a country playing a leading role in the South East Asian economic miracle. Unlike the other countries in the region, Thailand did not fall prey to the colonial ambitions of the French, Dutch or British. Nor was the country directly involved in the two Indochinese wars which devastated much of the region. Thailand retained its independence by selectively adapting its social and political structure. The Thais successfully played off the French and British with a succession of treaties, backing whoever was in the ascendant, rather than displaying any national loyalty. Thailand's links with the United States also began with trade, but the relationship was strengthened at the turn of this century by the American provision of foreign advisers. The real nature of Thailand's independence as the twentieth century has progressed is a complicated issue.

The dialectics of imperial tropical medicine and warfare have been used to discuss the modern history of malaria. It is ironic therefore that Thailand should be one of the world's major sites of drug-resistant *falciparum* malaria, at its most acute and deadly along her borders, despite the fact that the country has not been colonised by European powers or been the site of major warfare in recent times. Clearly there is more to the history of malaria than these two historiographical avenues.[6]

The post-World War Two control of malaria has been dominated by the World Health Organization's (WHO) Malaria Eradication Programme (MEP). This global effort to curb and then remove the spectre of malaria from the developed and the developing world fell foul of technical difficulties and the inherent prejudices of tropical medicine.

The issues of drug resistance illustrate the implicit imperialism and conservative ethnocentricism of Western medicine as embodied in the guardian of 'health for all', the WHO. This chapter deals with two specific incidents in the history of drug-resistant malaria. First, the response to the discovery of chloroquine resistance in Thailand by Dr Tranakchit Harinasuta. Second, the West's and Thailand's response to the drugs derived from the Chinese medicinal herb qing hao (*Artemisia annua L.*).[7]

These are, of course, examples of contested knowledge. In this case not a dispute between traditional medicine and Western medicine but the non-acceptance by the international scientific community of the results of Western medicine as practised in a developing country of South East Asia and in communist China.

The West could afford to be circumspect about drug-resistant malaria, and new means to combat the problem, but for Thailand and

China these were immediate public health problems. Non-acceptance by the West shows, first, the different health priorities of the developed and developing worlds and second, the control which the West has been able to exert over the developing countries by various means despite the end of the imperial era.

Yet there has been discernible progress in Thai self-confidence and action. In the 1960s the Thais were neither sufficiently confident in their own research nor sufficiently independent of foreign aid to move unilaterally on their malaria chemotherapy policy. As a result they asked for outside assistance in confirming what was to become a serious situation with potentially untreatable malaria. In the 1980s they moved independently to assess, license and use the Chinese drugs.

While the Chinese research may have been conducted under an ideology which the West chooses to discredit for political reasons, the same cannot so easily be said of Thailand.[8] The Thais had selectively adopted the curative and clinical methods of Western medicine without external pressure from direct colonial rule. Initially this selective technology transfer did not include the ethos of academic medicine and research. That began in a limited way after World War Two in a bid for intellectual self-sufficiency.

Thai researchers experienced difficulties exploiting the early results of their work and were constrained by linguistic and cultural differences. For instance, the preparation of material for publication was hindered by lack of knowledge of, and access to, publishing outlets.[9] If tropical medicine is the 'Cinderella' specialism in modern medicine, it would seem that work in this field by indigenous practitioners ranks even lower on the professional scale.

In this chapter the non-acceptance of the Thai physician Tranakchit Harinasuta's work serves as a parallel for the more recent Western dissent over the qinghaosu drugs. The chapter develops the themes of the historically determined, self-interested nature of Western pharmaceutical production, and the West's attempts to control the production of knowledge and the application of its results in developing countries.

Western medicine in Thailand

As Thailand maintained its independence, medicine was not part of foreign domination. The usual tensions between traditional healing and Western medicine are not found there. Western allopathic medicine was introduced by missionaries, but imported drugs, including quinine, were sold independently by pharmacists and peddlers.[10] The pragmatic, mainly Buddhist population used the clinical curative aspects of Western medicine as an additional system:

> not because of a conclusive scientific proof of theoretical correctness but rather for more 'practical' or empirical reasons, including immediate availability, convenience, low cost, high perceived effectiveness, satisfaction of the need to feel something is being done, appropriateness for the immediate social situation, and perhaps social prestige (including affiliation with a group perceived to be powerful, successful and benevolent).[11]

The selective interest in Western medicine was unsupported by an ethos of research and experimental investigation. The early Thai doctors merely practised what they had been taught. This caused significant problems for the first generation of Thai clinicians who developed an interest in research.

In 1888, as part of his attempts to carefully westernise aspects of Thai government, King Chulalongkorn (Rama V) ordered the construction of a permanent hospital in Bangkok, the Siriraj, to replace the temporary buildings erected during epidemics. His initiatives differed from the typical development of Western medical education outside Europe and America. In the colonial situation medical technology was imported and practised by outsiders.[12] Here it was the Thais themselves who were being trained in a system which allowed integration and assimilation rather than simple dominance.

Siriraj Hospital trained Thai students in Western medicine, the first group graduating in 1893. In 1917 the Medical School was amalgamated with Chulalongkorn University and granted its own degrees after 1928. In addition to the medical curriculum, based on the biomedical sciences and allopathic therapeutics of the West, courses in Thai remedies and Chinese *materia medica* were included. This policy reflected the Thai eclecticism and disregard for the dominance of any one system.[13] However, the scale of the operation was small, and the results were limited accordingly. The medical graduates of Chulalongkorn University (approximately twenty per year) were employed in the military and naval services, the Red Cross and private practice.

Dr Heiser, from the International Health Commission (IHC) of the Rockefeller Foundation, visited Thailand in 1916 on his world tour, and offered financial help and technical advice. Following this the IHC assisted in reorganising the medical school in 1923. The equation of improved rural health and economic growth implicit in the IHC's objectives served the interests of the Thai government, although it was able to maintain more control than China.[14] This acceptance of American Rockefeller aid represents Thai manipulation of foreign powers to meet their own ends.

In 1928 a medical register was established for qualified doctors, but was meaningful only in Bangkok. In 1935 an initiative to spread Western medicine into rural Thailand was instigated by the opening of a school in Chiengmai. The six-month course was designed to produce 'medical assistants'. Chulalongkorn University followed suit with a similar course. These assistants were licensed, and their permitted activities defined. Traditional healers were not excluded by these moves towards the regulation and control of medical practice. As members of a branch of the art of healing they were included in the 1936 Act for the Control of the Practice of the Art of Healing, covering Dentistry, Pharmacy, Nursing and Midwifery.[15] Nurses (initially all male) were trained at the Bangkok nursing home for Europeans which opened in 1898. Midwifery training for Thai women was offered from 1897 in a school under royal patronage until it was taken over in 1921, again by the Rockefeller Foundation.

After World War Two redevelopment plans for South East Asia included educational and technical fellowships.[16] By such means it was intended that the threat of communism could be kept at bay and stability maintained in the region. In the 1950s, under the Colombo Plan, medical graduates were eligible to apply for postgraduate study abroad.[17] As the undergraduate medical curriculum was based on those of medical schools in the West, the syllabus lacked any detailed focus on 'tropical diseases', or what were for the Thais the infectious parasitic diseases of their own country and the South East Asian region in general.

Under this scheme Chamlong Harinasuta came to the Liverpool School of Tropical Medicine in 1951 to study for a Ph.D. degree under Brian Maegraith. A year later he was joined by his wife, Tranakchit Harinasuta, who took the Diploma in Tropical Medicine and Health (DTMH) course and assisted her husband with his research. After their return to Bangkok in 1953 the Harinasutas worked in the Siriraj hospital where they had both been trained. After various false starts and a military *coup d'état*, they opened a Faculty of Tropical Medicine in the University of Medical Sciences (renamed Mahidol University) in 1960.[18] It provided postgraduate instruction in Thai for medical graduates and was closely modelled on the course at the Liverpool School.

In 1966 under the South East Asian Ministers of Education Organisation (SEAMEO) the Bangkok faculty began teaching in English. The DTMH course at the new Faculty of Tropical Medicine was opened to all SEAMEO member countries under a fellowship scheme, and to other medical graduates from around the world who might wish to study tropical medicine in the tropics. Courses leading to Master's and Ph.D. qualifications were also offered.

In addition to the teaching the faculty hoped to stimulate interest in research. At the time there were considerable worries in Thailand about the shortage of qualified doctors and the exacerbation of this problem by a permanent brain drain, particularly to the United States. In the early 1960s a group of medical graduates chartered an aeroplane and flew to America, taking jobs as interns: few returned home.[19] It was hoped that increased opportunities for postgraduate education and research in Thailand would keep practitioners in the country.

However, education beyond diploma level posed particular problems for the faculty in its early years. Developing the necessary self-confidence to conduct research and question accepted knowledge was culturally problematic. Thai students at all stages of the education system show great respect and reverence for their teachers:

> There is no doubt that the way in which people are taught in Asia, or at least in Thailand particularly, does not lend itself to inquiry or questioning ... suddenly as a postgraduate you are expected to start questioning everything and that is very difficult, so what people tend to do is find that transition difficult, and they just tend to copy.[20]

The emphasis on cure as the only valuable component of Western medicine created a tension in Thailand which is still apparent: doctors are 'interested in treatment that is all – diagnosis and treatment'.[21] While acceptance of Western therapeutics was widespread where it was available, the ethos of academic medicine was more difficult to foster and more problematic in its execution. A good example is publishing in the scientific medical press. Tranakchit Harinasuta recalled how:

> In the old days, you know, we had not been trained in research. We had not been trained in writing the report. Nowadays the new generation learn how to carry out the research and we have more contact with the West, and with the language too. In the old days we used the Thai. We use English textbooks but we write in Thai, we speak in Thai.[22]

These aspects of the development of Western medicine in Thailand made research difficult, but it was in the international arena that the issues of contested knowledge came to the fore. As the single greatest cause of mortality in Thailand it was perhaps fitting that malaria provided the first example of this tension.

Malaria in Thailand

> Malaria is known in Thailand by such descriptive terms as kai-chub-sern ('shivering fever'), kai-pa ('jungle-fever'), kai-nua ('northern fever'), and kai-dok-suk ('teak-flower fever'). The last two names have their derivation in the high incidence of malaria in Northern Thailand and its prevalence during the rainy season when the teak trees bloom. But it

> may be said that malaria is an ancient and familiar affliction of the Thai people in every region and season.[23]

In 1918 King Vajiravudh (Rama VI) created a Department of Health to supervise the medical and public health services of Thailand. The department was organised in divisions. Malaria was included among many other illnesses in the Division of Infectious Diseases Control.

In 1930, at the request of the Thai government, the Health Commission of the League of Nations sent a malaria expert, Dr Ludwik Anigstein. He advised that in the less prosperous areas of Thailand, the northern rural regions, malaria presented a 'serious social problem demanding a special preventative effort'.[24] The death rate from the disease was estimated to be in the region of 40,000 to 50,000 a year, with a case rate of 3 million to 5 million, where the population was over 18 million. Malaria was now perceived as the major cause of mortality and morbidity in Thailand. In response a Malaria Section was created in the Division of Infectious Disease Control in 1934, with plans to reduce the expense to the Thai economy caused by malarial sickness and mortality. Supplies of quinine and totaquine were distributed at cost price via village headmen, and anti-larval programmes were started in certain areas in the country's first attempts to deal with the problems of malaria at a national level.

The dislocation of World War Two exacerbated the malaria problem. In 1943, in response to the worsening situation, the Malaria Section was upgraded to a separate division. As everywhere, there was a shortage of anti-malarial drugs. The abandonment of control operations, the dislocation of civilians, including forced labour by the Japanese, and troop movements resulted in an increase in the incidence of malaria. Mortality averaged over 50,000 deaths annual and epidemic conditions occurred for the first recorded time in various provinces. By 1947 malaria was the leading cause of mortality with 297·1 deaths per 100,000 of the population. In 1948 the Malaria Section was reorganised by the Ministry of Public Health into a Division of Malaria Control. The country was divided into five administrative regions, and a malaria officer with a staff of twenty technicians was allocated to each region. The regions were subdivided into five sections each of which formed an operational unit.[25]

This national initiative was complemented by the Thai government's request for a malaria control demonstration project. At the May 1948 meeting of the WHO Expert Committee on Malaria it was announced that countries could apply to host these projects. The expert committee saw the demonstration projects as a means of promoting a new technology on a grand scale: the control of malaria by the use of residual, long-lasting insecticides, particularly DDT.

In the post-war era Thailand was quick to accept the help of anti-communist America's aid packages and the rhetoric and tools of WHO's malaria control/eradication programmes. In Thailand the programme came to be seen by outsiders as a demonstration of the power of Western medicine and the political value of aid. M. E. Griffith described the health education aspects of the programme thus:

> The most effective informational activity is, of course, the actual house-to-house contacts made during the house-spraying campaign. This activity carries equipment labelled with the seal of Thai–American cooperation directly into the homes of more than half of the population of Thailand, bringing also an immediate demonstration of the practical effectiveness of international cooperation.[26]

The conservative anti-communist Thai government considered the campaign as a means of achieving greater health among the people. By improving the quality of life it sought to maintain the *status quo*. The anti-malarial operations represented disease management on an unprecedented scale in Thailand.

Sarapee, in Chiengmai province, in the north of the country, was selected as the demonstration area. It was a natural choice. The Thai government had maintained a Malaria Unit there since 1930, and the disease was endemic. The WHO/UNICEF project lasted from August 1949 to December 1951. UNICEF supplied the insecticides, spraying equipment and transport as part of its Far East Programme.[27] WHO provided international staff and technical direction. Sarapee was a major rice-growing region, and the UN Food and Agriculture Organisation (FAO) was interested in the correlation between the decreasing rate of malaria transmission and the quantity of foodstuffs produced in such a malaria control area.[28]

Spraying with residual insecticides began in 1949 and had reduced the death rate to 30·2 per 100,000 by 1960. From 1951, following the success of the WHO/UNICEF demonstration team, the Thai government and Special Technical and Economic Mission (STEM) of the Foreign Operations Administration (FOA) expanded the house spraying operation to reach the homes of 5 million by 1957. In 1958 the Ministry of Public Health created an internal administration to supervise the National Malaria Eradication Project of Thailand (NMEP).

By 1975 the NMEP was in such difficulties that a return to malaria control rather than the previous aim of malaria eradication was considered to be the most realistic policy. From 1972 to 1978 the number of detected malaria cases rose from 92,409 to 329,388. In that year the border/mountainous areas of Thailand were designated as control areas. From 1979 the total number of cases began to decline.[29] In that year alone there were 30,000 fewer cases, but, as a proportion of this total fall, the number of cases of *falciparum* malaria did not follow the same trend and across the South East Asian region the *P. falciparum* parasite increased as the cause of malaria, becoming the predominant species in Burma, Kampuchea, South China, Thailand and Vietnam.[30] Since the drug resistance of *P. falciparum* has the most serious consequences, this trend caused increasing concern.

Solving public health problems with Western science seemed to offer no cultural problems to the Thai government, which provided national personnel and the necessary working expenses. As a package the WHO malaria control/eradication campaign did not cause tension between traditional and Western medicine. Some people whose houses were sprayed resented the interference but did not perceive it as aggression by outsiders. What it did represent was the opening up of rural Thailand to an experience of Western medicine, albeit delivered by indigenous people.[31] Thai staff worked with technical assistance from outsiders, in line with WHO's policies.

At the Malaria Conference held in Bangkok in 1953 the government reported that:

> Unquestionably the access of the malaria control program has done much to stimulate public thinking on health problems and to encourage public cooperation with other health programs. The general feeling evident in most sprayed villages is that health has been greatly improved and that much less time has been lost from school and work due to sickness.[32]

Unfortunately malaria outsmarted both the pragmatism of the Thai people and Western scientific methods of control.

Antimalarials after World War Two: a problem solved?

In tropical theatres of war, control of malaria is a military priority. Fears over a shortage of quinine and the dominance of the German chemical companies in the field of antiparasitic drugs stimulated allied interest in synthetic antimalarials after 1939. At the end of World War Two the collaborative effort of Britain and the United States in anti-malarial chemotherapy offered a range of synthetic drugs active against *vivax* and *falciparum* malaria, capable of achieving radical cure and chemoprophylaxis.

Allied success in malaria chemotherapy was due to serendipity, the opportunities offered by wartime urgency, and a more complete understanding of the life cycle of the malaria parasites.[33] The wartime efforts of Curd, Davey and Rose from ICI's Blackley laboratories resulted in the production of paludrine.[34] The American chemical company Winthrop and the Sub-committee on the Co-ordination of Malarial Studies developed chloroquine (SN-7618), a 4-aminoquinoline.[35] In this context the technical details of the research are less important than the overtly military ideology which diverted human and fiscal resources into dealing with an immense problem in as short a time as possible. Once the war was over, the emphasis on anti-malarial chemotherapy declined. In both Britain and America interest in compounds synthesised during the war continued. However, this was a winding-up process, finalising the potential of any compounds which had not yet been completely tested for relative efficacy, dosage and toxity.

The next major impetus to develop antimalarials was again connected with warfare. This time it was the US involvement in Vietnam from 1965 to 1975, and the development of resistance in South East Asia to first one and then gradually all of the known synthetic antimalarials. The Walter Reed Army Institute of Research (WRAIR) was actively seeking new synthetic antimalarials from 1963. It screened 250,000 compounds and came up with mefloquine. How much the effects of warfare, the consequent dislocation of people, and the environmental destruction, or the eradication policies increasing the drug pressure, may have contributed to the rise of resistance remains to be investigated. Here we are concerned with the initial Thai reports of chloroquine resistance and their reception, in contrast to similar reports of resistance from South America.

Despite the Thais' acceptance and development of Western medicine as part of their own education and practice, their research into chloroquine resistance was not accepted by the West. The degree of importance attached to this problem also differed: for the Thais malaria was an ever-present and immediate problem of public health. In Europe malaria represented an overseas problem which was passing to the public health departments of the newly independent ex-colonies. In America malaria, outside of a war in the tropics, was also a less important issue. Cancer and heart disease swallowed up research budgets and facilities in the West. Multinational pharmaceutical companies were curtailing their interest in producing new drugs for the tropics, the cost of which prohibited purchase by the people who needed them most.[36]

The public health priority that drug-resistant malaria posed for the Thai authorities led them to license and try to control the use of the new, cheaper Chinese qinghao compounds when they became available in the early 1980s. Thai medical personnel, concerned with the problem of drug-resistant malaria, investigated the potential of these drugs and considered the best way to incorporate them in their malaria control strategies. WHO, by contrast, seemed more concerned to endlessly repeat the work already done in China, and to develop a patentable compound of its own.

Development of resistance in Thailand and new antimalarials

Throughout each phase of the malaria control/eradication/control programme in Thailand synthetic anti-malarial drugs were used as an integral part of the exercise. However, house spraying with residual insecticides and not mass drug administration was the key method. The spraying was supplemented by the distribution of chloroquine drugs (aralen – chloroquine diphosphate and nivaquine – chloroquine sulphate) by malaria control field teams, through hospitals and other authorised treatment centres. Antimalarials could also be bought over the counter from drug stores.

The malaria survey teams administered the first dose of the prescribed treatment to people showing any symptoms of malaria (present or recent fever and/or splenomegaly). Sufficient tablets were issued to complete a full course of treatment. When professional supervision was not available, the assistance of some responsible village leader (priest, headman or teacher) or other official was enlisted to avoid misuse of the drugs. There was, however, no absolute guarantee of compliance with the drug regimen. This may have been a contributory factor in the rise of resistance, with fresh infections or reinfections coming up through a sub-therapeutic dose of the drug.

The distribution of antimalarials was not entirely altruistic, nor was cure of the disease the only aim. Observers regarded this aspect of the work as reaching:

> multitudes of people who greatly need and will follow out the treatment which would otherwise be unavailable to them. The provision of even this limited medical attention is also pronouncedly effective in public relations in the villages and aids greatly in securing public cooperation in the malaria control program.[37]

By 1954 approximately 500,000 chloroquine tablets had been administered by field teams to about 100,000 people, and 5 million tablets had been issued by the division through other channels.[38] A large stock of the drugs, supplied through the WHO Mutual Security Agency, was held in reserve against special problems.[39]

After the initial twice-yearly spraying the interruption in malaria transmission allowed the project to move into the consolidation phase. Automatic spraying was discontinued, and replaced with several years of protective surveillance. Any remaining malaria cases were treated clinically to safeguard all formerly malarious areas against the return of the disease during this phase of anti-malaria vigilance.

Reports submitted to WHO and the US Foreign Operations Mission (USOM) concentrated on the results of spraying. Spraying was initially capital-intensive. Equipment had to be purchased, including means of transport to reach rural areas. Health education material in support of the spraying programme was designed and created by the Thai–American Audio Visual Service, in addition to simpler methods like wall charts and leaflets. Vital to the whole enterprise was the recruitment and training at all levels of staff, from qualified scientists to village volunteers. The Thai government's policy of road building and provision of education as a means of combating anti-government insurgency, led by communist infiltrators, served the malaria control programme well.[40]

Progress reports suggested early in 1958 that in the coming three years the Thai government would be able to maintain the further activities of malaria prevention without external assistance.[41] However, by June that year, at the Malaria Eradication Conference in Bangkok, USOM committed itself to prolonging aid. This was attributed to 'technical difficulties' with spraying while anti-malaria vigilance was implemented. Among the 'difficulties' cited were the slow release of government funds when required, rapid turnover of staff, the migration of people (often non-immunes) into newly deforested areas for agriculture and tin mining, and the use of temporary housing unsuitable for spraying. These 'virgin' areas were concentrated in the regions where malaria had been endemic: the borders with Burma (now Myanmar), Laos and Cambodia.

Thailand's borders were inevitably difficult regions in which to achieve malaria control, for the countries on the other side had to share a similar commitment, and the means to realise it. The WHO-sponsored Anti-malaria Co-ordination Board, formed in 1956 at Phnom Penh, Cambodia, had participants from Thailand, Burma, Laos, Cambodia and Vietnam. The efforts on inter-country co-ordination were specifically directed towards protecting the border areas first, thus confining a country's malaria problems and assuring against cross-border transmission of the disease.[42] Despite this organisational framework, movements of people during the Vietnam War, and the influx of Cambodian refugees in the 1980s and of Karen refugees (from south-eastern Myanmar) in the 1990s, have exacerbated the problems of drug resistance.

Amid all this Thailand's NMEP continued. During the phase of vigilance, when the problems were coming to the fore, there was necessarily an increased use of antimalarials to combat malaria resurgence in the areas no longer sprayed every year. It may be that the as yet unnoticed rise of chloroquine resistance contributed to these technical and political difficulties.

The NMEP was not concerned with conducting research; even pertinent epidemiological work was considered wanting.[43] The vertical control package with its emphasis on vector elimination had no inbuilt research component accompanying the cans of DDT. Nor was the programme co-ordinated with other developments in medicine in Thailand, in particular with attempts to institutionalise and promote the study and teaching of tropical diseases. When Tranakchit Harinasuta delivered her paper at the UNESCO-sponsored conference on parasite science in Singapore in 1962 and announced a series of cases demonstrating chloroquine-resistant malaria parasites in Thailand, the results were a surprise both to the world's medical community and to the majority of the NMEP in Thailand.[44] It was not just the nature of the findings that caused concern but the production of that knowledge. Thailand was a developing country in terms of its economic status and its apparatus for medical research. Moreover, what medical science was being conducted was not the legacy of a colonial regime which might have given it some measure of kudos.

Contested knowledge: chloroquine resistance

When Harinasuta presented her paper in 1962 she was, of course, summarising studies of chloroquine resistant malaria which had been under way for several years. She recalls how the problem first came to light:

> When we joined the program [MEP] we used DDT as an insecticide to kill the vector and then we used chloroquine as a schizontocide to kill the parasite in the patient, we used it extensively in about 'fifty-six, 'fifty-seven in Thailand, and then there is a complaint from the doctors working in the rural area, in the endemic area, that chloroquine didn't work very well, and they claimed that it might be chloroquine resistant.[45]

These were only observations, and in her account the Thai practitioners working with the NMEP regarded a rise in a patient's temperature chart as an indication of drug resistance. She took the work a step further. In the late 1950s, at the Siriraj hospital, Harinasuta began to count malaria parasites against white and red blood cells:

> At that time no one did the count here, and I try to find out how to count malaria ... and I did the count at 7.00 a.m. and 3.00 p.m. and 11.00 p.m., three times a day, and I found that there were many patients where the parasites disappear completely but the fever is still here ... but when I asked any authority on malaria no one believed it.[46]

In addition to this scepticism she had problems maintaining contact with the malarious patients who owing to pressure on beds were discharged after the amelioration of their symptoms: precisely the time she needed to continue the investigation. This situation improved when the Bangkok Hospital for Tropical Diseases was built as the clinical adjunct of the Faculty of Tropical Medicine in 1960. Harinasuta was now able to keep the patients who came to the hospital with malaria, eventually employing some of them:

> They became our assistants, technicians, and I asked the patients to pull the weeds, gardening, I don't mind they pull one or two [weeds] but I gave them some money, a bit of money, to buy cigarettes, at that time they all smoked cigarettes, Coca-cola, coffee and something like this.[47]

In this way she was able to study the clinical manifestations of resistant malaria over a long period of time. This work was different from the observations made by the US workers who published similar arguments about drug-resistant parasites from South America in the *American Journal of Tropical Medicine*. There are key differences between the two studies, their publication and their reception. They reflect the differences between the practice of biomedicine in the West as opposed to biomedicine practised outside Europe and North America by indigenous people. Moreover, Harinasuta's clinical methodology was increasingly being pushed aside in favour of laboratory medicine. The knowledge that malaria parasites could develop resistance to synthetic antimalarials *in vitro* and in animal models had been determined in the late 1940s.[48] However, the development of resistance in regions of active anti-malarial activity to the drug endorsed by WHO's eradication campaign was a different matter.

In 1961 Donald V. Moore and Jack E. Lanier reported observations of 'two patients infected with *P. falciparum* who did not respond to chloroquine in the usual manner'.[49] There followed in the same volume a further paper by Moore, this time co-authored by Martin D. Young, which described 'a strain of *P. falciparum* originating in Colombia, South America, show[ing] a poor response to normal and above-normal doses of chloroquine'.[50] In both these studies the observations were chance observations, involving Americans who had returned from South America to the United States.[51] Moreover, the research was conducted in the scientifically credible atmosphere of the National Institutes of Health, Bethesda, Maryland, and the Microbiology Department of the University of Texas Southwestern Medical School. The work did not form part of a coherent study in the country where the resistant strains had developed. Nor was there necessarily any need for the US workers to deal with this finding as a practical priority, in the same way as the Thai situation warranted.

From the scientific literature it appears that the US workers' results were not received with the same scepticism as Harinasuta's findings. Publication by Moore, Lanier and Young in a mainstream, refereed medical journal also ensured rapid dissemination, and unspoken authority. By contrast Harinasuta presented her work at a conference and the paper was published as part of the symposium report. It was not so widely available, nor so widely cited, as the American work.[52] This points to the low value attached to academic medicine in Thailand and to the restricted opportunities available to a researcher in her position. Harinasuta described the reception of her paper at the UNESCO meeting in Singapore thus:

> Those attending the meeting were all the big shots in tropical medicine and parasitology, about one hundred of them. They wouldn't believe me, they told me to my face that they wouldn't believe it ... except two of them come to me and said, 'You better work at it' ... In fact they wouldn't get up in the meeting and say that they believed me, but they said go on with your work ... and in 1963 I have a chance to go around the world and I met all the world authorities on malaria and I told them about this, and some of them laughed and some of them smiled ... I said, 'This is the problem in Thailand, I don't care it is not the problem in the United States, this is a problem in my country.'[53]

When she returned home, Harinasuta continued the clinical work. A further paper in the *Lancet* in 1965 was prepared with the help of Dr H. A. Reid, from the Liverpool School of Tropical Medicine, enjoying the school's Far East connections in Bangkok.[54] Here Harinasuta *et al.* challenged WHO's technique for assessing chloroquine resistance in the field, arguing that the standard 'procedure would grossly underestimate the extent of chloroquine resistance'.[55] It was just this type of practical intimacy with the problem that the Thai workers were able to achieve, and which made the difference to their work.

A degree of scepticism in medicine is warranted 'because otherwise we would all be taking quack remedies all the time'.[56] However, the motivation of such scepticism is not necessarily uniform, or in the best interests of those who could benefit and have no voice. In 1964 Bruce-Chwatt wrote:

> It should be stressed that while many observations are reliable, not all

> reports coming from the field and claiming the presence of chloroquine resistance are of equal value. There is little doubt that some such statements are hasty and may have overlooked the simple fact that the drug was not given or not swallowed, or was vomited, or that the dosage was too low. It seems that 'chloroquine resistance' has the appeal of novelty and it is not easy to distinguish between a genuine drug-fastness and spurious claims caused by poor supervision of drug administration and/or blood examination.[57]

Other WHO scientists appear to have shared Bruce-Chwatt's views, this time with specific reference to Thailand:

> Several observations concerning alleged resistance of *P. falciparum* to chloroquine in Thailand and in neighbouring countries have been published. The investigations of this problem which were carried out by national and foreign staff did not follow, however, the pattern recommended by the WHO Scientific group on resistance of malaria parasites to drugs WHO Technical Report Series 296 (1965). The screening methodology recommended by the Scientific group is considered essential in order to confirm the existence of drug resistance.[58]

Did anyone consider that it might be the WHO methodology that was flawed rather than the results of the Thai studies? Or that the administration of drugs was not flawed but involved with the production of drug resistance? The Ministry of Public Health in Thailand, at least, was sufficiently convinced by Harinasuta's findings. In order to win the necessary support from overseas, the Thai government asked WHO to provide a team to assist in investigating the problem in certain selected areas.

What Dr Basu, a WHO specialist, found when he looked for it was an alarming rate of chloroquine-resistant malaria – up to 100 per cent of cases in some study areas.[59] An optimistic report in 1965 which suggested no 'insurmountable technical or operational problems' with the NMEP changed in 1966 to the view that the programme was at a standstill in large areas of the country covering 11 million of the population.[60] These were areas of the country where the lowland people were moving into the hills to work either in agriculture in recently deforested regions or in tin or gem mining.

In such regions the population were enjoying a rise in living standards which they wished to maximise by maintaining their ability to work, despite the uninhibited transmission of malaria. This situation was exploited by the unqualified drug store owners. A variety of antimalarials were on sale, and malaria patients were making use of them either by self-medication or on the advice of the drug store managers. Basu reported that, in a sample of cases, twenty-three out of forty-two people had chloroquine in their urine prior to drug administration by the investigative team.[61]

After acknowledging the presence of chloroquine resistance the report recommended:

> That the most important remedial measure is the total coverage by insecticidal spray operations in adequate doses and in sufficient cycles strategically spaced to beat resistance by intensifying the spraying campaign.

The problem was sidestepped and a race begun:

> This will bring down the need for the consumption of antimalarials and consequently reduce the potential to the selection of resistant strains. The prevailing resistant strains will be contained and eliminated in the absence of further transmission.[62]

The NMEP was advised to stop using chloroquine in areas of resistance for presumptive and radical treatment. Since the case rate was high and the people would seek treatment, it was recommended that a sufficient number of passive case-detection posts should be created where patients could receive treatment and blood smears could be taken. Access to the drug store probably remained much easier, however. Quinine was recommended as treatment for some of the cases. Given its side effects, which the synthetic antimalarials had been designed to remove, self-medication with choloquine from the local drug store was likely to prove a more attractive option, exacerbating, not reducing, the problem.

With WHO acceptance of the reality of chloroquine resistance in Thailand, the country became one of the major focuses of clinical research into resistant *falciparum* malaria. Harinasuta was invited to join the WHO scientific group on the chemotherapy of malaria. This committee described the RI, RII, RIII grading system, and established an international definition of resistance.[63] Harinasuta and her colleagues at the Bangkok Hospital for Tropical Diseases also investigated new drugs to combat chloroquine-resistant *falciparum* malaria as and when they became available, most notably sulfadoxine-pyrimethamine and later mefloquine alone and in combination with various other compounds.[64] Thailand seemed ideally suited to conduct this type of research, with a malaria research infrastructure comprising the Faculty of Tropical Medicine, the Malaria Division of the Ministry of Public Health and the South East Asian Treaty Organisation (SEATO) research laboratories.[65] Underpinning these physical structures was an ethos of taking what seemed useful from elsewhere and adapting it to national needs. Thus most recently the Thais have been using Chinese qinghaosu drugs which are licensed in Thailand, although their distribution is controlled, where possible.

As suggested before, the Thais were never constrained to look in one place for solutions to their problems. When the Chinese work on qinghaosu was published the Thais were willing to investigate its potential worth. This in spite of the fact that they had been fighting communist insurgence from China for years.[66] The West, as embodied in the WHO, seemed less able to overlook the ideological backdrop to this new anti-malarial. Indeed, Western reluctance to accept the Thais' work on chloroquine resistance has many parallels with the intransigence over qinghaosu, despite the acknowledged need for anti-malarial compounds which are active against multi-drug-resistant *falciparum* malaria.

Contested knowledge: the development of anti-malarial drugs in China and their position in the West

The debates over the qinghaosu drugs, and over the development of a usable malaria vaccine, are part of the cutting edge of current malaria research. The history of both these attempts at alleviating one of man's oldest diseases are difficult to access because access to useful records is restricted. Oral history is invaluable, but the aim here is draw a parallel with the work on chloroquine resistance.

China has a substantial malaria problem. It was estimated in 1949 that there were 30 million cases of malaria per year.[67] The number had been reduced by 1979 to around 2 million reported cases annually, as part of a nationwide attack on the five major parasitic diseases of China. The programme formed part of a 'conscious effort to radically alter the health structure by infusing political ideologies into health care' and was of course part of the communist revolution of 1949.[68] The 'barefoot doctors' scheme and the deliberate integration of Western and traditional Chinese medicine at the practice and research levels were part of the outcome.[69]

During World War Two China faced the possibility of losing its quinine supplies. In 1941 work with Sinine was published.[70] It was followed by the preparation Ch'ang Shan from the *Dichroa febrifuga Lour* plant, tested by the Institute of Materia Medica of the National Academy of Medicine, Shanghai, and the Pharmacological Laboratory of the National Institute of Health, Nanking.[71] Clinical trials were also undertaken at the Ta-Tu-Kou Steel and Iron Works Hospital and the First Hospital of Traditional Chinese Medicine, Chungking.[72] This research was picked up by workers outside China but made little impact, and interest died out.[73] The drugs were not included in review articles which summarised anti-malarial chemotherapy despite the fact that the papers were written in English and had been published in mainstream journals.[74]

The work did not stop in China. In the 1960s, when chloroquine-resistant malaria appeared, research was intensified. Thus the publication of the work of the Qinghaosu Anti-malarial Co-ordinating Research Group was the result of established practice and represented a revitalisation of traditional medicine for political, ideological and medical reasons.[75] Perhaps because of this background to the work, or perhaps because it suffered the same scepticism that surrounded Harinasuta's work in the early 1960s, the majority of malariologists in the West failed to take any appreciable interest in the work that was being done in China. The point should be made that in 1979 the situation of multi-drug-resistant malaria was not at the acute stage which it has reached today. However, the arrival of these drugs was not accorded the respect their potential indicated because the research came 'from as the Americans would say left field, not from the conventional approach'.[76]

In particular WHO failed to 'hit it off' with the Chinese and decided along with WRAIR to develop its own oil-soluble compound, Arteether, because it could be made according to good manufacturing practices and the Chinese products Artemisinin, Artemether and Artesunate were not. A new compound would also be patentable. Yet the net outcome of the policies of WHO's Chemotherapy of Malaria Committee is that:

> Here we are sixteen years after the first publication in the Chinese literature, we still don't know which is the right drug to develop, we still don't know how to use the drugs, we don't know whether we can delay the development of resistance to these drugs, or use them to delay the development of resistance to other drugs, which are very important questions, and we are in a Catch 22 position where nearly all the available research money for these drugs is going into a compound which has already been available for over ten years, and which does not appear to be the right drug anyway. There are no discernible advantages and only disadvantages when compared to Artesunate, which is already available.[77]

The West has taken a superior view of the work of the Chinese in the same way it did with Harinasuta's contributions. In between WHO (and all that it represents) and China are the pragmatic Thais, even if their pragmatism is driven by necessity rather than nicety. The West could afford to dally over the Chinese work; the Thais could not. The priority was clear. Resistance to the various mefloquine combinations had reduced an efficacy of 92 per cent to 30 per cent by 1990. The usefulness of quinine and the newer quinine-plus-tetracycline combination has also diminished. Qinghaosu drugs are not a panacea for multi-drug resistant malaria: 'it is now becoming increasingly clear from animal studies that were conducted by the American army themselves that the oil-soluble derivatives, artemether and arteether, are neurotoxic'.[78] The Thais have been working on the problems likely to result from non-compliance. Seven days are required for successful treatment, but because patients may feel well again after only two or three days they may fail to take the remaining medication, thereby increasing the risk of developing resistance to the compounds.[79] The Thais are trying to avoid this by controlling the distribution where they can, although where the problem of malaria is most acute, on the Thai–Cambodian and Thai–Myanmar borders, there is the least likelihood of success. The government Malaria Division is also trying to combat self-medication and encourage attendance at clinics by repeating its policy of changing the official line on malaria treatment in line with the results of trial studies.[80] However, they now rely on their own results and no longer require the confirmation of outsiders as once they did.

Contested knowledge?

Commercially produced Chinese and Vietnamese qinghaosu compounds:

> Are being used in an uncontrolled way in an increasing number of countries, because they are obviously successful, and they are very well tolerated and there are no discernible side effects when you take them, so they are very well accepted; and they are cheap, so they are now leaking out all over South East Asia and into Africa and South Amcrica, which is a disaster, because we will inevitably see resistance ... so market forces have led the way, and the scientific community and WHO and everyone has just been running behind trying to catch up.[81]

In the wake of the MEP came drug-resistant malaria. Drug-resistant malaria is no longer an issue because the world malaria map is dotted with its presence. By including her in the WHO Scientific Group the West could be said to have endorsed the work of Harinasuta, but not necessarily her claim to the primacy of the discovery. It seems that her clinical studies in Bangkok required 'reinforcement' by A. S. Alving, who also in 1962 reported at a conference in London 'That a chloroquine-resistant strain of *P. falciparum* had been isolated from an American Marine who had acquired his infection also in Thailand'.[82] The JHK strain was one of several used later by Alving and his co-workers in the much cited experimental work involving prison volunteers in the United States. The problem of drug-resistant malaria dominated the Seventh International Congress on Tropical Medicine and Malaria, held in September 1963: knowledge of resistance had passed into the corpus of mainstream tropical medicine.

Parallel to the reporting of chloroquine resistance in Thailand is the recent history of Chinese work on qinghaosu and the West's attitude towards the research. The Chinese proponents of the qinghaosu compounds have faced the same struggle for acknowledgement as Harinasuta did. It is not so much that this work has not been accepted as that it has had to be re-dressed before it could be made available to the people who need it. It is a story akin to Hans Andersen's tale of the emperor's new clothes.

Without the legacy of colonialism the Thais seem to have avoided tension between traditional medicine and their acceptance and practice of Western medicine. However, this had little effect on the way medical research from Thailand was received by the international scientific community. It is not necessarily the content of a body of knowledge that is contested, but the way that knowledge is created, by whom, and how it is disseminated, which are of equal importance. The issues around resistance and new anti-malarial compounds highlight the whole question of drug development and production for the tropics. Perhaps what is needed is a 'radical change in the whole background philosophy to drug development which is blinkered biased and out of date ... and suffers from a stultifying bureaucracy'.[83] A bureaucracy that has been able to contest knowledge not because of its content but because of where it came from.

Notes

1 Dr N. J. White, interview broadcast on the BBC 2 *Assignment* programme 'Fatal latitudes', 23 February 1993.

2 Resistance has been reported to the other human malaria parasites but this chapter refers to *falciparum* malaria.

3 Easily administered, i.e. a single dose or short course, three days, so that the best possible compliance can be achieved.

4 Drug resistance is defined as 'the ability of a parasite strain to survive and/or to multiply despite the administration and absorption of a drug given in doses equal to or higher than those usually recommended but within the limits of tolerance of the subject'. J. Karbwang and T. Harinasuta, *Chemotherapy of Malaria in South East Asia*, Bangkok: Ruamtasana, 1992: 48.

5 Qinghaosu Anti-malaria Co-ordinating Research Group, 'Antimalaria studies on Qinghaosu', *Chinese Medical Journal* 92 (1979): 811–16.

6 Most recently see W. F. Bynum and B. Fantini (eds), *Malaria and Ecosystems: Historical Aspects, Parassitoliga* (special issue) 36 (1994).

7 The active anti-malarial principle of *Artemisia annua L.* is qinghaosu. It is known in the West as artemisinin. T. T. Hien and N. J. White, 'Qinghaosu', *Lancet* 341

(1993): 603–8.

8 Various countries in the West have been happy to use Thailand's desire to remain free of colonialism and communism for their own ends, ignoring the fact that the military have a stranglehold over Thai politics. See Donald E. Nuechterlem, *Thailand and the Struggle for South East Asia*. Ithaca, N.Y.: Cornell University Press, 1965.

9 In 1979 the *South East Asian Journal of Tropical Medicine and Public Health* was launched by the Bangkok Faculty of Tropical Medicine to deal with this.

10 The French, British and Americans had missionaries in Thailand, the first medical missionary arriving in 1676.

11 P. Kunstadter, 'Do cultural differences make any difference? Choice points in medical systems available in north-west Thailand', in A. Kleinman *et al.* (eds), *Culture and Healing in Asian Societies*, Boston, Mass.: Hall, 1978: 185–218, at p. 209.

12 R. Jeffery, 'Recognizing India's doctors: the institutionalization of medical dependency, 1918–39', *Modern Asian Studies* 13 (1979): 301–26; K. D. Patterson, *Health in Colonial Ghana: Disease, Medicine and Socio-economic Change, 1900–55*, Waltham, Mass.: Crossroads Press, 1981: 11–32.

13 Thailand has various complementary indigenous systems of health care, often with a shared herbal pharmacopoeia. These systems represent the ethnic diversity of Thailand, especially in the northern parts of the country. The Chinese, who provided labour and dominated trade and commerce until the early twentieth century, brought with them their own systems of medicine.

14 E. R. Brown, 'Public health in imperialism: early Rockefeller programs at home and abroad', in J. Ehrenreich (ed.), *The Cultural Crisis of Modern Medicine*, New York: Monthly Review Press, 1978: 252–70.

15 R. H. Bannerman *et al.* (eds), *Traditional Medicine and Health Care Coverage*, Geneva: WHO, 1983: 306.

16 Commonwealth Consultative Committee on Economic Development in South and South East Asia, *The Colombo Plan for Co-operative Economic Development in South and South East Asia*, meeting September–October 1950.

17 *The Colombo Plan Technical Co-operation Scheme*, London: HMSO, 1954.

18 Chamlong Harinasuta, interview, 17 January 1995, Faculty of Tropical Medicine, Mahidol University, Bangkok, Thailand.

19 Kunying Tranakchit Harinasuta, interview, 9 January 1995, Hospital for Tropical Disease, Mahidol University, Bangkok.

20 Dr N. J. White, interview, 11 January 1995, Wellcome Research Laboratories, Faculty of Tropical Medicine, Mahidol University, Bangkok.

21 Kunying Tranakchit Harinasuta, interview, 10 January 1995, Hospital for Tropical Disease, Mahidol University, Bangkok.

22 *Ibid.*

23 WHO CDT Information Centre: Malaria Control in Thailand, by L. A. Kosol and M. E. Griffith, 1953: 1.

24 V. Thompson, *Thailand: the new Siam*, New York: Paragon Book Reprint Co., 1967: 703. See also L. Anigstein, 'Malaria and anophelines in Siam', *Quarterly Bulletin of the Health Organisation of the League of Nations*, 1 (1931): 233–308.

25 WHO CDT Information Centre: Report of Thai Government/WHO/UNICEF Malaria control demonstration project by Dr G. Sammasivan, Dr M. L. Bhatia, Dr Udom Pranich and Dr Vimol Notananda, 5 February 1953.

26 WHO CDT Information Centre: ICA health summary (2/1957), Malaria eradication in Thailand, by Dr M. E. Griffith: 7.

27 WHO CDT Information Centre: Communication to the Director, WHO, South East Asia Region from the Director-General, Department of Public Health, Thailand, 18 June 1949.

28 S. Litsios, 'Malarial control, the Cold War, and the post-war reorganization of International Assistance', *Medical Anthropology*, 17 (1996).

29 A. D. Brandling Bennett, E. B. Doberstyn and S. Pinichpongse, 'Current epidemiology of malaria in South East Asia', *South East Asian Journal of Tropical Medicine* *and Public Health* 12 (1981): 289–97, at p. 293.

30 T. Harinasuta, K. E. Dixon, D. A. Warrell and E. B. Doberstyn, 'Recent advances in malaria with special reference to South East Asia', *South East Asian Journal of Tropical Medicine and Public Health*, 13 (1982): 1–34.

31 Before World War Two, Western medical care in rural areas was available either from mission stations or from a limited number of government medical officers. Mission stations vaccinated against smallpox and offered some basic training in midwifery, surgery and anaesthesia. In 1930 there were medical officers in forty-five of the seventy-nine provinces. See Thompson, *Thailand*: 716.

32 WHO CDT Information Centre: SEA/MAL/3 Malaria Conference, Bangkok, Thailand, 21–4 September 1953, Report submitted by the Government of Thailand, p. 6.

33 H. Power, 'Malaria drugs and World War II: the role of the Liverpool School of Tropical Medicine in the development of antimalarials', forthcoming.

34 D. G. Davey, 'Researches on the chemotherapy of malaria' I, 'The biological approach', *Glasgow Medical Journal*, 28 (1947): 67–72; F. H. S. Curd, 'Researches on the chemotherapy of Malaria' II, 'The chemical approach', *ibid.*: 73–9.

35 For a brief history of the development of chloroquine see G. R. Coatney, 'Pitfalls in a discovery: the chronicle of chloroquine', *American Journal of Tropical Medicine and Hygiene*, 12 (1963): 121–8.

36 W. Peters, 'Problems with presently used antimalarials', in W. Wernsdorfer and P. Trigg (eds), *Modern Design of Antimalarial Drugs*, Geneva: UNDP/World Bank/WHO, 1983: 3–16.

37 WHO CDT Information Centre: Malaria Control in Thailand, by L. A. Kosol and M. E. Griffith, 1953: 22.

38 *Ibid.*

39 Described as itinerant labour, irrigation and other large-scale construction projects, agricultural colonies, prison camps and other malaria-susceptible groups – the military. WHO CDT Information Centre: SEA/MAL/3, Malaria Conference, Bangkok, 21–4 September 1953, Report submitted by the Government of Thailand: 13.

40 D. Wit, *Thailand: another Vietnam?* New York: Scribner, 1968.

41 WHO CDT Information Centre: A projection of the Malaria control programme in Thailand operated by the Thai Ministry of Public Health assisted by the USA Operations Mission 1954–58.

42 WHO CDT Information Centre: ICA health summary (2/1957), Malaria eradication in Thailand, by Dr M. E. Griffith: 8–9.

43 WHO CDT Information Centre: Notes by Dr G. Gramiccia on visit to Thailand 4–17 December 1964.

44 T. Harinasuta, S. Migasen and D. Bunnag, 'Chloroquine resistance in *P. falciparum, UNESCO First symposium on Scientific Knowledge of Tropical Parasites,* UNESCO: Singapore, 1962: 148–53.

45 Harimasuta, interview, 19 January 1995, Hospital for Tropical Diseases, Mahidol University, Bangkok.

46 *Ibid.*

47 *Ibid.*

48 A. Bishop and B. Birkett, 'Drug resistance in *P. gallinaceum* and the persistence of paludrine resistance after mosquito transmission', *Parasitology* 39 (1947): 125–37; J. Williamson and E. M. Lourie, 'Acquired paludrine-resistance in *P. gallinaceum*' I, 'Development of resistance to paludrine and failure to develop resistance to certain other antimalarials', *Annals of Tropical Medicine and Parasitology* 41 (1947): 278–91.

49 D. V. Moore and J. E. Lanier, 'Observations on two *P. falciparum* infections with an abnormal response to chloroquine', *American Journal of Tropical Medicine and Hygiene* 10 (1961): 5–9 at 5.

50 M. D. Young and D. V. Moore, 'Chloroquine resistance in *Plasmodium falciparum*', *American Journal of Tropical Medicine and Hygiene* 10 (1961): 317–20, at p. 317.

51 In the first paper the condition was erroneously diagnosed as relapsing *vivax* malaria. Only when the blood slide was routinely used for a teaching demonstration was it realised that the parasites were *P. falciparum*. The case was investigated further and later rediagnosed as malaria resistant to chloroquine.

52 Neither the London nor the Liverpool School of Tropical Medicine has a copy of the *UNESCO First Symposium on Scientific Knowledge of Parasites*. The *Science Citation Index* for 1964 shows five and six citations for Moore and Lanier (1961) and Young and Moore (1961) respectively, Harinasuta (1962) has only one citation and that is in a publication by W. Peters of the Liverpool School, who is quite likely to have had contact with the Faculty of Tropical Medicine in Bangkok. In his major monograph *Chemotherapy and Drug Resistance in Malaria* (London: Academic Press, 1970) Peters appears to have accepted her findings. See 10.

53 Harinasuta, interview, 10 January 1995, Hospital for Tropical Diseases, Mahidol University.

54 T. Harinasuta, P. Suntharasamai and C. Viravan, 'Chloroquine-resistant *falciparum* malaria in Thailand', *Lancet* II (1965): 657–60.

55 *Ibid.*: 659.

56 Harinasuta, interview, 17 January 1995, Faculty of Tropical Diseases, Mahidol University.

57 L. J. Bruce-Chwatt, 'Changing tides of chemotherapy of malaria', *British Medical Journal*, I (1964): 581–6, at p. 582.

58 WHO CDT Information Centre: SEA/MAL/50, Field visit report on malaria eradication programme, Thailand, Dr G. Gramiccia, 5–18 April 1965, p. 8.

59 WHO CDT Information Centre: SEA/MAL/55 Rev. 1, Assignment report on resistance of *P. falciparum* to chloroquine in Thailand (WHO project SEARO 7), by Dr P. C. Basu, 24 June–22 August 1965.

60 WHO CDT Information Centre: SEA/MAL/58, Assignment report on malaria eradication in Thailand WHO project: Thailand 65 by Dr G. L. Adan, September 1962–October 1965: 8.

61 WHO CDT Information Centre: SEA/MAL/55 Rev. 1, Assignment report on resistance of *P. falciparum* to chloroquine in Thailand (WHO project SEARO 7) by Dr P. C. Basu, 24 June–22 August 1965.

62 *Ibid.*: 23.

63 WHO, *Chemotherapy of malaria*. Report of a WHO scientific group, Technical Report Series, No. 375, Geneva: WHO, 1967.

64 T. Harinasuta and C. Viravan, 'Sulphormethoxine (Fanasil) and combinations of sulphormethoxine (Fanasil) and chloroquine or pyrimethamine (Daraprim) in the treatment of chloroquine-resistant *falciparum* malaria in Thailand', paper presented at the eleventh Pacific Science Congress, Tokyo, August 1966.

65 When this alliance was dissolved the laboratories remained and were renamed Allied Forces Research Institute Medical Science (AFRIMS).

66 J. Race, 'The war in northern Thailand', *Modern Asian Studies* 8 (1974): 85–112.

67 Z. Ahou, 'The malaria situation in the People's Republic of China', *WHO Bulletin* 59 (1981): 931–6.

68 P. K. New and M. L. New, 'The links between health and the political structure in new China', *Human Organization* 34 (1975): 237–51 at 238.

69 M. M. Rosenthal, 'Political process and the integration of traditional and Western medicine in the People's Republic of China', *Social Science and Medicine* 15A (1981): 599–613.

70 S. Liu, Y. Chang, T. Ch'uan and S. Tan, 'The new antimalarial drug Sinine: a preliminary report', *Chinese Medical Journal* 59 (1941): 575–7.

71 T. Q. Chou, F. Y. Fu and Y. S. Kao, 'Antimalarial constituents of the Chinese drug Ch'ang Shan *Dichroa febrifuga Lour*', *Journal of the American Chemical Society* 70 (1948): 1765–7.

72 C. F. Tsu, 'Chang Shan in the treatment of malaria', *Journal of Tropical Medicine and Hygiene* 49 (1947): 75–7; H. Chi and F. Lan-Chou, 'Studies on malaria in new China', *Chinese Medical Journal* 77 (1958): 533–51.

73 J. B. Kiepfli, J. F. Mead and J. A. Brockman, 'An alkaloid with high antimalarial activity from *Dichroa febrifuga*', *Journal of the American Chemical Society* 69 (1947):

1837; F. A. Keuhl, C. F. Spencer and K. Folkers, 'Alkaloids of *Dichroa febrifuga Lour*', *Journal of the American Chemical Society* 70 (1948): 2019–3; F. G. Henderson, C. L. Rose, P. N. Harris and K. K. Chen, 'Dichroine, the antimalarial alkaloid of Ch'ang Shan', *Journal of Pharmacy and Experimental Therapeutics* 95 (1949): 191–200; J. W. Fairburn and T. C. Lou, 'A pharmacological study of *Dichroa febrifuga Lour,* a Chinese antimalarial plant', *Journal of Pharmacy and Pharmacology* 2 (1950): 162–77.

74 See, for example, W. C. Cooper, 'Summary of antimalarial drugs', *Public Health Reports* 64 (1949): 717–32. Cooper worked at the Laboratory of Tropical Disease, NIH, Bethesda, Md.

75 The names of some of the contributing institutions indicated the background to this work: Institute of Chinese Materia Medica, Academy of Traditional Chinese Medicine; Institutes of Biophysics and Organic Chemistry, Academia Sinica; Academy of Combined Traditional Chinese and Western Medicine, Shandong Province.

76 Harinasuta, interview, 9 January 1995, Hospital for Tropical Diseases, Mahidol University.

77 Dr N. J. White, interview, 26 January 1995, Wellcome Research Laboratories, Faculty of Tropical Medicine, Mahidol University, Bangkok.

78 *Ibid.*

79 Professor Tan Chongsuphajaisiddhi, interview, 9 January 1995, Faculty of Tropical Medicine, Mahidol University, Bangkok.

80 White, interview, 11 January 1995, Wellcome Research Laboratories, Faculty of Tropical Medicine, Mahidol University.

81 White, interview, 26 January 1995, Faculty of Tropical Medicine, Mahidol University.

82 Peters, *Chemotherapy and Drug Resistance in Malaria*: 10.

83 *Ibid.*

GUIDE TO FURTHER READING

General

Arnold, David (ed.) *Imperial Medicine and Indigenous Societies*. Manchester: Manchester University Press, 1988.

Bannerman, R. H., J. Burton, and Wen-chieh Ch'en, eds. *Traditional Medicine and Health Care Coverage: a Reader for Health Administrators and Practitioners*. Geneva: World Health Organization, 1983.

Brockway, Lucile H. *Science and Colonial Expansion: the Role of the British Royal Botanic Gardens*. New York and London: Academic Press, 1979.

Bynum, W. F., and Roy Porter (eds) *Companion Encyclopedia of the History of Medicine*. London: Routledge, 1993.

Chakrabarty, Dipesh. 'Postcoloniality and the artifice of history: who speaks for "Indian" pasts?' *Representations* 37 (1992): 1–26.

Etherington, Norman. *Theories of Imperialism: War, Conquest and Capital*. London: Croom Helm, 1984.

Headrick, Daniel R. *The Tentacles of Progress: Technology Transfer in the Age of Imperialism, 1850–1940*. Oxford: Oxford University Press, 1988.

Hessenbruch, Arne (ed.) *Reader's Guide to the History of Science*. London: Fitzroy Dearborn, 1996.

Horton, Robin. 'African traditional thought and Western science.' *Africa* 37 (1967): 50–71 and 155–87.

Howard-Jones, Norman. *The Scientific Background of the International Sanitary Conferences, 1851–1938*. Geneva: World Health Organization, 1975.

Kuper, Adam. *The Invention of Primitive Society: Transformations of an Illusion*. London: Routledge, 1988.

Landy, David (ed.) *Culture, Disease and Healing: Studies in Medical Anthropology*. New York: Macmillan, 1977.

Lindenbaum, Shirley, and Margaret Lock (eds) *Knowledge, Power and Practice: the Anthropology of Medicine and Everyday Life*. Berkeley, Cal.: University of California Press, 1993.

MacLeod, Roy, and Milton Lewis (eds) *Disease, Medicine, and Empire: Perspectives on Western Medicine and the Experience of European Expansion*. London and New York: Routledge, 1988.

Nandy, Ashis (ed.) *Science, Hegemony and Violence: a Requiem for Modernity*. Delhi and Oxford: Oxford University Press, 1988.

Said, Edward W. *Orientalism*. Harmondsworth: Penguin Books (1978) 1985.

Stocking, George (ed.) 'Colonial situations: essays on the contextualization of ethnographical knowledge.' *History of Anthropology* 7 (1991): 3–8.

Science and Empire Newsletter. Joint publication of NISTADS (New Delhi) and REHSEIS (Paris).

India

Arnold, David. *Colonizing the Body: State Medicine and Epidemic Disease in Nineteenth-century India*. Berkeley and Los Angeles: University of California Press, 1993.

Bala, Poonam. *Imperialism and Medicine in Bengal: a Sociohistorical Perspective*. New Delhi: Sage, 1991.

Catanach, Ian. 'Plague and the tensions of empire: India, 1896–1918' in *Imperial Medicine and Indigenous Societies* (ed.) David Arnold. Manchester: Manchester University Press, 1988.

Chandavarkar, Rajnarayan. 'Plague panic and epidemic politics in India, 1896–1914' in *Epidemics and Ideas: Essays on the Historical Perception of Pestilence* (ed.) Terence Ranger and Paul Slack. Cambridge: Cambridge University Press, 1992.

Guha, Ranajit (ed.) *Subaltern Studies*.

Harrison, Mark. *Public Health in British India*. Cambridge History of Medicine (ed.) Charles Webster and Charles Rosenberg. Cambridge: Cambridge University Press, 1994.

Klein, Ira. 'Plague policy and popular unrest in British India'. *Modern Asian Studies* 22 (4 1988): 723–55.

Kumar, Deepak (ed.) *Science and Empire: Essays in Indian Context, 1700–1947*. Delhi: Anamika Prakashan, 1991.

Kumar, Deepak. *Science and the Raj, 1857–1905*. Delhi and Oxford: Oxford University Press, 1995.

Prakash, Gyan. 'Science "gone native" in colonial India.' *Representations* 40 (1992): 153–78.

Sangwan, Satpal. *Science, Technology and Colonisation: an Indian Experience, 1757–1857*. New Delhi: Anamika Prakashan, 1991.

Africa

Chirimuuta, Richard, and Rosalind Chirimuuta. *AIDS, Africa and Racism*. Second edition, London: Free Association Books, 1989.

Feierman, Steven, and John M. Janzen (eds) *The Social Basis of Health and Healing in Africa*. Berkeley and Los Angeles: University of California Press, 1992.

Gallagher, Nancy E. *Medicine and Power in Tunisia, 1780–1900*. Cambridge: Cambridge University Press, 1983.

Janzen, John M., and Gwyn Prins (eds) 'Causality and classification in African medicine and health.' Special issue of *Social Science and Medicine* 15b (1981).

Lyons, Maryinez. *The Colonial Disease: a Social History of Sleeping Sickness in Northern Zaire, 1900–40*. Cambridge: Cambridge University Press, 1992.

Vaughan, Megan. *Curing their Ills: Colonial Power and African Illness*. Cambridge: Polity Press, 1991.

Vaughan, Megan. 'Healing and curing: issues in the social history and anthropology of medicine in Africa.' *Social History of Medicine* 7 (2 1994): 283–95.

East Asia

Bowers, John Z. *When the Twain Meet: the Rise of Western Medicine in Japan.* Baltimore: Johns Hopkins University Press, 1980.

Croizier, Ralph C. *Traditional Medicine in Modern China: Science, Nationalism and the Tensions of Cultural Change.* Cambridge, Mass.: Harvard University Press, 1968.

Farquhar, Judith. *Knowing Practice: the Clinical Encounter of Chinese Medicine.* Boulder, Colo.: Westview Press, 1994.

Kleinman, Arthur K. *Patients and Healers in the Context of Culture: an Exploration of the Borderland between Anthropology, Medicine and Psychiatry.* Berkeley: University of California Press, 1980.

Kuriyama, Shigehisa. 'Between mind and eye: Japanese anatomy in the eighteenth century' in *Paths to Asian Medical Knowledge* (ed.) Charles Leslie and Allan Young. Berkeley: University of California Press, 1992.

Nathan, Carl F. 'The acceptance of Western medicine in early twentieth century China: the story of the North Manchurian Plague Prevention Service', in *Medicine and Society in China* (ed.) John Z. Bowers and Elizabeth F. Purcell. Philadelphia: Wm F. Fell for the National Library of Medicine and the Josiah Macy, Jr, Foundation, 1974.

Ohnuki-Tierney, Emiko. *Illness and Culture in Contemporary Japan: an Anthropological View.* Cambridge: Cambridge University Press, 1984.

Owen, N. G. (ed.) *Death and Disease in South Asia: Explorations in Social, Medical and Demographic History.* Singapore: Oxford University Press, 1987.

Sivin, Nathan. *Traditional Medicine in Contemporary China.* Ann Arbor: Center for Chinese Studies, University of Michigan, 1987.

Thomson, James C., Jr. *While China Faced West: American Reformers in Nationalist China, 1928–37.* Cambridge, Mass.: Harvard University Press, 1969.

Watanabe, Masao. *The Japanese and Western Science.* Translated by O. T. Benfey, Philadelphia: University of Pennsylvania Press, 1990.

Zito, Angela, and Tani E. Barlow (eds) *Body, Subject and Power in China.* Chicago: University of Chicago Press, 1994.

The Americas

Birn, Anne-Emmanuelle. 'Local health and foreign wealth: the Rockefeller Foundation's public health programs in Mexico, 1924–51.' Sc.D., The Johns Hopkins University, 1993.

Cueto, Marcos (ed.) *Missionaries of Science: the Rockefeller Foundation and Latin America.* Bloomington, Ind.: Indiana University Press, 1994.

Ettling, John. *The Germ of Laziness: Rockefeller Philanthropy and Public Health in the New South.* Cambridge Mass.: Harvard University Press, 1981.

Kunitz, Stephen. *Disease and Social Diversity: the European Impact on the Health of Non-Europeans.* New York: Oxford University Press, 1994.

Solórzano, Armando. 'The Rockefeller Foundation in Mexico: nationalism, public health, and yellow fever.' Ph.D., University of Wisconsin–Madison, 1990.

INDEX